Morphogenesis and the Crisis of Normativity

Social Morphogenesis

Series Editor:

MARGARET S. ARCHER
Centre for Social Ontology, University of Warwick, Coventry, UK

Aims and scope:

To focus upon 'social morphogenesis' as a general process of change is very different from examining its particular results over the last quarter of a century. This series ventures what the generative mechanisms are that produce such intense change and discusses how this differs from late modernity. Contributors examine if an intensification of morphogenesis (positive feedback that results in a change in social form) and a corresponding reduction in morphostasis (negative feedback that restores or reproduces the form of the social order) best captures the process involved.

The series consists of 5 volumes derived from the Centre for Social Ontology's annual workshops "From Modernity to Morphogenesis" at the University of Lausanne, headed by Margaret Archer.

More information about this series at http://www.springer.com/series/11959

Margaret S. Archer
Editor

Morphogenesis and the Crisis of Normativity

Springer

Editor
Margaret S. Archer
Centre for Social Ontology
University of Warwick
Coventry, UK

This volume IV follows the book "Social Morphogenesis", edited by Margaret S. Archer, which was the first book in the series published in 2013 http://www.springer.com/social+sciences/book/978-94-007-6127-8, the volume "Late Modernity", edited by Margaret S. Archer, published in 2014 and the volume "Generative Mechanisms Transforming the Social Order", edited by Margaret S. Archer, published in 2015.

ISSN 2198-1604 ISSN 2198-1612 (electronic)
Social Morphogenesis
ISBN 978-3-319-28438-5 ISBN 978-3-319-28439-2 (eBook)
DOI 10.1007/978-3-319-28439-2

Library of Congress Control Number: 2016939118

Printed on acid-free paper

This Springer imprint is published by Springer Nature
The registered company is Springer International Publishing AG Switzerland

Independent Social Research Foundation

With thanks to the ISRF for its ongoing funding of the Centre for Social Ontology under whose auspices this annual volume of the Book Series on Social Morphogenesis is published

Contents

1 **Introduction: Does Social Morphogenesis Threaten the Rule of Law?** 1
Margaret S. Archer

Part I The Great Normative Transformations

2 **The Great Normative Changes of the Twentieth Century** 31
Douglas Porpora

3 **Reflexive Secularity: Thoughts on the Reflexive Imperative in a Secular Age** 49
Philip S. Gorski

4 **Emergence, Development and Death: Norms in International Society** 69
Colin Wight

5 **The Normative Texture of Morphogenic Society: Tensions, Challenges, and Strategies** 87
Andrea M. Maccarini

Part II Morphogenesis and the Decline of Normative Consensus

6 **In Letter and in Spirit: Social Morphogenesis and the Interpretation of Codified Social Rules** 113
Ismael Al-Amoudi

7 **Anormative Social Regulation: The Attempt to Cope with Social Morphogenesis** 141
Margaret S. Archer

8 Joint 'Anormative' Regulation from Status Inconsistency: A Multilevel Spinning Top Model of Specialized Institutionalization 169
Emmanuel Lazega

9 The Fragile Movements of Late Modernity 191
Mark Carrigan

Part III Morphogenesis and What Makes for Changes in Normativity

10 The Relational Understanding of the Origin and Morphogenetic Change of Social Morality 219
Pierpaolo Donati

11 Collective Practices and Norms 249
Tony Lawson

12 Ethics from Systems: Origin, Development and Current State of Normativity 279
Wolfgang Hofkirchner

Chapter 1
Introduction: Does Social Morphogenesis Threaten the Rule of Law?

Margaret S. Archer

The Problem

Do shared values promote social stability and social integration, or is it the other way round? Is it rather that social stability fosters normative consensus about the legitimacy of the rule of law, the appropriateness of prevailing rules and attachment to existing conventions? This question has a long history in the philosophy of law and the sociology of development, whose respective thinkers often took different positions during the Twentieth century. What they did agree upon was that the lack of social change was conducive to both an unchallenged rule of law and to shared values embedded in established custom and common beliefs. In short, morphostasis was the precondition of a harmonious relationship between legal validity and normative consensus in society – whichever way round it was held to work.

When novel practices become rife – at work, in the family, through geographical mobility, a multinational global economy and the digitalization of the life-world in general – is it possible to establish a new corpus of laws, norms and rules, given that intense morphogenesis denies the durability of any new stable context? This spells a crisis for normative regulation, for social integration and for social stability alike, which is the theme of this volume.

These three factors, 'social normativity', 'social integration' and 'social regulation' (NIR)[1] are ineluctably interdependent. What legal philosophers and social

[1]This is a specific instance of the more general maxim SAC, where adequate explanations need to make reference to Structure, Culture and Agency. Here N = C, I = A and R = S.

M.S. Archer (✉)
Centre for Social Ontology, University of Warwick, Coventry, UK
e-mail: margaret.archer@warwick.ac.uk

M.S. Archer (eds.), *Morphogenesis and the Crisis of Normativity*,
Social Morphogenesis, DOI 10.1007/978-3-319-28439-2_1

theorists can differ about (though this is not always the case) is which of the three has causal primacy, if any.[2] In the beginning, what was always the case in both disciplines was joint endorsement of the imperative: 'NIR must cohere'. As social change increased and intensified throughout the twentieth century, fundamentally NIR came apart in the two sets of hands. A critique of this 'fragmentation' is what basically unites the contributions to the present volume. They can be read partly as diagnoses of the loss of NIR as morphostasis gave way to morphogenesis, and partly as prognoses about the possibility of its restoration in morphogenic society.

Legal Validity and Social Solidarity: Their Common Anchorage in Normativity

Law is not true or false but 'valid' or 'invalid' and social solidarity is not true or false but rather existent or non-existent. In both cases, the task for theorists was similar: to establish upon what legal 'validity' and social 'solidarity' turned, that is, what accounted for their bindingness? The answers were not dissimilar until the period with which we deal, roughly 1980 onwards. In shorthand, the joint response was 'shared normativity', or what I once called 'The Myth of Cultural Integration' (Archer 1985), fostered by the early anthropologists, i.e. a common cultural conspectus amongst those sharing much the same life, resources and knowledge as one another. In this respect, Parsons and Kelsen can be considered as twin giants who placed the same holistic importance on shared normativity as the *a priori* for social solidarity as for legal validity.

On the one hand, Parsons' elaborate theory, built by climbing on Durkheim's shoulders, retained as its corner stone the necessity of shared normativity in any functioning social unit. However, this ceased to be problematic within his 'normative functionalism' – unlike the 'pathologies of the division of labour' that had so exercised Durkheim and prompted him to emphasise the urgency of remedial measures in the form of practical social policy interventions. Instead, to Parsons, the operation of a 'central value system' was postulated as unquestionably and universally unifying the *goals*, *means* and *norms* of different parts of any

[2]Hans Kelsen, generally regarded as the father of legal normativism, was not so far removed in his thinking from Emile Durkheim. To Kelsen, social normativity was foundational to social regulation and the three tasks of law (co-ordination, co-operation and distribution). Legal validity could never be a matter of coercion, that is, the acts of 'predatory regimes' whose use of power spelt social malintegration. Durkheim strongly tended to see the degree of social integration as pivotal to the harmony of the three properties but held that re-establishing their harmonious relations at the end of the Nineteenth century necessitated working on all three: teaching common civic morals to restore normative uniformity; introducing common education and occupational associations to re-animate social integration; and abolishing inherited wealth to buttress democracy and render social regulation acceptable.

social system and thus integrating it: culture consisted 'in patterned or ordered systems of symbols which are objects of the orientation of action, internalized components of the personalities of individual actors and institutionalized patterns of social systems' (Parsons 1951: 327). Integration of the social system derived from each sub-system being permeated by the same fundamental values – which is a functionalist version of Kelsen's *grundnorm* – and was maintained by the homeostatic feedback mechanisms operating between them – also akin to Kelsen's cascading derivative process by which each norm acquired its validity from a more basic one and thus ensured legal morphostasis (as deviations would be illegitimate descendants).

Hence, Parsons' three major social subsystems were always held to be compatible with one another, meaning that the normative order was postulated as *constitutive* as well as *regulative* of the integrated social order and its legal rules. This defence of NIR's complementarity earned Gouldner's critical riposte that Parsons 'never seems to ask about the conditions under which moral values *will* be held in common'. To Gouldner, Parsons failed to acknowledge that power differences (among others) are likely to be conducive to differences in moral values and will thus, within his own assumptions, undermine the stability 'of relationships in which they exist' (Gouldner 1971: 242). Consequently, Parsons was chastised for considering cultural values as shared (when much is imposed), as binding (when so many interpretations of convenience can always be made), and as producing consensus (when the differential accentuation of particular components can generate severe conflict), but never, until his days as a 'Marxist outlaw', did Gouldner challenge the existence of a *central value system.*

On the other hand, Kelsen's ultimate concern with the source of the 'ought' meant to him that the validity of any part of the legal order depended upon being able to trace back its grounding in the *basic norm* as the ultimate power-conferring source, creating a chain in which the validity of subsequent norms could be deemed legitimate descendants. For example, if imprisonment is held to be a legal act, its validity derives proximately from the criminal code, '[a]nd if one asks about the basis of validity of the criminal code, one arrives at the state constitution, according to whose provisions the criminal code was enacted by the competent authorities in a constitutionally prescribed procedure' (Kelsen 1992:57). Press further, and one is enjoined to undertake further regress: 'One may come across an earlier constitution, and finally the first constitution, historically speaking, established by a single usurper or a council, however assembled. What is to be valid as norm is whatever the framers of the first constitution have expressed as their will' (Kelsen ibid 1960: 196f).

Radical morphogenesis raises three problems that are illustrated by the contentious case of 'French Revolutionary law'. First, since three revolutionary Assemblies rapidly succeeded one another, why should the 'will' of the *Constituante*, as the earliest, take precedence over those of the *Législative* or the *Convention*? After all, political successors always claim to have made changes that are advances on their predecessors; sometimes they could be right. At this point, Kelsen introduces a second criterion; a legal order has validity only 'If its norms are *by and large* effective, i.e. actually obeyed and applied' (Kelsen 1960: 219). But none of the three Assemblies lasted sufficiently long to be termed 'effective', being quickly displaced by the Consulate and then the First Empire. Second, were *Liberté, Fraternité and Egalité* to be considered as constituting the (new) revolutionary *grundnorm*, if that is not an oxymoron? In any case, this slogan is hardly persuasive given that much Napoleonic legislation traduced all three normative principles. That might have been one reason why Kelsen later came to treat the ground norm as an imaginary rather than a substantive assumption, a logical necessity for establishing the chain of validity-conferring events, but itself empty of content and thus unhelpful where intense socio-legal change is concerned. Lastly, if efficacy finally trumps origins in validating a legal order, it would seem that regress can only stop if and when there is a *successful* and *durable* seizure of political rule. French history proves obdurate, for it can well be maintained that the Code Napoléon was more effective than either Napoleon or *Bonapartisme* were durable. Moreover, since that which legally endured also underwent significant modifications; should these be dismissed as being alien to the normative will of the first Emperor – or to that of the Revolutionary Assemblies – or to those of the *ancien régime* Monarchs?

Problems such as these led many to voice a critique that parallels but exceeds Gouldner's criticisms of Parsons' inattention to changing interpretations of a normative corpus because of power struggles over particularistic interests. For example, Peter Koller maintains,

> I do not see how the basic norm could explain the law's normative validity, if it is designed as a merely imaginary assumption that is completely void of any substantial content, whether moral or prudential. Second, the efficacy of a normative system, combined with such an empty basic norm, does not enable us to distinguish a legal order, whose norms are deemed to be binding on its addressees, from the commands of a predatory regime that are enforced in an organized way, but are not regarded as binding by the subjects. In order to cope with this problem, Kelsen states that the basic norm shall not be presupposed in regard to systems which have no enduring efficacy, presuming that predatory regimes will not endure a long time (Kelsen 1960: 49). However, this reply is not only highly indeterminate, but also empirically contestable. (Kollner 2014: 164–5)[3]

Another way of putting this point from the comparison explored here is that 'efficacy' was the dummy for Kelsen's concept of validity, just as 'adaptation' underwrote Parsons' concept of functionality. Both theorists fared best when historical social scenarios were quietly morphostatic and did not have to confront problems of radical social change.

[3]Recourse was made to International Relations to solve this problem as a further form of regress, which is not historically persuasive and fails to acknowledge that such IR were always matters of contestation in the past.

Normativity in Changing Times

The previous section dealt with how the legal order was held to derive its validity from social normativity, conceptualized at the level of the Cultural System (C.S),[4] where the Law and Culture (of the land) reinforced one another through negative feedback *under* conditions of considerable and lasting stability (an enduring morphostatic relationship). This prompted the sociologist Stephen Turner to voice a general critique by introducing the difficulties presented by the incidence of morphogenesis. How could the argument about the continuity of normative underpinning of continuous legal validity 'be made to square with the variations of actual normative behaviour and that recognition that what counts as normative comes and goes historically in close relation to social change and varies by community?' (Turner 2010: 45). In stressing the difficulties presented by changes in historical normativity (only some of which are at the C.S level) in conjunction with normative variations across communities, he raises, in my terms, the separate issue of the Socio-Cultural (S-C) variability of the norms endorsed by various groups within a community that can rarely be presumed to be consensual. Different social and ideational interests on the part of distinct groups fuel conflictual socio-cultural efforts – of persuasion, censorship, manipulation and mystification – to convince others in order to advance their own cause. In other words, we are brought back to the cultural domain being *relationally contested*, in the same way that the social order has been represented in my previous contributions to this book series.

Already by supplementing the *normative origins of law* by the *efficacy of law*, as co-determinants of legal validity, Kelsen had inserted a major sociological consideration: what makes obedience to the law *binding* if it originates in coercion and operates through coercion?[5] H.A.L. Hart's (1963) revisionist position (which represents a weaker version of Gouldner's stance towards Parsons), does make a tentative move towards differentiating between legal orders as bodies producing 'power-conferring rules' (C.S.) upon subordinate agencies and conventional rules of conduct and their associated social pressures (S-C), but does not make sufficient use of it. Instead, the two are clamped too tightly together meaning that his two-part approach to legality only works if the two types are assumed to be mutually reinforcing. (That is, if the C.S. and the S-C are, or somehow come into alignment with one another.) Thus, when confronting a lack of social consensus in which certain sections of a population contest legal obligation, the power-conferring rules of legitimate legal agencies 'establish public authorities by endowing some people

[4]The C.S. refers to all items logged into the Universal Archive of the Cultural System that have the dispositional capacity of intelligibility, without depending upon a knowing subject at any given time. Relations between such items are *logical* ones. S-C refers to the Socio-Cultural level of relations between *people* and their attempts to persuade, manipulate or mystify others into holding or not challenging their views (Archer 1988). I will return to this distinction later in the chapter.

[5]It is the failure to give a satisfactory answer to this question that usually leads to Kelsen being characterized as advancing a 'sanctions theory'.

with appropriate powers to change the legal order through the creation and repeal of its norms, settle individual conflicts through binding decisions, and enforce legal obligations by coercive means' (Koller 2014: 166). This is also held to be advantageous in accounting for why more developed societies require a legal order to supplement conventional social norms (Hart 1994: 89f.).

My reservation is that this account explains only the normative bindingness of rules to those who accept them, which forms part of Raz's objections (1990: 53ff.), but those who dissent from either the 'creation' or the 'repeal' of legal norms find themselves once more subjected to the commands of a 'predatory regime'. The one thing that will not have been settled is social conflict, supposedly resolved by new 'binding decisions', because nothing makes such a settlement a matter of obligation rather than a response to coercion. Since one important driver of legal philosophy[6] is to differentiate valid legal orders from the various forms of Mafiosi coercion, this will not do; because both the C.S. and the S-C are simply held together by force alone.

One attempt to rescue the general thrust of this argument about what makes the law's claim to be normatively binding is Koller's argument that *both* the legal *authorities* must claim moral legitimacy for their directives and *also* their *addresses* must find these claims morally acceptable. Here, he follows Elster's argument (1989), maintaining that conventional norms gain acceptance and application amongst their addressees, along with other components of the Myth, and that the population acts in accordance with one 'conventional morality'. In this manner, the S-C is once more assumed to be homogeneous. Ideational deviations pertain to self-interested individuals alone and not to objective divides between interest groups and the ideas they endorse to promote them versus the counter ideas of their opponents. That is, until such coherent Cultural Systems are admitted to lose their effectiveness as social differentiation develops.

On a very large scale map the journey taken by legal Normativism could be marked off into three stages delineating historical changes in the relationship between normativity and the legal order, that is, between the components of NIR.

(a) In the beginning there was held to be a unitary and unifying normative source underwriting legal validity and hence obligations, one binding upon societies' members that bonded them cohesively via the hierarchical chain from which subsidiary legal injunctions were consistently derived.
(b) With the advent of growing social differentiation in modernity, the *legitimacy* of norms was at first complemented and then partially overtaken by consideration of the *actuality* of norms. The legal order was increasingly held to turn upon a *minimal acceptance by legal subjects* of binding guidelines for action in what could crudely be termed the 'democratic defence of validity' (Ross 1968 :82f.), one endorsed variously by Hart, Raz, Dworkin and Habermas.

[6]Because this volume is concerned with normativity and social change, I dwell almost exclusively upon the legal normativists within the philosophy of law. This is not to deny that other schools of legal philosophy have plenty to contribute to this book's theme as some contributors show.

(c) The augmentation of (supra-functional) social differentiation and multiculturalism led contemporary legal thinkers to accept and explore normative divergences between the *authorities* and the *addressees* of the law, without whose complementarity the legal order lacked stability – *bindingness* had become 'shaky'.

As social differentiation does develop – at first as functional differentiation and later as pluralism and multiculturalism – the next question is: 'What then happens to legal normativity under intense morphogenesis?' Once morphogenesis engages, it challenges the possibility that both the 'authorities' and the 'addressees' can claim moral legitimacy on *compatible ideational grounds*. The (new) problem is that the 'interplay between the two claims, *which are often not in harmony*, is of decisive importance for the persistence of a legal order both as to its normative validity and its social effectiveness' (Kollner 2014: 172 my italics).

Their lack of complementarity (harmony) threatens the 'proper functioning' and 'temporal stability' alike of the legal order because:-

> a high degree of *convergence* between the 'authorities' and the 'addressees' is certainly an ideal situation ... This situation, however, does not occur frequently. Usually, there are more or less significant tensions between the participants' claims to the law's legitimacy that may reflect divergent views of political morality between the law's authorities and addressees as well as within either group. Let us assume the extreme situation where the claims *diverge* so much that the participants are divided into a number of competing groups who cannot even reach partial agreement on the most basic moral requirements the law ought to satisfy in order to be acceptable to most of them. In that case, *the law's existence is shaky*, if one can say that a legal order exists at all: at any rate, *its normative force will be questionable, and it will lack both effectiveness and temporal stability*. (Koller 2014: 172 my itals)

The failure to be effective and stable characterizes the legal order as morphogenesis engages and morphostasis diminishes. However, Koller vascillates about legal contestation, even in modernity. On the one hand, he argues that '[a]s a rule, legal norms emerge in some way when there is a special need for them, i.e. when social groups that have a voice become dissatisfied with the current state of affairs and are able to push their interest via a legal regulation onto the public agenda' (2014: 173). In other words, his support for the consensuality of the conventional S-C level is retracted and the shaping of the legal C.S. no longer draws upon it but is moulded by contestation. On the other hand, Koller maintains that 'even when the emerging legal regulation may replace some previous conventional norms, it usually relies on the actual existence of many conventional norms. In fact, no legal order would function in a proper way without the support of many conventional norms' (Ibid). This have your cake and eat it argument is somewhat reminiscent of Lewis Coser's attempt in *The Functions of Social Conflict* (1956) to square manifest social contestation with on-going functional integration, thus endorsing *normative* functionalism but also furnishing it with a mechanism accounting for evolutionary 'adaptation'.

Moreover, the argument exactly parallels the recent one over the role of 'habits' or 'habitual action', during the last quarter of a century of rapid morphogenetic social change. My argument (Archer 2007, 2010, 2012) that new opportunities (new jobs, new technologies, new skills, new locations) rendered habitual action, acquired in family, neighbourhood and school, increasingly inappropriate as guidelines to social action in the late twentieth century, was met by an identical riposte. In a nutshell, the novel competencies required to meet the novel (and often unavoidable) challenges of acquiring new skills and occupying new openings, were held to be developed *on the basis of existing habits* (Elder-Vass 2007), thus ensuring continuity in the life-worlds of succeeding generations. It still puzzles me what past forms of habitual action serve as a platform for the young to engage in software programming, to enter international stock market trading, financial services or drone warfare.

Nevertheless, Kollner's argument concludes in an analogous manner *vis åvis* the C.S and the S-C levels: 'As a result, legal and conventional norms are closely interrelated and interdependent, both causally and conceptually. This particularly applies to the relationship between law and conventional morality, because a legal order *acquires its normativity from its compatibility with the prevalent conventional morality*' (Koller 2014: 173 my italics). In other words, this chapter began with Kelsen's top-down derivation of legal validity from its anchorage in the supposed groundnorm. Koller has completely inverted that argument by grounding the normativity of the legal order from the bottom up in 'the prevalent conventional morality'. Social scientists (let alone political leaders) can only ask what this supposed 'conventional morality' is that could be deemed 'prevalent' today – amidst not only multi-culturalism, but terrorism, corporate malpractice, decline of the family, the banishing of religion from public life, the demise of ideology and so forth.

One defensive solution is for certain sociologists to abandon, as they surely must, the notion of one 'conventional morality', commanding global S-C endorsement and to substitute the more modest proposition that different collectivities endorse and enforce the distinctive beliefs and normative practices of their groups, thus reinforcing different 'conventions'. For example, Elder-Vass introduced the general claim that 'norm circles', that is, a group of people identified in terms of coalescing supportively around a given norm and, as emergent entities, having the causal power to reinforce the dispositional conformity of individual 'members' to it by augmenting their sense of obligation (Elder-Vass 2010). To talk in terms of 'norm circles' does entail an unstated acceptance of the social fragmentation of normativity itself. Hence, C-S relational influence is broken down into a plethora of 'norm circles' (Elder-Vass 2012).

However, given his familiar acknowledgement of the diachronic need for analytical and morphogenetic histories of emergence but also his 'clean break' with the past (Archer 2015) and exclusive focus upon the synchronic, 'norm circles' never provide an account of the origins of the normativity that is taken as given in his approach. As Jamie Morgan pertinently comments, '[o]ne might reasonably ask how the cultural norm circle accounts for the origins of cultural norms, for the nature of their dissemination and for the complexity of their interrelation ... [and] why does one belief or cultural component become 'culture' rather than another?' (Morgan 2014: 135) Elder-Vass leaves us without answer. Instead, we are given a series of applications of this approach to *inter alia* 'practical norm circles', 'knowledge norm circles' and 'linguistic norm circles' (persuasively challenged by Sealey and Carter 2014). But, what is their interplay and how does this contribute to our understanding of cultural (or sub-cultural) normativity? In short, this is an account of the emergent effects of integration in small groups. It is confined to ('I'), since it lacks an account of where the norm in question ('N') came from and what form of regulation ('R') it results in. Otherwise, it merely tells us that strong group integration promotes normative conformity which, as a general proposition, does not appear to be controversial.

Self-Imposed Restrictions in Legal Normativism and Social Interpretavism for Dealing with the Legal Order in the Context of Social Morphogenesis

The large canvas upon which the legal philosophers had sketched and tried to refine solutions to the problem of normativity and explored its sources is the expansive meeting place between society's culture and society's legislation. Although some of the better known explanatory ventures have been found largely wanting here, this is not because – in the tribal warfare between disciplines – the social theorists are held to have done better. Discontent with both stems from the fact that those briefly and inadequately introduced above are more preoccupied with vindicating their philosophical positions than with advancing substantive concepts, propositions or theories about socio-legal processes of development, especially when confronted by intensive social change.

In the following section I have tried to distil these self-denying philosophical ordinances into three main points, dealing with the legal normativists and the critique of them by social theorists.

Resilient Holism

Undoubtedly, the *alpha* of legal normativism is the foundational and lasting conviction that the 'bindingness' of the legal order is something special and irreducible. The legislative facts to be explained are always intrinsically normative and their 'validity' has to be presumed and incorporated into any explanation, such as where they came from or how they started or what maintains them. Omit this key feature and proffer an account, for example, of 'legal behaviour' or 'knowledge about the law', as sociologists do, and it is immediately discounted as being about something other because it is non-normative. Without reference to the binding fact of legal validity, any such explanation offered by social theorists is held to be necessarily deficient because of its 'failure to include the specifically normative component of the norm – the thing that makes it binding and therefore a genuine norm' (Turner 2010:195). To the legal normativist it would parallel a discussion of any religious liturgy without reference to what 'makes it sacred'. I will call this the presumption of the intrinsically normative character of legal social regulation. This presumption also turns out also to be inescapably holistic.

Another way of putting the matter is that every legal 'ought' derives from its rooting in a form of collective intentionality, not far removed from Durkheim's *conscience collective*.[7] Obviously, collective intentionality depends upon some kind of collective: tribe, community or, most usually, a 'group'. However, latter day normativists (of whom Wilfrid Sellars is the foremost) are quite reasonably reluctant to take external and empirical evidence for the existence of any group as defining its membership (who are the members of a university: its employees, its graduands, its alumni, its benefactors, its external examiners etc.?). If the 'group' is defined according to any of these criteria (or all of them), then some of those considered to belong to it may not feel that they do. To Sellars, someone who has no internal 'sense of belonging to the group' cannot have anything more than a 'truncated understanding of ought' (1997 [1956]: 205). Normativity and Integration are tied closely together. This argument is intended to dispose of more than the undeniable fact that any 'community' may normatively proscribe stealing or adultery, but some are nonetheless thieves or adulterers. That would be to subscribe to what I dub a 'democratic majority' view of legality and since it is simply another version of aggregative individualism, he finds the majority view wanting as the source of the 'ought'.

Instead, Sellars insists upon genuine 'participation' or subjective belongingness to 'the group'. When that is the case, the group is 'internalized' as 'us', in what Plural Subject theorists have characterized as 'we thinking' or the 'we mode' of thought. For Sellars this, in turn, constitutes a change in consciousness, a development of or inclusion in the psychic unity *of* a group (as distinct from a group mind). 'Internalization' is akin to having adopted the group's 'Generalized Other' in G.H. Mead's terms. But it exceeds Mead's source of social conformity because this change of consciousness gives rise to a new form of intentionality by producing a collective intentionality that is binding on members (1997 [1956]: 203). It is shared and binding, but is binding because shared. In nascent morphogenic society, the trouble is that less and less is shared.

[7] This excludes 'custom' or 'convention', which might be reducible to what everyone just does in some community. It would thus be susceptible of reduction to aggregate Individualism which is unacceptable because there is no necessity to include any 'ought' in its explanations. For instance, some early food gathering tribe may have lived on fruit and nuts, not because they subscribed normatively, as a body, to vegetarianism but because there were few alternative food stuffs or knowledge about them as alternative edibles.

The Link with Plural Subject Theory

In a nutshell, the simple fact that 'we' make statements about 'our' shared intentions (beliefs, goals, identities and actions, agreements and acceptances) has become the lynch-pin for understanding and explaining our 'collective intentionality' itself as that of the Plural Subject. From these grammatical origins, theories of 'joint', 'collective' or 'plural' thought and action have been developed by prominent analytical philosophers (including Michael Bratman, Margaret Gilbert, John Searle and Raimo Tuomela).[8] Most of them hold that the theories they have advanced on the basis of 'we thinking' do the biggest of jobs: nothing short of re-defining the subject-matter of social science and its appropriate mode of explanation. That mode is very congenial to legal normativists.

How does the fact that people often say 'we think' provide a springboard for the conceptualization of human sociality and the explanation of the societal order, and especially the regulative order? Analytical philosophers are not homogeneous in how they construe 'we think', but for all it provides the key to major aspects of the social: to 'co-ordination' for Bratman, to 'co-operation' for Searle, to 'commitment' for Tuomela and to 'obligation' for Gilbert. All variously see 'we think' as being deontic – the generic source of 'rights', 'duties' 'obligations', 'authorizations', 'requirements', 'permissions' etc. and this is how the springboard to the socio-legal works at all levels.[9]

In sum, 'collective intentionality' in the form of the Plural subject promises no less than to solve the problem of the sources of normativity. In their re-working of this concept '[g]roup wills supply both a standard and a regression stopper – a source of normativity that is primal in the sense that it produces norms without reference to norms' (Turner 2010: 120). In so doing, and working initially from everyday examples (walking together or regularly sharing lunch), they advance a thoroughly normative theory that they venture to be universal and therefore applicable to all

[8]Space precludes a detailed discussion of each of these thinkers, who differ in important ontological ways, but can be found in Pierpaolo Donati and Margaret S. Archer, 2015, Chap. 2 'The Plural Subject versus the Relational Subject'.

[9]Bratman alone resists such ambitions. Searle states his ontological aim as being: '[t]o construct an account of social and institutional reality' (2010: 60 and 1993). Tuomela considers he is writing about 'the conceptual resources and philosophical prerequisites that a proper understanding and explaining of the social world requires' presenting 'almost a philosophical "theory of everything" in the social world relying on the 'we-perspective' (2010: vii–viii). Gilbert's claim is that 'analysis of our concepts of "shared" action" discovers a structure that is constitutive of social groups as such ... going for a walk together may be considered as a paradigm of social phenomena in general.' (1996: 178). Later on, she amplifies this statement: 'I believe that the concept of joint commitment is a fundamental social concept – perhaps *the* fundamental social concept' (1996: 366). Most of these authors have written subsequent books spelling out the macroscopic implications of the Plural Subject, such as Searle's 2010, *Making the Social World*: *The Structure of Human Civilization* (see also 1995) and Gilbert's 2006 *A Theory of Political Obligation*.

times and places. Thus, such theories are, in principle, claiming to cope with intensive morphogenesis and not to depend upon enduring morphostasis.

Given that contributors to this volume are seeking to address this last problem, then Plural Subject theory should potentially be of considerable interest to us too. However, what militates against this are three main reservations that make us reluctant to adopt it. The first is the most severe deterrent because the 'presentism' of this approach, means that the social relations forming the Plural Subject are without past or future and thus never can confront morphogenesis or, for that matter, any other account of 'changing times'.

The accounts given are almost exclusively *present tense*. In none do the examples of social relations given have a history. 'We think' is discussed without any diachronic account of how 'we' came to 'think' such and such or to be in a position to do so. Furthermore, in the present tense, the resulting joint actions are not acknowledged to entail relational dynamics. Searle's cooks who regularly make béarnaise sauce together (1990) simply continue pouring and stirring in a frozen time frame; one or the other never suggests that pouring more slowly or stirring faster might enhance their co-operation or the end product. Yet, joint action is rarely non-reflexive, non-discursive and free from learning. These are the aspects of ordinary social relations through which the future is forged in the present through incremental – or innovative – changes. Alternatively, they can also result in growing boredom and a future preference for shop-bought sauce. In other words, outcomes are never allowed to be generative or degenerative: those regularly walking together never start buying boots and joining a hiking club, nor do they conclude that the local walks are becoming monotonously repetitive.

Second, the practice of reflexivity is almost completely ignored. Since many of the examples these authors give involve joint action that takes time to accomplish and may result in failure (two people trying to start a car together) and none deny that 'I think', it is curious that neither party attempting to get the car going ever seems to volunteer reflexive suggestions about how it might be better done. After all, if one of these works, 'we' might come to think differently; just as 'we' might come to think differently about forms of regulation!

Third, in Plural Subject theorizing emergent properties are excluded,[10] but their absence makes for huge difficulties (which do not concern us here, but see Donati and Archer 2015) except that they also characterize legal normativism and this affinity accounts for some of the latter's main difficulties. As I have maintained, normativist legal philosophy is unapologetically Holist in its social ontology. I will illustrate this by returning to Sellars. As we have seen, he is (rightly) opposed to aggregate Individualism, hence no enumeration of personal intentions (supposing these to be unproblematic) can add up to a collective intention. So what would? Turner puts this question in terms of a 'missing ingredient'. Any intention 'in a collective or 'we' form, needs to have some additional property, call it S, that makes it actually collective or shared ... But to use a collective intention in an explanatory

[10]Gilbert alone makes the occasional reference to 'supervenience'.

way – for example, to explain a norm that is binding on members of a community – something needs to be shared in fact... What sort of facts might there be about S?' (2010: 125). Some might try to evade this question, though Sellars is not one of them. Searle is.[11]

In specifying what he considers to be the 'missing S', accounting for sharedness, we have already seen Sellars endorsing the psychic unity arising from 'feelings of belongingness' to a group. From amongst the Plural Subject advocates, Sellars seems closest to Tuomela, to whom We-mode thinking entails various interconnected concepts in addition to we-mode intentions (such as, 'We will perform joint action X together'). The most important of we-mode reasons is collective commitment to the group's '*ethos*', which 'glues' members together. The 'central assumption' and, thus, the core meaning of 'we think' to Tuomela 'is that the members of a group share an ethos, E, that consists of contents such as goals, beliefs, values, standards and norms' (2010: 18), which they should accept, satisfy, maintain and promote. In this argument, S = Ethos. Unfortunately, E itself is problematic when it stands as the predicate of what is shared – and the feelings associated with it.[12]

If the 'we mode' hangs upon behaving towards the group 'ethos' in the above ways then its acceptability turns upon the answers to two questions : (i) What kinds of intra-group relations are held to bring about and sustain this conformity to the ethos? (ii) Is there a *consistency of contents* making up the group 'ethos' such that members can be said to share them, where sharing stands for all the forms of normativity held in common as listed above? These are two separate questions: (i) is posed at the Socio-Cultural level and is about the extent of intragroup consensus and (ii) at the level of Cultural Systems is about the logical coherence of the ideas involved (Archer 1988). Yet neither such consensus nor such coherence can ever be

[11]The 'sense of togetherness', which he holds to be important, is not entailed by Searle's 'we think'; because he agrees someone can be misguided or mistaken in thinking it. Thus, he admits that 'collective intentionality in my head can make a purported reference to other members of a collective *independently of the question whether or not there are such members*.' (1990: 407 italics added). In that case, the 'we' is wrongly projected because there is no 'we' to which 'we think' or 'we intend' refers or can refer. Thus, he admits that 'I may be mistaken in taking it that the "we" in "we intend" actually refers to a we' (1990: 408). It is therefore in order to ask what makes 'we intending' something necessarily plural? The response of Pettit and Schweikard seems unavoidable: 'Not the fact that a number of people instantiate it, since Searle allows that I may instantiate such a state in the mistaken belief that others do so too. So what then? We see no answer in Searle's work and find his position on this issue inherently obscure.' (2006: 31–2).

[12]If emergence is allowed, then an alternative approach to 'sharedness' becomes possible. Donati and Archer (2015) maintain that *The Relational Subject* can orient his or her actions (goals, intentions, commitments) to the emergent goods and evils they themselves generate (trust, commitment, common projects and certainly togetherness) and their opposites as relational evils. In short, *relational subjects can achieve a 'we-ness' without our needing to invoke 'we thinking' as a necessary mechanism or mediatory process*. Indeed, we ourselves explicitly denied that the workings and effects of 'we-ness' entailed (i) sharing the same beliefs or coming to do so (Bratman); (ii) positing that we have the same thoughts in our heads (Searle); (iii) having achieved a mutual agreement and sharing a common ethos (Tuomela); or (iv) arriving (explicitly or tacitly) at a joint commitment (Gilbert).

taken for granted (Archer and Elder-Vass 2011) and they can vary independently of one another. This distinction is central to the present volume and will be used to introduce Part III.

Sociological Critiques Based on Methodological Individualism also Depend Upon Morphostasis

'[H]istorical questions about the emergence, character and success of legal orders were for Weber questions that could be entirely separated from considerations of legal validity themselves' (Turner 2010: 73). Turner agrees and seeks to naturalize normativity as a matter of learning and experience and thus to debunk its reification at the hands of the legal normativists, but he does so as a methodological individualist. Stephen Turner is a Weberian in this respect. He wants to accomplish this by refocusing upon *legitimation* (a property resulting from social interaction) rather than *legitimacy* (a property belonging to norms themselves), and to re-justify 'empathy' (*verstehen*) as crucial to the sociological enterprise in the legal field. Although empathy has always had its defenders as well as its detractors, Turner jumps quickly over these disputes by maintaining that 'something very significant has happened in the intervening years that has altered dramatically the status of empathy' (Turner 2010: 175). This is:-

> [T]he discovery of mirror neurons in monkeys and the subsequent development of inquiries into empathy and the mirroring systems of human beings. Mirror neurons activate both in the performance of actions and in the perception of actions. They enable the brain to operate on a dual-use basis, so that the neurons used for acting are also used for what Weber would call the direct observational experience of a meaningful action such as chopping wood... And having a location in the brain changes the status of empathy – it ceases to be an intellectual process bound up with the error-prone folk language of intentionality, and becomes a fact of science with a discoverable set of features located in specific neuronal processes. (Turner 2010: 175–6)[13]

By this route, Turner naturalizes empathy. The norms that the legal normativists had always maintained were indispensable for understanding the meanings used and applied in the world – and therefore entailed an ineluctable excursion into their special territory that precluded naturalism – can be sloughed off because now susceptible of explanation in norm-free terms. They become 'empathetic projections that are confirmed, sustained, corrected, and improved upon '*through interaction with others*' (Turner 2010: 178 italics added). By making empathy impossible to eliminate as part of social interaction, Turner has effectively produced an argument paralleling the legal normativists position towards norms. Predictably, the latter reject this, but more to our point, does it serve to ground a substitute sociology of *non-normative legal legitimation*?

---

[13]Some supporting scientific references accompany this passage.

It seems to me that there are three objections that our contributors make. First, Turner asserts that when some action is made empathetically intelligible, this is 'final in the sense that there is no further explanation of it' (Turner 2010: 179). In that case, since there is no reference to intelligibility being dependent on the structural context (which makes understanding 'cashing a cheque' depend upon referring to how banks work[14]), or its embedding in the cultural system (concept-dependence), then *intelligibility* rests on its inter-agential comprehensibility alone. In other words, it abrogates the SAC requirements in being purely agential. And this could well mean that those subjects claiming mutual comprehension could be living in cloud cuckoo land inhabited by 'ghoulies and ghosties'.[15]

Second, Turner blocks any corrective route out of this situation by disallowing any reference to the regulative role played by the objective world in curtailing our wilder fancies. Instead, 'intersubjectivity of the sort produced by mutual comprehension based on empathy plus feedback produces as much 'objectivity' in this case as is to be had. And universal intersubjective agreement ... is as much as there is to 'Objectivity' (Turner 2010: 178). Truth obviously departs, but are we thus to say that 'gravity' and its causal effects upon us did not exist before our mutual comprehension of it? And what is Turner going to say to those who are unconvinced by the explanatory role assigned to 'mirror neurons', that is, where there is no mutual comprehension?

Third, if there is no further explanation required once some action is held to be empathetically understandable, then the 'only evidence of it being a success is indirect – through the success of our interactions' (Turner 2010: 183). But in what does their success consist? If this consists in attaining mutual comprehension alone, the argument becomes circular. Were two points of view both understandable and yet their protagonists locked in disagreement, what would be considered the 'success of their interaction'? Because action is always required, are those 'preparatory meditations' (William James), 'musements' (Peirce) or reflexive deliberations through which courses of action are evaluated and determined deemed irrelevant to one course being selected? I raise this because our reflexive internal conversations are far from being transparent to the empathy of others.

Finally, in winding up his book, Turner who has leaned heavily upon the human capacity to learn and especially to understand those similarly situated, recognizes that the latter does not mean 'sharing a framework' although empathy does depend on having 'these same things' in common. Ultimately, he rests his case for our ability to empathize upon Weber's statement that we 'understand what a person is doing ... on the basis of the facts of the situation, *as experience has accustomed us to interpret them*' (1978 [1968]:5, cited on p. 183 my itals). That, in common with

[14]In Mandelbaum's classic example (1973).

[15]Certainly Turner also refers to correction by 'feedback' here, but because he does not specify feedback from what, this does not necessitate contextual or conceptual referents and could be satisfied by fanciful references from those persons involved to equally weird referents they find mutually acceptable.

the corpus of arguments from the philosophers of legal normativity, *presupposes morphostasis*. It assumes that the 'facts of the situation', human experiences of them and the 'accustomed' interpretations based on these remain *stable*, that is sufficiently unchanging for us to have learned how others understand them. With intensive morphogenesis, these assumptions no longer hold[16]; the traction they once provided for legal philosophy and the sociology of *verstehen* have gone. The experiential has gone evanescent where the social order is concerned.[17]

That they no longer give such traction is the challenge of this volume, for neither approaches examined can be of assistance. In Volume II (2014, Ch. 1) I discussed the difference made once historic 'social stability' gave way but could be superseded by new forms of emergent 'stabilization'. Yet even if this were proved to be correct, such novel processes would not underwrite unchanging 'facts of the situation' or repetitive human experiences such as to permit 'accustomed interpretations'.

Normative Morphogenesis

Because normativity in all its aspects forms part of societal culture, normative morphogenesis since 1980 can be analysed from within the framework already developed for cultural change and stasis (Archer 1988: 203–273). The millennial period marks a decisive shift away from the characteristics of later modernity – as registered in science, religion and ideology – in terms of both the *logical relations between ideas* at the level of the Cultural System (C.S.) and at the Socio-Cultural level (S-C) in terms of the *ideational relationships between people.*

The hallmark of cultural relations in modernity was one of 'competetive contradictions' between the respective corpuses of ideas activated critically and conflictually by opposed groups for purposes of legitimation. Consequently, the situational logic of action was that of *elimination* from the time of the great Age of Ideology onwards and, although never fully successful in achieving this goal, it generated institutional polarization and normative cleavage among the population: State versus Church, Right versus Left, Unions versus Employers, Us versus Them etc. To

[16]Exactly the same was true of Mead's 'Generalized Other'. One can only admire his honesty in admitting that once social institutions exceed a certain size it becomes dubious if individuals can continue to take the roles of the other: '[T]he community may in its size transcend the social organization, may go beyond the social organization which makes such identification possible. The most striking illustration of that is the economic community. This includes everybody with whom one can trade in any circumstances, *but it represents a whole in which it would be next to impossible for all to enter into the Attitudes of others*' (Mead 1934: 326–327 italics added). *Mind, Self and Society.*

[17]In any case, the experiential represents the confines of reality in empiricism and not to Critical Realists whose stratified social ontology of the social also includes the 'actual' and 'real' levels, inaccessible to human experience.

account for the transformation in the contemporary period it is necessary to outline major changes in (a) the constitution of the C.S., in (b) the ideational outlooks predominant within the S-C and in (c) the interplay between the two. This interplay became transformed from the aggressive and overt situational logic of elimination, grounded in 'competetive contradictions' to a much looser situational logic of action based upon 'contingent complementarities'. These represented the opportunity for agents to make what would by *synthesizing* compatible cultural items. (Although what was made of opportunities was never independent of differences in power and resources characterizing the positions from which different groups started out at this new T^1.)

To stress 'contingent complementarities' needs highlighting because it is not the increase in variety *alone*[18] that has supreme importance, as in approaches which accentuate the increasing speed in the accumulation of knowledge (such as Rosa's 'acceleration theory' 2003), which basically emphasizes that there is a growing amount to know. That is simply a statement about the speed of accretion rather than a theory of the growth of knowledge. Such fast aggregation may – and probably does – result in ideational *bricolage*, but it is directionless, and thus not equivalent to (C.S.) cultural elaboration, much less to morphogenesis precisely because it relies entirely upon contingency.

Conversely, to detect and develop a 'contingent complementarity' entails (at least) two cultural items that are *logically* compatible and whose detection and exploitation lead to purposeful developments (which can prove to be dead-ends). Successful synthesis adds to variety, enhances the prospect of yet more novel elaboration in the same direction and so contributes to shaping one morphogenetic trajectory in the growth of knowledge, which may or may not be trivial and can be benign or noxious according to the purposes for which it is used – or abused. Syntheses and synergies are part of the cultural structure (that is never just a heap of items), which confronts *all* agents at T^1, though some active agents may themselves have been responsible for developing them and others can already be aligned against them.[19]

The three sections of this book deal sequentially, with changes in the C.S., the S-C and relations between them, which cumulatively means they deal with the three phases of this new and unfinished morphogenetic cycle that has not yet reached T^4. Because our substantive concern is specifically with the normative order, this means that the components of the C.S. examined and explained are normative and the focus is upon their coherence (N); those of the S-C concern social integration (I); and their interplay should result in an account of nascent tendencies in social regulation (R), involving laws, rules, regulations and conventions.

[18]We emphasized in the first of these Volumes (Archer (ed.) 2013: 3–4) reasons why 'variety' could not be enumerated and thus have confined ourselves to statements of 'more' or 'less' of it.

[19]This is why it is *always important* to insist that the delineation of morphogenetic phases is *analytical* and depends on the research question in hand.

Working in that order, the first question is what has altered about the composition of the C.S. that justifies characterizing the relations between its component items as 'contingent complementarities'? Formally, I have maintained that the fundamental answer is a huge increase in *variety*, and in this case *normative variety*. As 'new items (pure and applied theories) are lodged in the system, the probability increases that the fund of undetected complementarities (either between novel items themselves or between these novelties and older items) also increases, though not in any fixed proportion . . . [Yet], although the detection of any particular contingent complementarity remains indeterminate, a higher *rate* of discovery appears to be an empirical fact' (Archer 1988: 265). However, the question remains, what accounts for this unprecedented growth in normative *variety*?

In Part I, the contributors dwell upon certain major factors and how each prompts synthesis or synergy (recalling that these processes generate *further variety* over time[20]). All of these stem in one way or another from second-order effects of globalization. In detailing and encapsulating some of the 'great normative changes' leading from the end of the Twentieth century, Doug Porpora sets the scene by stressing how chains of morphogenetic cycles, initiated by social movements, paved the way as precedents and exemplars for the development of the next – from Civil Rights to the Women's movement and on to the LGBTQ – such that 'we can think of cultural milieu as the result of iterated morphogenic cycles building on each other' (Chap. 2: 16). All of these were globally influenced and had global repercussions; for example, of the 17 nations in which gay marriage is now (January 1st 2015) legal, every instance is a millennial change. In particular, the 'virtue of tolerance', which is synthetic by definition, has displaced principled religious opponents and introduced the 'Macro-Moral Disconnect', meaning a retreat of the deontic from public life as religion is increasingly confined to the private domain. More generally, it clearly signals the expulsion of morality from public life.

Philip Gorski fills in the religious theme by accentuating the significance of diasporic movements, or what I had more generally termed 'migration' in order to cover scientific morphogenesis as well. In either case, geographical movement and mixing 'amplifies deviations from their starting points and generates novelty. Thus the transfer of ideas is never the replication of those ideas in a new environment, for literal copying is possible only when the two domains are practically identical. Instead, the transferred ideas have to be synthesized with the properties of their new field of application and this itself is innovatory' (Archer 1988: 260–261). Gorski illustrates the above statement for world religions, as diaspora disconnects them from their original geo-local or regional 'centres' and their cultural particularities. The peripheral and mobile groups become more homologous with the new environments in which they embed themselves. However, their reconnection to and incorporation of elements (ideas and artifacts) from their new locales does not leave

[20] '[T]he central argument is that synthesis is the generic consequences of contingent complementarities refers strictly to the work performed on two consistent elements . . . and the results of these endeavours which they then offer back to the Cultural System' (Archer 1988: 258).

the local mechanisms of cultural production unchanged. This interchange introduces the *reflexive imperative* as part of the embedding process, but nothing confines the outcomes of such religious reflexivity to a retreat into fundamentalism as some kind of default setting.

What we have not examined is the current disembedding of the diasporic and its re-embedding into a new 'contingent complementarity'; namely the revival of the old Islamic Caliphate, bringing together today's disenchantment – both material and ideational – of Muslims in the developed world and those opposed to this part of the world from the middle east. To revamp an old ideal in order to confront contemporary circumstances is itself a novelty and an illustration of the fact that 'ideas never die', but can be re-animated from the C.S. provided there are current S-C agents committed to renewing their social salience.

In dealing with international relations, Colin Wight is acutely aware that 'norm emergence', often spearheaded by 'norm entrepreneurs', such as Martin Luther King, had an effect not only on civil rights in the U.S. but also on anti-apartheid in South Africa. As he puts it, his examples all highlight 'how domestic actors can influence international practices, but the process goes both ways and norms can diffuse at the international level and become accepted and adopted in domestic contexts' (Chap. 4: 67). Similarly, a shared international experience, such as the dropping of the atomic bombs on Hiroshima and Nagasaki, changed the social context of all nations and provided traction for the adoption of a new transnational norm to restrict nuclear proliferation. These instances are multiplied by technology, specifically the new digital, polymedia repositories of the C.S. for information (including mutual surveillance), without it being the case that this fosters a consensus developing around them at the national S-C levels.

Finally, Andrea Maccarini brings the foregoing contributions together by asking the general question 'how 'unbound' is morphogenesis going to be from normativity itself, from its prompts and restraints?' (Chap. 5: 77). It is necessary to probe at this level of generality because the preceding contributors could indeed be perfectly correct for the domains examined, without any of them warranting a generalization that answers Maccarini's question. Indeed, he himself convincingly examines various strategies by which different groups seek to evade or confront new attempts at *control* or *justification* in normative terms. Therefore, *qua* examples, such variations could count against any general tendency in normative change. Not so in the second half of his chapter where he gives a frighteningly realistic reason for contemplating the full retreat of normativity as we have known it! Not 'tolerance' (repressive or otherwise), not multiple forms of 'embedded' diaspora, and not a more gloomy prognosis for international relations, but a practice that is already upon us: the demotion of an unknown but potentially large proportion of the human race to the status of *disposable* people. This refers to the moving percentage of *unenhanced* human persons. Transhumanism is no longer merely an idea from Mary Shelley's febrile mind, but is already an established medical practice and one that has also recruited a host of ideational advocates.

We confront its impact as a real novelty, but with a high probability of growing. I will simply list some of the potential impacts of transhumanism to give some notion of their range: Christian theology would be sorely challenged by its Redeemer not 'being a man like us in all things but sin', for to whom or what would 'us' refer?[21] How would the great historical legislators, statesmen, generals, writers, and popular leaders fare in the humanities? Would science to date represent the limited achievements of an 'unenhanced' species? Would the same be the case for renowned sportsmen and women and the records they set? And where would that leave the social sciences, without their 'fixed' benchmark in common humanity? Perhaps, what would be challenged as much as any of the above is the nature of law, for how could the universalization of normativity survive against the bifurcation into one law for the *ubermensch* and another for the *untermensch*, however much benificence was credited to the former?

Part 2 moves on to consider Socio-Cultural integration (S-C) and the importance that both Weber and Lockwood (1964) attached to any instance of its independent variation from the Cultural System. In this case, when both forms of integration were high, it accounted for the smooth operation of the law versus the manifestation of discordant normative interpretations of it, when the state of the two varied from one another. In a nutshell, when the C.S. level was highly integrated (i.e. displayed considerable logical coherence) and co-existed with a correspondingly high level of S-C integration (i.e. absence of conflictual divisions in the population), these constituted the conditions for morphostasis – of law and normativity in this case. Conversely, in this far reaching and prescient use of Critical Realism's stratified social ontology, the reversal of these conditions was propitious for morphogenesis. This is a very blunt summary for clarity of presentation. Ismael Al-Amoudi gives us a more sophisticated version, tailored to our specific concern with normativity, but also introduces the importance of the differential distribution of power at the onset of social interaction in T^2–T^3.

He begins by noting that the codification of rules is always fundamentally incomplete because they can never fully foresee and therefore specify the range of actions prescribed and proscribed by law or the precise contexts of their application. The interpretation of any law is, therefore, always mandatory in times and circumstances of morphogenesis or of morphostasis, though more demanding in the former. Al-Amoudi neatly distinguishes between those interpretations according to the 'letter' of the law, compared with those that appeal to its 'spirit'. He asks what is required for a given population to arrive at a consensual, harmonious interpretation of codified rules and how these requirements bear upon late modernity with its low social integration, contextual discontinuity and steep differences in power? His response is that consensus on the 'letter' presupposes only minimal social integration (all that needs to be shared at the S-C level is a common language and understanding of basic interaction, such as making a payment), but it does depend upon high system integration (C.S), one that is free from the contradictions which dogged rules governing bureaucracy and those governing taxation in medieval society. Conversely, for consensus on the 'spirit', high social integration

[21] There are obvious parallels for the founding figures of other world religions.

is a necessary condition. This is an incisive analysis but Al-Amoudi's original contribution comes in showing how with intense and concurrent morphogenesis the most powerful agents can make the best use of the opportunities offered and take the most advantage of the literal applications (e.g. loopholes or 'what is not forbidden is permitted') of the codified laws.

Clearly, by themselves neither high nor low integration at the social (S-C) or system levels (C.S.) actually *do* anything; they form the context. Agents and actors are needed for real *doings*, whether these concern active contestation of the normative context from below or involve its design, redesign and enforcement from above. The next two chapters provide a nice complement to Al-Amoudi's.

Mark Carrigan takes the prevailing low level of social integration (S-C) and its simmering disgruntlement and considers it in relation to both the 200 years-old recipe for bringing relief – the social movement – and the personal effects of the new reflexive imperative in the context of the digitalization of cultural abundance. The two are linked because a social movement can serve as the carrier for a personal cause, whilst allowing such personal concerns to find a more effective course of action in shared projects. However, the escalation of digital opportunities is double edged: it means both that an increased reflexivity is a pre-requisite for the use of this 'escalation in cultural abundance' but also that it represents a 'digital overload', crowding out what matters to someone by the urgency with which the media impose 'presentism', distracting subjects from discerning those elements that merit follow-though in the light of their nascent concerns. The ease of assembly of a public demonstration fosters 'fragile movements', prone to a short life expectancy because appealing to a brittle expressivism rather than fostering a collective reflexivity in which 'we' deliberate upon about effective forms of collective action for 'us'.

Margaret Archer deals, instead, with the prevalent low level of system integration (C.S.) characterizing the proliferation of legislation at international, regional, national, and institutional levels and suggests that the intensification of morphogenesis has resulted in legal clashes and complexity which still cannot keep up with the regulation of morphogenetic novelty. The 'solution' is argued to be a marked retreat from law as the instrument of legal regulation with its intrinsic normativity and increasing resort being made to 'anormative bureaucratic regulation', that performs the tasks of increasingly complex social coordination without reliance upon normative assent from the subjects in question. This manoeuvre depends upon low social integration but serves to reduce it still further. In short, anormative rules advance as the key source of social order when S-C solidarity is wanting and traditional C.S. legal instruments are failing devices for directing social co-ordination as morphogenesis continues to intensify.

Emmanuel Lazega agrees but takes the argument a stage further by showing how business leaders are and try to be the beneficiaries of anormative regulation by shaping the bodies, agencies and practices that execute it, to the detriment of democratic decision-making. 'The staggering number of specialized, unvoted, and taken for granted rules . . . that organize society based on both public administrative law and private standards has created a situation in which the institutions of electoral democracy are strongly challenged by a new political economy' (Chap. 8: 144). This he illustrates through his empirical network analysis of how, as mediators or brokers, the international law firms have colonized global law through their acquired powers of arbitration. The specific example he traces is the generation of anormative rules, procedural rather than substantive in kind, and hence unintelligible outside this circuit of legal expertise. These regulate a key aspect of intellectual property, namely the conferral of Patents that are central to contemporary capitalism. He substantiates these propositions by examining the building of a new institution, a Unified Patent Court for Europe, which does not yet exist, through the secondary socialization of established national judges at a collegial Forum. What they learn is to prioritize the procedural rules upon which they can concur, even or especially when they are at variance on their substance. Such a meso-level outcome thus escapes any need to seek legitimation by the electoral system.

If these four chapters are read consecutively, readers will note that the authors are in considerable agreement, but in a gloomy accord. They have ranged over the macro-, meso- and micro-levels and none has adduced grounds for hoping that the seeds of eudaimonia lie in any of these social strata. What we have all traced in our different ways is the durability of the existing distribution of power at T^1 and its extraordinary adaptability during T^2–T^3. Given the retreat from normativity, which most of us have accentuated, along with detecting few realistic prospects for an increase in social integration, we have found little reason to hope for arrival at a very different T^4 in the immediate future.

Part 3 Pierpaolo Donati's chapter goes down the same track. Given pluralization, (multiculturalism etc. see his 2008) he maintains that the 'impersonal morality' of the law and of social conventions is in demise and with it 'the normative cement constituted by shared values and norms is breaking down' (Chap. 10: 184). Although in full agreement that current norms express the power relations between the agents and actors involved, he is more concerned than any of us *with the morphogenesis of normativity itself* than with the fate of the normative in other domains during intense morphogenesis.

The burden of his analysis is that Social Relations are themselves nomos-building. In other words, normativity arises from the Socio-Cultural level. This must be correct because, in itself, no amount of (logical) complementarity between any pair of C.S. elements does anything at all; it remains inert until activated from the S-C by active agents who note it, regard its exploitation as conducive to their concerns and hence try to develop it.[22]

The process of nomos-building that gradually raises the level of social integration, generically depends upon the emergence of relational goods from *sociality* (specifically solidarity and subsidiarity engendering trust) generated by couples and small groups – such as the 'Social Streets' – voluntary associations etc. (see Donati and Archer 2015). This raises three issues that may prove controversial.

[22]This is exactly my own view of the elaboration of the Cultural System, where I defended the proposition that 'There is elaboration of the CS due to the S-C level modifying current logical relationships and introducing new ones' (Archer 1988: 227–269).

First, is his claim that *relationality* is the *source* of moral value ('it is the properties and causal powers of reciprocity that define what is good or bad.'). This he illustrates with regard to the 'Social Streets' where 'the relation that inspires associative agency is the value to be pursued, independently of its utility, efficacy, or efficiency. In these social practices, what matters is not the material goal that can be achieved (for instance, the maintenance of a common good like a public garden in the neighbourhood) as such, but 'the sociality behind it', i.e., the sociality among the neighbours who produce it' (Chap. 10, 205).[23] We can certainly dispense with 'utility, efficacy, or efficiency' in that small-scale, face-to-face example of reviving conviviality but, as we say in English, 'that's not the way to run a railway'. Sociality is undoubtedly a mechanism generating relational goods and evils, but where bigger and more impersonal undertakings are concerned – such as the safety and punctuality of train services – it is at least questionable that 'sociality' should or could trump the other three considerations because it partly depends upon them; if passengers are to get to work, see their dispersed families, or attend meetings of their voluntary associations. In such cases, could we not reverse the aphorism and say 'sociality lies in front' of the efficiency of such services and cannot therefore be independent of them?

Second, and empirically, can relational subjects become sufficiently resilient to opposed vested interest groups promoting the incongruent norms of competitive consumerism through a digitalized invasion of the life-world and a debased substitution of superficial 'friendship' for real relationality as engendered by the social media? Donati's basic response is to insist upon an ontological justification, that sociality is of (greater) moral worth because it nurtures human flourishing. Epistemologically, however, the above forms of S-C manipulation can lead any number of subjects to conclude otherwise, and is this too not 'nomos-building', whatever our ethical judgement upon these results?

Third, the chapter is pitched at the meso-level and Donati himself has expressed doubts concerning macro-institutional entities, explicitly including the judicial system, coming to constitute Relational Subjects because such institutions are 'are normatively obliged to act according to formal, public criteria and involve individuals whose personal qualities, ideas, cultures and social origins differ greatly from one another' (Donati and Archer 2015: 191–2). Yet, they can block the upward percolation of alternative norms from the meso-level and, some would argue that they can systematically prevent the generation and articulation of humanistic norms and practices at the meso-level itself. Tony Lawson is one who argues precisely that.

Lawson presents a non-trivial case of enduring morphostasis and seeks 'to explain the unreasonable persistence of certain of the practices of modern economics', (Chap. 11: 244) namely its attachment to abstract mathematical modelling detached from economic reality, which endures meaning that 'The crisis in the economy is essentially ignored' (Chap. 11: 225). He questions how this is possible.

[23]We have rehearsed some of the pros and cons raised by this proposition in the conclusion to Donati and Archer (2015), especially pgs 327–331.

Lawson retains his commitment to an explanation in terms of his logical 'positioning formula' (X counts as Y in C) with social Darwinism supplying the generative social mechanism. All the same, the interesting substantive analysis he provides does translate smoothly into the morphogenetic framework and developments of it presented in our previous volumes (especially Maccarini 2015). He does not give his reasons for preferring this explanatory framework and in what respects he deems it to be of superior power. It could be that he does not recognize (or accept) that the M/M approach can deal with his conundrum. Nevertheless, to account for the strange detachment of mathematicised economics, we are in agreement that 'to provide a full explanation it is necessary to determine how the relevant set of norms became accepted in the first place and how challenges to its position/status are repelled' (Chap. 11: 225).

The historical overview of the 200 years during which mathematical modelling became accepted in economics does seem a classic case of the relational contestation of which I have given many examples in science (Archer 1988, 2013). Its attainment of hegemony is convincingly explained by Lawson through the coalescing of those escaping Nazi rule by moving to the U.S. and then seeking protection from McCarthyite witch-hunts from their redoubt within abstruse mathematics. The irrealism of modeling was a good form of self-protection; but, in Lakatos' terms, it was also a 'degenerating paradigm shift', hence its durability and lack of challenge needs explaining. This is also to be accounted for by the successful actions of what I term a vested interest group (commandeering posts, journals, awards etc.). Why did this endure? Lawson maintains 'for much the same reasons as they were able to rise to prominence in that earlier period: they can and do nothing to challenge the status quo'. Inaction is a form of action and one I view, as does Lawson, as sparing governmental policy from serious criticism. In short, there is no serious disagreement between the two explanatory frameworks over the analytical history of this degenerative development.

However, allow me briefly to signal three points at which the M/M approach could provide added value in explaining the persistence of modelling in economics. First, by showing that such inaction is not an aberration, advantageous for the dubious dealings of the multi-nationals and the digitalized finance sector because the abstracted indifference of economists represents their self-immobilization as a source of critique. This is not a peculiarity; a notable precursor was the retreat of Soviet social scientists into 'laboratory empiricism' that protected both them and the régime. Second, that faced by economic crisis these econometricians conform very closely to Maccarini's (2015) description of one defensive response to morphogenesis and its challenges, namely to form an 'enclave' insulating itself from the surrounding environment. Third, there are the associations of Heterodox economists, existing in all developed countries, as weak Corporate agents. Yet why, have they mostly proved so poverty-stricken in articulating an alternative? One answer worth exploring is that in terms of 'contingent complementarities' they have not identified a complementary item in the C.S. to partner their critique and to draw them away from mathematical modelling. The nucleus of one exists in, for example, Stefano Zamagni's work on the co-operative economy, but the Anglo-Saxon world lacks any equivalent to the fifteenth century civil economy of some Italian city states to resonate with them and then give salience to this alternative.

Working from Socio-Biology and on a much bigger canvas, Wolfgang Hofkirchner sets out to provide an alternative route away from the capitalist neo-liberal hegemony in which norms are stripped away from moral values, a process that simply entails a competitive concern to establish and maintain forms of anormative co-ordination conducive to the durability of global financialized capitalism. It gives no side glance towards co-operation that promotes social integration and offsets its continuing decline; one that could now presage systemic breakdown, as the current situation of Greece in relation to the EU may portend.

However, it is one thing to advocate a new 'integrativism', based on an emergent ethics; a global embracing of moral re-humanization and its preferability to the 'moral disconnect' – ironically shared by neo-liberalism and post-modernism alike. Yet, from where is it to come? Hofkirchner does not merely assert that the values he calls 'the new cosmopolitanism' is 'an idea whose time has come' (Chap. 11: 249), and does not shrink from locating it in the tradition of Catholic Social Teaching, most proximately in Pope Francis's new Encyclical, *Laudato sí*. The development of its main theme, 'integral ecology', remains to be worked out, partly in terms of complementary institutional forms and particularly in terms of the *realpolitik* needed to introduce them. It courts the dangers of Latino populism but, nevertheless, since the '99 %' originated within the most developed parts of the world, there is a real foundation for a nascent collective and relational subject to devote its meta-reflexivity to the tasks of delineating those institutional transformations required for a break though to a co-operative 'system of a higher order'. The stabilization of intensifying morphogenesis would require normative emergence but this would necessarily have to be on-going, given the tendency of morphogenesis is for 'variety to generate more variety'. Equally, continuous ideational elaboration would need to be matched by continual structural elaboration; social and system integration have to remain synchronized, just as must 'solidarity' and 'subsidiarity' if they are to become mutually supportive and remain so as morphogenesis continues.

Conclusion

At the beginning of this Introduction I noted the conviction of modernity's 'normativists', in both legal philosophy and social theory, that 'NIR must cohere': namely, a necessary condition of an orderly society was that normativity, integration and regulation must be mutually reinforcing. What we have shown is that this coherence itself required a more fundamental condition to be met: that of *societal morphostasis*. Once morphogenesis engages and intensifies, the components of NIR cohere less and less. They do so for different reasons and with different consequences, but the common denominator is that they become mutually unsupportive. This is the conclusion arrived at by taking this volume as a whole. It is justified by extrapolating three separate propositions about (N), (I) and (R) and then juxtaposing them. There is not space to present a properly argued justification here, but perhaps what follows can be regarded as a robust hypothesis about 'Morphogensis and Normativity' that warrants consideration.

(i) Where (N) is concerned, intensified morphogenesis has entailed a retreat from public, deontic normativity in the developed world.

There are other ways of putting this: that the Macro-Moral Disconnect has expelled not only religion from public life but any form of universalistic moral vision; macroscopic normativity is then confined in a contradictory fashion to the private sphere; in so far as the binary division between the public and private is breached, then the 'communities' doing so are presumed to be homogeneous; given the differences between them, 'tolerance' becomes the highest public virtue, its manifestation in everyday practice is 'political correctitude' and in regulative policy it is 'anormativity'.

(ii) Where (I) is concerned, the increase in accessible cultural variety serves to decrease social uniformity and, in consequence, social integration.[24]

This proposition deals with the ideational domain alone, with how 'contingent complementarities' are exploited and developed to generate new items of cultural novelty. It needs to be supplemented by introducing the durability of vested *material* interests; those originally (T^1) best placed in terms of wealth, repute and power also take most advantage of the new ideational opportunities available and thus retain competitive benefits over others (during T^2–T^3). Consequently, social integration diminishes still further because *inter alia* the latter can no longer resort to strong and durable social movements for redress.

(iii) Where (R) is concerned, social regulation becomes increasingly preoccupied with co-ordination and attends to fostering co-operation and redistribution only in so far as these are needful for coordinating different societal sectors.

Obviously, anormative regulation effectively denies normativity and represents the complete reversal of the views shared by the leading thinkers with whom this Introduction began; neither a *grundnorm* nor a central value system serves to underwrite orderliness in the global social order. Juxtaposing these three propositions shows the components of NIR pulling further and further away from one another – a formula for mess and distress rather than orderliness and stability.

Thus, Morphogenesis sets a challenge for today's social scientists, as a process that once engaged, will not cease. Either we can suffer and wallow along with our fellow human beings in the current T^2–T^3 phase, dedicating our work to documenting its disorderliness, destructiveness, unfairness, inhumaneness and other iniquities. If that route is taken, it is a normative choice based on the normative assumption that the more these features are accentuated, the more morally repugnant they will appear. Or, on the grounds of this presumed repugnance, social science

[24] As I wrote in Archer (1988: 244).

can venture into deliberating about what is fundamental to eudaimonia and begin the great adventure in conceptualizing a possible concrete utopia for T^4 – which is, of course, a highly normative exercise. There, morphogenesis itself may defeat us; we need our anchorage in common humanity in order to contribute to the well-being of the human family, but transhumanism can haul up our anchor – and that of humankind – leaving us without a mooring in nature or a natural kind.

References

Archer, M. S. (1985). The myth of cultural integration. *British Journal of Sociology, 36*(3), 333–353.
Archer, M. S. (1988). *Culture and agency: The place of culture in social theory*. Cambridge: Cambridge University Press.
Archer, M. S. (2007). *Making our way through the world: Human reflexivity and social mobility*. Cambridge: Cambridge University Press.
Archer, M. S. (2010). Routine, reflexivity and realism. *Sociological Theory, 28*(3), 272–303.
Archer, M. S. (2012). *The reflexive imperative in late modernity*. Cambridge: Cambridge University Press.
Archer, M. S. (2013). Social morphogenesis and the prospects of morphogenic society. In Archer (Ed.), *Social morphogenesis*. Dordrecht: Springer.
Archer, M. S. (2015). How agency is transformed in the course of social transformation: Don't forget the double morphogenesis. In M. S. Archer (Ed.), *Generative mechanisms transforming the social order*. Dordrecht: Springer.
Archer, M. S. & Elder-Vass, D. (2011). Cultural systems or norm circles. *European Journal of Social Theory*, 1–23.
Bratman, M. E. (1993). Shared intention. *Ethics, 104*(1), 97–113.
Coser, L. (1956). *The functions of social conflict*. New York: Free Press.
Donati, P. (2008). *Oltre il multiculturalismo*. Roma-Bari: Laterza.
Donati, P., & Archer, M. S. (2015). *The relational subject*. Cambridge: Cambridge University Press.
Elder-Vass, D. (2007). Reconciling Archer and Bourdieu. *Sociological Theory, 25*, 4.
Elder-Vass, D. (2010). *The causal power of social structures: Emergence, structure and agency*. Cambridge: Cambridge University Press.
Elder-Vass, D. (2012). *The reality of social construction*. Cambridge: Cambridge University Press.
Elster, J. (1989). *Solomonic judgements*. Cambridge: Cambridge University Press.
Gilbert, M. (1996). *Living together*. Lanham: Rowman and Littlefield.
Gilbert, M. (2006). *A theory of political obligation*. Oxford: Oxford University Press.
Gouldner, A. (1971). *The coming crisis of western sociology*. London: Heinemann.
Hart, H. A. L. (1963). *Law, liberty and morality*. Oxford: Oxford University Press.
Hart, H. A. L. (1994) [1961]. *The concept of law*. Oxford: Oxford University Press.
Kelsen, H. (1960). *Reine Rechtslehre*. Vienna: Deuticke.
Kelsen, H. (1992). *Introduction to the problems of legal theory*. Oxford: Clarendon.
Koller, P. (2014). On the nature of norms. *Ratio Juris, 27*(2), 155–175.
Lockwood, D. (1964). Social integration and system integration. In G. K. Zollschan & H.W. Hirsch (Eds.), *Explorations in social change*. Boston: Houghton Mifflin.
Maccarini, A. (2015). Turbulence and reational conjunctures: The emergence of morphogenic environments. In M. S. Archer (Ed.), *Generative mechanisms transforming the social order*. Dordrecht: Springer.
Mandelbaum, M. (1973). Societal facts. In J. O'Neill (Ed.), *Modes of individualism and collectivism*. London: Heinemann.

Mead, G. H. (1934). *Mind, self and society*. Chicago: University of Chicago Press.
Morgan, J. (2014). What is progress in realism? An issue illustrated using norm circles. *Journal of Critical Realism, 13*(2), 115–138.
Parsons, T. (1951). *The social system*. London: Routledge and Kegan Paul.
Pettit, P., & Schweikard, D. (2006). Joint actions and group agents. *Philosophy of the Social Sciences, 36*(1), 18–39.
Raz, J. (1990) [1975]. *Practical reason and norms*. Oxford: Oxford University Press.
Rosa, H. (2003). Social acceleration: Ethical and political consequences of a desynchronized high-speed society. *Constellations, 10*(1), 1–33.
Ross, A. (1968). *Directives and norms*. London: Routledge and Kegan Paul.
Sealey, A., & Carter, B. (2014). Response to Elder-Vass: Seven ways to be realist about language. *Journal for the Theory of Social Behaviour, 44*(3), 268–281.
Searle, J. R. (1990). Collective intentions and actions. In P. R. Cohen, J. Morgan, & M. E. Pollock (Eds.), *Intentions in communication* (pp. 401–415). Cambridge, MA: MIT Press.
Searle, J. R. (1995). *The construction of social reality*. London: Penguin.
Searle, J. R. (2010). *Making the social world*. Oxford: Oxford University Press.
Sellars, W. (1997) [1956]. *Empiricism and philosophy of mind*. Cambridge, MA: Harvard University Press.
Tuomela, R. (2010). *The philosophy of sociality*. Oxford: Oxford University Press.
Turner, S. (2010). *Explaining the normative*. Cambridge: Polity.
Weber, M. (1978) [1968]. In G. Roth, & C. Wittich (Eds.), *Economy and society: An outline of interpretive sociology*. Berkeley: University of California Press.

Part I
The Great Normative Transformations

Chapter 2
The Great Normative Changes of the Twentieth Century

Douglas Porpora

Given the focus of the present volume on normative morphogenesis, this chapter canvasses some of the great normative transformations of the twentieth century. What were those changes and who or what effected them? These are the basic questions this chapter will address. As a follow-up, it will further ask where these changes leave us now and the extent to which they all cohere within the contemporary condition we have been calling morphogenic society.

What do we even mean by normative change? Well, change in norms – and by extension, values. Values may be clear enough, although difficult to define. "'Values,'" Anne Swidler (2001) tells us in *Talking of Love*, placing the word within quotation marks lest we mistake it for something real, "are usually seen as the ranking of options on a hierarchy of preferences."

As I say elsewhere, Swidler's definition of values is exceedingly thin and emotionally barren, as if lifted from the pages of a treatise on rational choice theory. Not what one would expect from a doyenne of cultural sociology. We hold some values more strongly than others, which is why we have a rich vocabulary for labeling them: commitments, concerns, passions, ideals, interests, and so on. Preferences also is a word we use to label our values, but it is one of the weakest. I more than just prefer that justice be done, that my wife thrives, or that the earth abides. When we speak of values, as Collins (1984) notes, we are speaking about things about which we are emotionally engaged. Values refer to what we love, what we stand for, for what we are willing to sacrifice, even die.

What about norms? Norms are rules, but a certain kind of rules. Whereas in their chapters in this volume, Al-Amoudi (2016) and Lawson (2016) regard all rules as simultaneously regulative and constitutive, I continue to follow Searle (1970) in distinguishing regulative from constitutive rules. In terms of that distinction, the

D. Porpora (✉)
Department of Anthropology, Drexel University, Philadelphia, PA, USA
e-mail: porporad@drexel.edu

M.S. Archer (eds.), *Morphogenesis and the Crisis of Normativity*, Social Morphogenesis, DOI 10.1007/978-3-319-28439-2_2

norms I will discuss here are all regulative rules telling us how we should behave. That designation, however, remains too broad. The *should* invoked by regulative rules is a mixed bag. There is the *should*, for example, of rationality that enjoins us to avoid contradictions or belief without adequate warrant. That kind of norm will not occupy us. Nor will I be addressing the purely regulative rules without moral valence that Archer (2016) discusses in her chapter in this volume. While along with Archer a number of other contributors to the volume – Donati (2016), Gorski (2016), and Maccarini (2016) – also address what Maccarini calls the neutralization of moral norms, it is norms that remain value-laden that I will be addressing.

Even value-laden norms are a mixed bag. At the bottom of the totem pole perhaps stand rules of etiquette. Arising in their formal guise as rules of gentility that did and still do represent in part markers of social class membership (Elias 1978), etiquette can also be regarded, along the lines of Goffman (1963), as ways of showing deference or respect to others as sacred objects. As such, etiquette certainly does belong to our inquiry, and we will address ourselves here to changes over the twentieth century in the rules of etiquette.

More value-laden are the norms that span the overlap between morality and legality. Not all that is immoral is illegal, and not all that is illegal is immoral. As Donati (2016) tells us in his paper, while most people in the West continue to consider incest immoral, there is a move now in Germany to decriminalize it. Conversely, marijuana-use remains illegal in many places but is not generally considered immoral. Still, our strongest proscriptions – as against murder – are both immoral and illegal. In any case, along with etiquette, it will be norms of morality and legality that will be my object in this chapter.

As in my appeal to cases in the previous volume, I make no claim here that the cases I am assembling are exhaustive or even necessarily the most important of their kind. They are at least important changes in the ways we morally and legally conduct ourselves and consequently understand who we are. These changes, I group as follows:

- Etiquette
- The Secular Revolution
- Human Rights
- Racial Civil Rights
- The Women's Movement
- The LGBTQ Movement

To get some overall handle on these changes, let us imagine ourselves at the beginning of the twentieth century. At that time, automotive transport was still a rarity, and the telephone was just coming into wider public use. Etiquette manuals instructed men to hold doors open for women, who did not have the vote and whose exclusion from many sources of employment effectively subordinated them to men (fathers or husbands) in much the manner earlier of Jane Austen's novels.

Rudyard Kipling had just penned *The White Man's Burden* to commemorate the American conquest of the Philippines, and much of the world still resided in colonies. In the United States, polite society called African Americans "colored" for fear of offending with the word black. In much of the country, those so designated were restricted to their own restaurants, water fountains, and rest rooms. In the American south, lynchings were common. Other kinds of prejudice, such as anti-Semitism, abounded throughout the world, expressed in ethnic jokes and much worse.

Throughout the countries of the West, divorce was rare and legally restricted. Full rights to divorce did not come to England until the Matrimonial Causes Act of 1973. In the United States, it was only 1969 that California became the first state to pass a no-fault divorce law. People married early, and single girls found pregnant were either married or shipped off for abortions, which, in the United States was only widely legalized by the Supreme Court in the Roe v. Wade decision of 1973. The word queer had just come into vogue as a designation for homosexuality, the practice of which, several decades earlier had come to be called "the love that dare not speak its name." Indeed, Oscar Wilde had issued his *Ballad of Reading Gaol*, commenting on his imprisonment in England for gross indecency.

The Scopes "Monkey" Trial was still 14 years in the future, but a Christian fundamentalist reaction to growing secular humanism was already brewing. It would be another 60 years before Roman Catholics would experience the reforms of Vatican II, and the U.S. presidential election of John F. Kennedy in 1960 was made problematic by widespread suspicion that as a Catholic, Kennedy would take orders from Rome.

Europe and the United States were industrialized, and factory-based industry constituted a major source of employment. Social democracy was strong in Europe, and even in the United States, the American Federation of Labor had been around already for 15 years. However, family farming as well still claimed over 40 % of the labor force.

At the beginning of the twentieth century, there was no United Nations, nor even a League of Nations. Instead, as Wight (2015) tells us in his paper, nations confronted each other in what was virtually an anarchic state of nature, punctuated at most by shifting alliances. There was international trade, but nowhere of the dimensions we now associate with globalization. Instead, in many countries for many industries, tariff protections remained. National publics were insular. While now, about one third of Americans hold passports, as late as 1990, that figure was under 3 %. Even now, foreign news attracts much less attention among Americans than domestic matters. The isolation was even greater before.

Before the mid-twentieth century, there was no universal talk of human rights. The basic concept goes back at least as far as the *Magna Carta* and, in the modern period, was popularized first in the form of the natural rights spoken of by the British social contract theorists and the *philosophes* of the French enlightenment. Both the American and French revolutions were founded on this basis. In the nineteenth century, the establishment of the *International Committee of the Red Cross* and the first of the Geneva Conventions did broach the subject at an international level. Yet it was not until after the two world wars that human rights talk became more hegemonic in the modern world system.

With this contextual background behind us, let us turn to what are at least some of the great normative transformations of the twentieth century. We begin with what is perhaps mostly symptomatic of deeper transformations: Changes in Etiquette.

Changes in Etiquette

Etiquette may not be the most profound of the norms that bind us, but the rules that constitute it are perhaps most pervasive in our lives and hence reflective of multiple social dimensions. Dealing with both self-presentation and deference to others, etiquette was a focus of study by Goffman (1963) and before him by Elias (1978), who even more specifically was concerned with the great transformations in etiquette that resulted in our modern sensibility.

How do we study etiquette and changes in it? Goffman examined etiquette manuals, as of course did Elias. We are fortunate now to have a new study in such a vein by Seth Abrutyn and Michael Carter (2014), who compare the first (1922), the fifth (1937), and the eighteenth (2011) editions of Emily Post's etiquette manuals.

Abrutyn and Carter are specifically concerned with what they consider a decline of Durkheimian collective consciousness in America, by which they mean a loss of firm moral consensus at the level of manners. This breakdown, they demonstrate, shows up in the etiquette manuals. What Abrutyn and Carter track in effect is a growing heterogeneity over the course of the twentieth century in American culture.

At the beginning of the twentieth century, Abrutyn and Carter argue, the etiquette manuals portrayed American culture as a single, monolithic whole, epitomized by the American upper class. As was the case for Erasmus's *Handbook on Manners for Children* studied by Elias, the etiquette manuals of the early twentieth century were perused by those anticipating upward mobility. The norms the manuals advanced were not, however, depicted relativistically as just the ways of a particular class, however, dominant, but, as in the moral realism of Erasmus's rulebook, as the objectively proper way all civilized beings should comport themselves.

Implicitly, then, those at the top of the hierarchy were conceived as upholding that which was objectively right, what befits "the long, slow progress of social intercourse in the upward climb of man from the primeval state" (Post 1922: 6; Abrutyn and Carter 2014: 9). Accordingly, in contrast with the 18th edition of the manual, the first edition, consistent with the treatise of Erasmus, focuses on the shame occasioned by very particular transgressions. Strong adverbs of frequency – *always* and *never* – are much more frequently employed in the first than in the 18th edition. Thus, "the groom's presents to his ushers are always put at their places at the bachelor dinner" (Post 1922: 233; Abrutyn and Carter 2014: 12). Similarly, "the hostess never leaves her post" (Post 1922: 180; Abrutyn and Carter 2014: 12).

There is over time likewise a diminution in the strength of modal verbs. Abrutyn and Carter (2014: 14) observe that *must* appears over 500 times in the first edition as in "one inexorable rule of etiquette is that you must talk to your next door neighbor at a dinner table" (Post 1922: 155). In contrast, the 18th edition uses the word *must* only 65 times. Instead, the 18th edition favors the weaker modal, *should.* With growing tentativeness about the particular, what Abrutyn and Carter notice more generally between manuals, is a growing abstraction in what etiquette is deemed to be about. As the 18th edition puts it, "Being considerate, respectful, and honest is more important than knowing which fork to use" (Post et al. 1937/2011; Abrutyn and Carter 2014: 9).

The 18th edition is further distinguished by attention to the emergent forms of interaction occasioned by new technology. Thus, there is advice on how to "unfriend" someone on Facebook; when and how to use a cell phone in public; and online dating (Abrutyn and Carter 2014: 8, 17).

Abrutyn and Carter (2014: 10) further observe a decline in gender differences between the first and 18th editions. At my own expense, Archer will be amused to hear that according to the 18th edition, for a gentleman, "it is still inappropriate to wear a hat in a house." On the other hand, the 18th edition makes no special note of hat tipping in deference to women. Hat tipping or removal is rather described as a sign of respect to any other, male or female (Abrutyn and Carter 2014: 10). Providing some vindication for me, however, Abrutyn and Carter cite a section from Dresser's (2005) etiquette manual entitled, "Hats Off – Not!" which observes how fluid hat rules have become. Yea!

How do we explain the observed transformations in the rules of etiquette? Following the morphogenetic/morphostatic (MM) approach (see Archer 1995), to which most of us in these volumes subscribe, the changes seem largely although not totally unintended consequences of actions in changing contexts pursued for other or larger purposes. Certainly, the rules arising around new digital technologies are occasioned by those new technologies themselves, which present new social dilemmas for actors to negotiate. In Marxian terms, a change in the material infrastructure led to a change in the cultural superstructure.

Other changes in etiquette – and certainly their greater fluidity today – reflect deeper structural changes, in particular the diminished hegemony of once dominant WASP sensibility. With the civil rights movement, the women's movement and so on, multiculturalism has become a core social value and with it a greater acknowledgement of at least a degree of relativism, that there often is no single right way of conducting oneself, that proper conduct may vary from subculture to subculture.

The growing abstractness Abrutyn and Carter observe in the understanding of etiquette itself seems to signal a second cycle of a morphogenetic process. It can be understood, that is, as an agentic response to the structural and cultural changes wrought by a previous cycle as the abstraction seems an attempt to recapture coherence across the fragmentation produced by previous changes.

The Secular Revolution

I once knocked back on her heels a very good, atheistic student. When I asked her from whence she derived her morals, she replied it is all common sense. What gave this student pause was my counter suggestion that what she was calling common sense was the cultural legacy of Judaism and Christianity. I continue to think this assessment correct: Regardless of one's religious belief, most of us in the West inherit our morality from religion, which is not to say we could not have arrived at the same moral place via other routes. Still, given the close tie between religion and morality, I consider the secular revolution here.

The Secular Revolution may seem an odd phrase. Going back to Comte and perhaps before, secularization has been thought by social scientists to represent a natural process, captured by what has been called the "secularization thesis," the thesis that, with modernization, religion will inevitably fade away. Although there have been multiple factors expected to lead toward this end, among them certainly have been liberal enlightenment culture and the growth of science.

In contrast with that account, *The Secular Revolution* is a collection of essays edited by Christian Smith (2003) arguing that secularity in the twentieth century has been not entirely a natural process but also the political work of certain elites, such as the rising intelligentsia. Does my use of that title as a heading signal my support for this thesis? I do think the thesis true, but I adopted the heading for another reason that I will explain shortly.

The whole secularization thesis is currently up in the air as Phil Gorski and Altınordu Ates (2008) tell us in a great piece in the *Annual Review of Sociology* and on which I draw in this section. Whereas it once was almost taken for granted, then disputed and slated for rejection, the secularization thesis is now being rethought in more complex and sophisticated ways.

To introduce some of the complications, over the long debate about it, understanding of secularization has varied. Is it a macro-thesis about the withdrawal of religion from large-scale societal functions or a similarly macro-level decline in religious authority and discourse? Alternately, is it rather a more micro-level thesis about the fading of religious consciousness among individuals? If the latter, given that religiosity is a multidimensional quality, has religiosity faded equally along all dimensions? Here Gorski and Ates warn against what they call an overly pastoral view of the question, which emphasizes practices associated with collective worship. Those practices might decline, they say, without a similar decline in religious belief or religious ethical practice. As there is in other words what Davie (1994) termed "believing without belonging," it may well be that it is only organized religion that is in decline and not religion per se.

Of course, as Gorski and Ates further say, we are not even quite sure how religious people were along all dimensions in the past so that it is difficult to say over the *longue durée* whether what we observe today is a cyclical slump or a secular decline. Certainly, Gorski and Ates show, the pace of any decline in religiosity has varied across space and time and been given – locally at least – to periodic reversals.

Fortunately, for our purposes here, we can sidestep many of these issues. In the first place, taking the advice of Gorski and Ates, we can distinguish between secularization per se and de-Christianization. Whether or not there has been an overall decline in religiosity along certain dimensions, there is more agreement that there has been such decline specifically in Christianity.

Second, however non-uniform religious decline may have been across the *longue durée*, there is much more consensus, Gorski and Ates tell us, that there has been a sharp decline in Christianity within the period on which I focus, that is, the twentieth century. The decline has been particularly noticeable in Britain and the United States, the latter long-noted for its historically high rates of religious observance. Some of the fall-off in the United States has been fairly recent. In particular, over the past 20 years, the percentage of the religiously unaffiliated in the United States, what are sometimes called "the nones," has doubled, now comprising 16 % of the population (Pew 2012). Membership decline in mainline Protestant denominations has been particularly steep but now seems also to be affecting Evangelical churches. The United States would also show drastic drops in Catholic membership were it not for a steady influx of Catholic immigrants.

Throughout the twentieth century, there have been other periods of sudden Christian decline in both America and Britain. There have been, for example, such declines after both world wars. In Britain, Callum Brown (2001) attributes another such drop to the 1960s counter-culture, which also seems to have had like effect in the United States.

I borrowed the phrase *Secular Revolution*, I can now say, to refer to this sudden de-Christianization (and, seemingly, also de-Judaization) in the twentieth century, but the question remains as to its cause. Has it been due to larger tectonic forces or to the deliberate agency of particular elites and movements? It seems both. As Gorski and Ates (2008: 61) suggest, along with non-agential forces of secularization, there have been agents who have actively tried to abet them, just as there have been non-agential forces operating against secularization and agents who have for their part tried to abet those counter-forces. We thus seem to have here a complex and fluid situation in which multiple mechanisms are operative and in which the outcomes reflect their momentary balance.

To bring this all back to our inquiry, what does such secularization have to do with moral change? I think two main things. The first relates to a complaint I have with introductory texts on the philosophy of ethics, about which I have written before (Porpora 2001; Porpora et al. 2013). My complaint is philosophers' tendency to reduce religious ethics to what they call *divine command theory*. Divine command theory stipulates that religious people, oblivious to the *Euthyphro* dilemma, consider what they take to be moral as that which God commands, simply because they are God's commands. Philosophers accordingly ignore alternate sources of religious morality, originating either in cosmogonic understandings of who we are in the universe (e.g., equal children of God) or in a divinized ideal of the good such as elucidated by Feuerbach (1989).

My complaint notwithstanding, it is likely that philosophers have tended to emphasize divine command theory because historically, theologians aside, divine command theory describes how common people have thought of morality. If so, then we might expect a modern decline in religious authority to result in a decline within the general population of the tendency think about morality as what God commands. In contrast, as blind obedience fades as a moral motivation, people look for more reasoned warrants for their moral principles and, not finding them, abandon those prescriptions that fail the test. We can thus see how we might have arrived in the twentieth century with what has been called the *permissive society* with all that label entails: The sexual revolution; free love; use of artificial contraception; abortion rights; gay rights; etc.

Further, as divine command theory fades in purchase, so does, among the general population, any *deontological* approach to ethics. In its stead, consistent with the general trend toward instrumental rationality (see Weber 2012; Horkheimer and Adorno 2007) is a greater reliance on the logic of moral utilitarianism. Indeed, the work of Jonathan Haidt (e.g., 2013) seems positively to equate moral rationality with moral utilitarianism. We thus arrive at a point where in America, even torture comes to be discussed – at least in the secular arena – entirely in terms of moral utility (Porpora et al. 2013).

I could continue with the above line of thought, but we must move on. As I wrote in our previous volume, a second consequence, I believe, of the demise of religious authority or of religious discourse is a loss of moral grounding (see also Porpora 2001; Taylor 1992). Simply put, the variety of ways in which religion once grounded morality has not been adequately replaced. Thus, while we may retain as legacy the morality of our religions, we find we are without the resources now to justify that morality. Thus, along with the loss of a fuller moral vocabulary (Bellah et al. 2007; Luckmann 1997; Porpora et al. 2013), we get a postmodernist swing (hardly just among intellectuals) toward moral relativism.

The Human Rights Movement

We observe now worldwide a full-fledged human rights culture or even what some have called a regime (Rabossi 1990; Dunn and Wheeler 1999). It encompasses lawyers, journalists, politicians, and the public (Nickel 2007). It is enshrined in such international accords as the *Universal Declaration of Human Rights*, and the subsequent declarations of political, social and economic rights. Worldwide, wrongs are opposed and heeded in the name of human rights. Human rights are spoken of even by those who oppose or transgress human rights when defending themselves in international opinion.

Human rights talk thus represents a salutary and remarkable discursive hegemony. How did we get here? One lesson of the human rights movement is that change can take a long time. Although the roots of rights talk can be traced back even further, we can certainly find their cosmogonic origin in Judaism and Christianity as we saw, in the opening lines of Thomas Jefferson's *Declaration of Independence*: "All men are endowed by their creator with certain inalienable rights."

Jefferson's reflections were part of a trend. Human rights talk was generally bolstered during the eighteenth century enlightenment by the writings of the social contract thinkers, most notably John Locke, who influenced Jefferson, and, some (see Hunt 2008) argue, by the growth of the novel, through which people developed greater empathy for each other. Then, along with the American Revolution, which made Jefferson's words famous, there was the French Revolution, considered one of the pivotal moments in the development of a modernist sensibility (Mayer 2002), that featured the "rights of man."

We can think of cultural milieux as the result of iterated morphogenetic cycles building on each other. Thus, building on a diffuse moral climate in which the concept of rights was coming into focus, there were already in the nineteenth century organized social movements that much more intentionally promoted human rights. These constituted the kind of norm entrepreneurs of which Wight speaks in his chapter. Chief among them was the movement led by Henry Dunant that in 1863 established the *International Committee of the Red Cross*. Although today we think of the *Red Cross* mainly in terms of disaster relief, its efforts led to the first Geneva Convention in 1864.

Another three Geneva Conventions followed in the twentieth century, the fourth convention after World War II in 1949. Further and most prominently, the charter of the United Nations (UN) affirms the "dignity and worth of the human person" and in 1948, the United Nations General Assembly adopted the Universal Declaration of Human Rights (UDHR). A major reason for the UDHR was the world's horror at the Holocaust and a felt need by UN member states that the articulated concern for human rights in the UN charter was insufficiently strong.

Both the UN and the UDHR were instruments of world leaders, particularly Franklin Roosevelt, who sought a successor to the *League of Nations*, and his wife, Eleanor, who chaired the commission that drafted the UDHR. Here, then, we observe agency as well, but it is not agency at a grassroots level but rather of a structurally highly placed sort.

For all its contemporary importance, the concept of human rights reflects the problem I identified at the end of the last section. As political theorist Jack Donnelly (2002) says, human rights rest on a social decision to act as if they exist. But are human rights simply a reification? On what foundation does all our talk of human rights rest?

For some, like Michael Ignatieff (2003), ignoring the question of foundations is a pragmatic decision. It is enough for Ignatieff that we agree on what is right or good. No need to reach agreement on why we agree. I doubt that Ignatieff is right, but that dispute is an issue for another time. Our space here permits only our notice of how currently without foundation is secular talk of human rights.

The Black Civil Rights Movement in America

In 1909, sociologist W.E.B. Du Bois joined with other black activists to form the *National Association for the Advancement of Colored People* (NAACP), several co-founders of which were Jewish. Jews in particular gave the NAACP much support.

One of the principal victories for the NAACP came in 1954 with the Supreme Court decision in *Brown v. Board of Education* against the racial segregation of public schools. Closely following in 1955, Rosa Parks refused to relinquish her seat to whites on a public bus. Parks, it should be noted, was not just an isolated individual, irate at injustice. Irate she was, but she was also secretary of the Montgomery Alabama chapter of the NAACP and had been trained in non-violent resistance at the *Highlander Center* in Tennessee (where I also was excited to spend a day training for service learning). The struggle against racial injustice was thus an instance in which social change was agentically motored intentionally from below by grassroots social movements.

And prominent among the change agents in that movement was religion (as it was also, it might be said, in India and South Africa). I have already mentioned the strong involvement of Jews in the American civil rights movement. Prominent as well were churches, particularly the Black Protestant Church. If the protest of Rosa Parks culminated one morphogenetic cycle against past injustice, her arrest began another. In response to Parks's arrest, local black ministers, among them Ralph Abernathy and Martin Luther King, organized what became the *Southern Christian Leadership Conference* (*SCLC*) to lead a boycott of city buses. In December 1956, the boycott led to a federal ruling in U.S. district court – *Browder v. Gayle* – declaring segregation on Alabama buses unconstitutional.

As Doug McAdam (2012; see also Wikipedia 2014) has observed, however, there was not just one civil rights movement but multiple. Along with *NAACP* and *SCLC*, there was the Student Nonviolent Coordinating Committee (*SNCC*) and the Congress on Racial Equality (*CORE*), which together formed the "big four" civil rights organizations.

It was not, however, all just grassroots social movement efforts. As indicated, U.S. federal courts played a large role as did the executive branch of the government. Roosevelt had hosted Booker T. Washington in the White House, and Eisenhower in 1957 sent troops to enforce de-segregation in Little Rock, Arkansas. Among other things, under John F. Kennedy, Attorney General Robert F. Kennedy sent federal marshals to Alabama to protect the *Freedom Riders*. In 1965, President Lyndon Johnson signed the *Voting Rights Act* into effect. Thus, while the African American civil rights movement was largely an agentic struggle, like the human rights movement more generally, it involved actors in multiple positions of the social structure and, as Lazega (2015) reminds us in his paper, of actors tied to other actors in complex social networks.

Not only that. By the time of the Civil Rights Movement, 86 % of households had television. Thus, the 1963 March on Washington was the first event to be broadcast around the world (Al-Muslim 2014; Kashar 1996).

The Women's Movement

As *Wikipedia* tells us, the women's movement has included a whole range of issues: reproductive rights; domestic violence; maternity leave; equal pay, women's suffrage; sexual harassment; and sexual violence. At this point, there are different ways to tell this story. One, again, is to emphasize morphogenetic cycles and to see how the civil rights movement served as a precedent for the furthered rights of women.

Another way to tell the story is to highlight the role of economic and technological change. The economic changes have to do with what in the United States became the postwar bust circa 1972. The bust was preceded by a boom. The United States had emerged from the Second World War without the internal destruction that afflicted most of the remaining industrialized world. Thus, the United States became a towering economic giant, supplying the world with industrialized goods. Accordingly, the United States exited the war not only free of lingering depression but also in a state of economic boom.

During the boom, a family could still be comfortably supported by a single income earner. Thus, it was a time when on American television series, husbands like Ralph Kramden could proclaim how a "man's home is his castle" and oppose their wives going out to work. Women therefore generally remained economically dependent on their husbands.

For a variety of reasons, the boom ended around 1972 and since that time, with what regulation theorists (see, e.g., Jessop 2007) call a change in the *regime of accumulation*, wages in real dollars have stagnated. Over the initial protests of the developed world's Ralph Kramdens, it became economically necessary for wives to enter the labor force. That entry exposed women to myriad injustices in the work place – from unequal pay to sexual harassment – and changed the power dynamics at home. Thus, here in M/M fashion, a change in material conditions would eventually result in deep cultural changes.

But normative changes were brewing from other sources as well, among them a constellation of forces or conjuncture tending toward what would become the permissive society. The erosion of religious taboos in the 1960s, particularly among the young, I have already mentioned. That effect was amplified, however, by a postwar baby boom that made the young the defining generation of the age, effecting a veritable youth culture. Simultaneously, partly because of the economic boom and partly due to other factors, college education was – at least in the United States – becoming not only much more widely accessible but among the middle and upper middle class increasingly normative.

That development in turn pushed up the age of marriage, resulting in a growing normative acceptance of pre-marital sex. Whereas even in the past pre-marital sex may have been practiced more widely than acknowledged, births out of wedlock were societally unacceptable. As the development of the pill in 1960 greatly reduced that possibility, the cultural impulse toward permissiveness was bolstered. The greater sexual freedom for both men and women led in its turn to further changes in relations across the sexes, resulting simultaneously both in greater female empowerment and further female exploitation.

As women entered the workforce, they came to imagine themselves not just as wives and mothers but also as teachers, lawyers, physicians and pursuers of other careers. The multiplicity of female roles on offer made scheduling reproduction problematic in a way it had not been before. Women saw themselves in possession of the right to decide how and when to reproduce. That shift coincided with a new uncertainty within the medical profession, which in the wake of the Thalidomide controversy, was no longer sure about the boundary between therapeutic and criminal abortion. The result was that abortion was transformed from a question that was narrowly medical to one that was broadly political (Luker 1985).

That result was again not just a natural occurrence. The *Zeitgeist* in this direction was nurtured by normative entrepreneurs who organized female "consciousness-raising groups," which in turn, echoing what C. Wright Mills (1970) termed the *sociological imagination*, proclaimed "the personal is political." That principle would extend beyond the issue of reproduction to such issues as workload within the home and equal pay outside. And ultimately here too we have to do not just with agency at a grassroots level but ultimately at the highest political levels as well as with the U.S. Supreme Court decision Roe v. Wade. Academia also played its role with a burst of academic feminist work that made its way into popular culture.

As brought home by accounts of gang rape on American university campuses, the fight for women's equality is far from over. The fight so far has nevertheless had broad cultural ramifications, not just in redefining womanhood but in the process of contributing to a fundamental postmodern destabilization of what it means to have and to represent a self-identity. That destabilization in what is most central to us is centrally at issue in the final change we will consider.

The LGBTQ Movement

With the LGBTQ movement we are dealing centrally with what Maccarini (2016) describes as norm neutralization or *denormativization*. In particular it is the disappearance of the stigmas attached to non-normative sexuality that we are witnessing. As the very acronym suggests, the LGBTQ movement is an amalgam of lesbians, gays, bisexuals, transgendered folk – and now with the Q – even those just questioning how they wish to identify. The questioning itself is significant on three counts. First, as I suggested just above, it signals the destabilization in our idea of the self, first inaugurated by the women's movement but carried further by so-called *Queer* theory and readings of Foucault that have lent so much to what still remains of a postmodern sensibility. It is a sensibility that reduces the ontology of selfhood to less coherent phenomenology (see Porpora 2015).

There is unfortunately no space to expand much on the previous cryptic statement except to note its bearing on the second and third ways the Q is significant. The second way is that much of the movement has to do with challenging the normativity of human classifications and the way they putatively stifle certain personal identities. As important as that question is, however, it has been posed within Queer theory in a way that reduces selves to how they experiences themselves, so if someone experiences herself as multiple, then she actually is multiple ontologically. The problem with that account, as I have argued elsewhere (Porpora 2001, 2015), is that, morally our care extends to the single self that confronts us as a Thou in Buber's (1971) sense and not to a legion of Lacanian subject positions. My fear then with Queer theorization is its destabilization and dislocation of the object of moral concern.

The third way the Q is important is that it signifies the postmodern political instability that extends even to the LGBTQ movement itself. The fact is that gays in particular are not wont to accept the bisexual identity, seeing in it rather a failure to commit to a wholly gay identity.

Wikipedia helpfully informs us that as in the case of other movements we have canvassed, the roots of the LGBTQ movement go way back with even Jeremy Bentham in the United Kingdom arguing along utilitarian lines that as a victimless crime, homosexual relations should be legalized. It was long after, however, before such movement bore much fruit. Thus, as has now been popularized by the movie, *The Imitation Game*, as late as 1952, Alan Turing was arrested for homosexual relations conducted within his own home.

If the LBGTQ movement emerged with new force thereafter, it was in the United States due partly to the riots at the Stonewall Inn in Greenwich Village, New York and partly to the way in which the AIDS crisis both reinvigorated activism and greater public empathy for the gay community (Altman 1988). In both cases, the gay and lesbian movement built on the precedence of earlier rights movements and in turn served as yet another precedent for the extension of the movement to bisexuals, the transgendered, and the questioning. We thus again have chains of M/M cycles, crowned finally by action at higher political levels.

Conclusions

Let us begin with how far we have come. Today, in the United States, no longer do we refer to black people as colored. Although racism is still definitely with us, at the same time it no longer is unusual to see racially mixed couples kissing – or more – on television. Compared with 1900, the television itself is new as are home and hand-held computers and the Internet. Not only do we regularly see racially mixed couples on television but also now openly gay and lesbian figures. In the United States and Europe both abortion and divorce are widely legal. Western Europe now is very de-Christianized, and Christianity appears to be weakening even in the United States. The world has now been largely decolonized, fostering a postmodern post-colonial discourse in the academy. Worldwide, we have experienced a process that Carrigan (2016) calls "communicative escalation," fostered by the Internet and globalization. We also have a United Nations and a worldwide regime of human rights – at least in terms of talk.

How did we get here? Whatever contribution this paper makes comes from juxtaposition, from, that is, comparing all the capsule narratives side-by-side to abstract some general elements of normative change. There are a few such common elements I want to propose. First, normative changes are complex phenomena, involving multiple mechanisms. Certainly, they involve human agency – in some respects intentional and in some unintentional. The agency involved, moreover, is multiply placed. At the grassroots level, it involves what may begin as isolated norm entrepreneurs who combine forces to form social movement organizations. The successful movements, however, eventually involve changes in formal rules that come from the higher placed agency of government officials. So agency is involved in different ways at different structural levels.

From Al-Amoudi's (2016) paper we gain an interesting insight on the nature of that agency. Al-Amoudi reminds us of Wittgenstein's point that the articulation of rules must always come to an end and beyond that we are left with unarticulated interpretation. That unarticulated background of interpretation forms the reservoir out of which rules are extended, transformed, transcended and otherwise reinterpreted and reformulated.

Along those lines, we see repeatedly not just within each individual narrative but also across them chains of M/M cycles, ways particularly in which one movement's success becomes a precedent for another's evolution. There has been in particular a building from human rights in general to racial civil rights specifically and from there (as well as from other sources) to women's rights and from women's rights (again from other sources as well) to the expanded rights relating to lesbians and gays, to bisexuals and the transgendered.

Contexts consist of both cultural and structural features. We observed, for example, purely cultural elements that rule certain social placements for women or people of color or the transgendered. A placement, however, has meaning only relative to other placements to which it is related. Thus, the cultural rulings as to placement immediately establish structural relations that confront actors as objective givens.

Among the givens we have encountered in the narratives have been unjust relations; technological changes – such as the pill or reproductive technologies – that altered relations; and changes in the capitalist order such as those that have weakened the economic viability of the family unit, which in turn also altered relations among family members. The givens also include certain cultural latencies in religion – liberationist latencies already there in the culture (see Archer 1988) waiting to be drawn on by religious social movements.

Other cultural elements involved in the narratives take diverse forms. I spoke above of latencies, of elements of culture that for a long time go unattended without thereby disappearing from the cultural stock. In some cases, these elements take the form of deep sensibilities, what Reed (2011) considers parts of broad, historically specific cultural landscapes. Such landscapes take a long time to develop and to breakout, if they do at all, in a strong sense of Zeitgeist. We saw that before human rights would become the object of a concerted movement, it was preceded by a long gestation period during which a certain cultural sensibility was established. It was only against that landscape, arguably, that the intentional movements could succeed.

In our annual face-to-face Workshops multiple participants asked me to say something about where in the end I thought we are moving morally. Archer in particular asked me to comment on what I (Porpora et al. 2013) recently termed the macro-moral disconnect. The macro-moral disconnect is how my colleagues and I recently termed a general failure of both individuals and of public discourse to address macro-moral matters – like war, torture, the use of drones – in moral terms, the tendency instead to reframe moral considerations in terms of prudential considerations. Certainly, that tendency coincides with the general tendency toward norm neutralization Maccarini (2016) cites and the tendency toward purely instrumental regulations observed by Archer (2016).

Part of what is going on was suggested by Donati (2016) and Gorski (2016). Donati speaks of a move away from deontological forms of morality in favor of pure moral utility and cites as an example the recommendation of the Ethical Council of the German Federal Government to decriminalize incest. It is almost as if the council were taking its advice from Haidt, who, as noted, symptomatically seems to equate moral rationality exclusively with a logic of moral utility. It is a logic my colleagues and I also saw operating in the American debate on torture that ensued after the revelations from Abu Ghraib. In the elite liberal press, the argument was either framed in purely prudential terms – whether or not torture works – or, if left as a moral issue then approached almost exclusively in the moral utilitarian terms of the ticking bomb – one tortured terrorist versus a million dead citizens. My colleagues and I found that one had to go to the religious press – both left and right – to find the appeals to human sanctity that might contend with utility.

I speak here as in the last volume very deliberately of a liberal sensibility. Maccarini asked in discussion whether what I am describing applies just to the West. I do not think so, but I also do not think it applies to the West as a whole. Rather I agree with Hofkirchner's (2016) suggestion that there is developing worldwide a global cosmopolitan conscience.

Hofkirchner opposes this global cosmopolitanism to what he calls a contrasting culture of moral indifference, but I actually think the two interpenetrate. The reason is that the morality of cosmopolitan culture tends to be exceedingly thin. Not only does it tend, as Donati (2016) suggests, to abandon deontological logic, but as Donati further suggests – and Gorski (2016) with him, its tendency is so to valorize personal freedom and autonomy that respect and tolerance become its cardinal virtues. Of course respect and tolerance are to be commended, but not everything – torture, for example, should be tolerated. Thus, Donati warns against what he calls the *Foucault Trap*, where personal autonomy itself becomes a mechanism of oppression. I think it a warning worth heeding.

References

Abrutyn, S., & Carter, M. J. (2014). The decline in shared collective consciousness as found in the shifting norms and values of etiquette manuals. *Journal for the Theory of Social Behaviour*. doi:10.1111/jtsb.12071.

Al-Amoudi, A. (2016). In letter & in spirit: Social morphogenesis and the interpretation of codified social rules. In M. Archer (Ed.), *Morphogenesis and the crisis of normativity*. Dordrecht: Springer.

Al-Muslim, A. (2014). *Fundamentals of interaction*. http://interactivefundamentals.journalism.cuny.edu/2008/10/16/the-media-and-the-civil-rights-movement/.

Altman, D. (1988). Legitimation through disaster: AIDS and the gay movement. In E. Fee & D. M. Fox (Eds.), *Aids: The burden of history* (pp. 301–315). Berkeley: University of California Press.

Archer, M. S. (1988). *Culture and agency: The place of culture in social theory*. Cambridge: Cambridge University Press.
Archer, M. S. (1995). *Realist social theory: The morphogenetic approach*. New York: Cambridge.
Archer, M. S. (2016). Anormative social regulation: the attempt to cope with social morphogenesis. In M. Archer (Ed.), *Morphogenesis and the crisis of normativity*. Dordrecht: Springer.
Bellah, R., Madsen, R., Sullivan, W. M., Swidler, A., & Tipton, S. M. (2007). *Habits of the heart: Individualism and commitment in American life*. Berkeley: University of California Press.
Brown, C. (2001). *The death of Christian Britain: Understanding secularisation, 1800–2000*. New York: Routledge.
Buber, M. (1971). *I and thou*. New York: Touchstone.
Carrigan, M. (2016). The fragile movements of late modernity. In M. Archer (Ed.), *Morphogenesis and the crisis of normativity*. Dordrecht: Springer.
Collins, R. (1984). The role of emotion in social structure. In K. R. Scherer & P. Ekman (Eds.), *Approaches to emotion* (pp. 385–396). Hove: Psychology Press.
Davie, G. (1994). *Religion in Britain since 1945: Believing without belonging*. Oxford: Blackwell.
Donati, P. (2016). The *relational* understanding of the origin and morphogenetic change of social morality. In M. Archer (Ed.), *Morphogenesis and the crisis of normativity*. Dordrecht: Springer.
Donnelly, J. (2002). *Universal human rights in theory and practice*. Ithica: Cornell University Press.
Dresser, N. (2005). *Multicultural manners: Essential rules of etiquette for the 21st century*. Hoboken: Wiley.
Dunne, T., & Wheeler, N. (1999). *Human rights in global politics*. Cambridge: Cambridge University Press.
Elias, N. (1978). *The civilizing process, vol 1, the history of manners*. New York: Pantheon.
Feuerbach, L. (1989). *The essence of Christianity*. New York: Prometheus.
Goffman, E. (1963). *Behavior in public places: Notes on the social organization of gatherings*. New York: Free Press.
Gorski, P. (2016). Reflexive secularity? Thoughts on the reflexive imperative in a secular age. In M. Archer (Ed.), *Morphogenesis and normativity*. Dordrecht: Springer.
Gorski, P., & Ates, A. (2008). After secularization? *Annual Review of Sociology, 34*, 55–85.
Haidt, J. (2013). *The righteous mind: Why good people are divided by politics and religion*. New York: Vintage.
Hofkirchner, W. (2016). Ethics from systems: Origin, development and current state of normativity. In M. Archer (Ed.), *Morphogenesis and the crisis of normativity*. Dordrecht: Springer.
Horkheimer, M., & Adorno, T. (2007). *Dialectic of enlightenment*. Stanford: Stanford University Press.
Hunt, L. (2008). *Inventing human rights: A history*. New York: Norton.
Ignatieff, M. (2003). Human rights as politics and idolatry. In M. Ignatieff & Gutman (Eds.), *Human rights as politics and idolatry* (pp. 53–100). Princeton: Princeton University Press.
Jessop, B. (2007). *Beyond the regulation approach: Putting capitalist economies in their place*. New York: Edward Elgar.
Kashar, S. (1996). *The civil rights movement: A photographic history 1954–68*. New York: Abbeville.
Lawson, T. (2016). Collective practices and norms. In M. Archer (Ed.), *Morphogenesis and the crisis of normativity*. Dordrecht: Springer.
Lazega, E. (2015). Joint 'Anormative' regulation from status inconsistency: A multilevel spinning top model of specialized institutionalization. In M. Archer (Ed.), *Morphogenesis and the crisis of normativity*. Dordrecht: Springer.
Luckmann, T. (1997). *The moral order of modern societies: Moral communication and indirect moralizing*. Budapest: Collegium Budapest, Institute for Advanced Study.
Luker, K. (1985). *Abortion & the politics of motherhood*. Berkeley: University of California.
Maccarini, A. (2016). The normative texture of Morphogenic Society: Tensions, challenges, and strategies. In M. Archer (Ed.), *Morphogenesis and the crisis of normativity*. Dordrecht: Springer.

Mayer, A. (2002). *The furies: Violence and terror in the French and Russian revolutions*. Princeton: Princeton University Press.
McAdam, D. (2012). Occupy the future. *Boston Review*. http://www.bostonreview.net/forum/occupy-future/what-should-sustained-movement-look.
Mills, C. W. (1970). *The sociological imagination*. New York: Penguin.
Nickel, J. (2007). *Making sense of human rights*. New York: Wiley-Blackwell.
Pew Research Center. (2012). Nones on the rise. *Pew Research Center Survey*. 28 June–9 July.
Porpora, D. (2001). *Landscapes of the soul: The loss of moral meaning in American life*. New York: Oxford.
Porpora, D. (2015). *Reconstructing sociology: The critical realist approach*. New York: Cambridge.
Porpora, D., Nikolaev, A., May, J., & Jenkins, A. (2013). *Post-ethical society: The Iraq war, Abu Ghraib, and the moral failure of the secular*. Chicago: University of Chicago Press.
Post, E. (1922). *Etiquette in society, in business, in politics, and at home*. New York: Funk & Wagnalls.
Post, E., et al. (1937/2011). *Etiquette, project gutenberg*. www.gutenberg.org/ebooks/author/5466.
Rabossi, E. (1990). La Theoria de la Derechos Humanos Naturalizado. *Revista del Centro del Estudias Constitucionales, 5*, 159–175.
Reed, I. (2011). *Interpretation and social knowledge: On the use of theory in the human sciences*. Chicago: University of Chicago Press.
Searle, J. (1970). *Speech acts: An essay in the philosophy of language*. New York: Cambridge.
Smith, C. (2003). *The secular revolution: Power, interests, and conflict in the secularization of American public life*. Berkeley: University of California Press.
Swidler, A. (2001). *Talk of love: How culture matters*. Chicago: University of Chicago Press.
Taylor, C. (1992). *Sources of the self: The making of modern identity*. Cambridge: Harvard.
Weber, M. (2012). *The theory of social and economic organization*. New York: Martino Fine Books.
Wight, C. (2015). Emergence, development and death: Norms in international society. In M. Archer (Ed.), *Morphogenesis and the crisis of normativity*. Dordrecht: Springer.
Wikipedia. (2014). *The African-American civil rights movement 1954–1968*. http://en.wikipedia.org/wiki/African-American_Civil_Rights_Movement_(1954-68).

Chapter 3
Reflexive Secularity: Thoughts on the Reflexive Imperative in a Secular Age

Philip S. Gorski

Is the modern world becoming more secular? And, if so, in what sense? Four decades ago, these were settled questions in the social sciences (Wilson 1985; Tschannen 1991). The world was becoming more secular. About this, there was virtual unanimity. At least within Western Europe, various indicators of religiosity were clearly declining – church attendance, belief in God and so on. And since Western Europe was presumed to be the leading edge of modernization, it was assumed, the rest of the world was bound to follow (Dobbelaere 1981; Acquaviva 1979). To be sure, there were still disagreements about the details, about the key mechanisms of modernization, say, or the proper definition of secularization. Still, there was broad consent about the general principle – a few even called it a law – that modernization was bringing about secularization.

And then came a long string of "empirical anomalies": liberation theology in Latin America, the Solidarity movement in Poland; the Moral Majority in the USA; the Islamic Revolution in Iran; and Hindu nationalism in India, to name only the best known. Even so, it was another decade and a half before José Casanova drew the now obvious conclusion: secularity does not entail the privatization of religion after all. "Public religions" were not only surviving in the modern world, Casanova contended, they were prospering (Casanova 1994).

Then came another batch of counter-evidence. Outside Europe, the confident predictions of secularization theory were being routinely violated. "The rest" was finally catching up with "the West." But religion was alive and well in the rapidly modernizing regions of the "global South." Whether it was Pentecostal revivals in Brazil, "Qigong fever" in China or the Gulen movement in Turkey, signs of

P.S. Gorski (✉)
Departments of Sociology and Religious Studies, Yale University, New Haven, CT, USA
e-mail: philip.gorski@yale.edu

M.S. Archer (eds.), *Morphogenesis and the Crisis of Normativity*,
Social Morphogenesis, DOI 10.1007/978-3-319-28439-2_3

"religious vitality" were everywhere.[1] Some survey researchers even spoke of a "global resurgence of religion" (Toft et al. 2011). The debate continued. But secularization theory was now on the defensive.

The renewed debate over secularization also sparked deeper reflections about the meaning of "secularism" and "secularity." Perhaps religion isn't going away. But secularism probably isn't either. Perhaps modernity doesn't entail secularization. But it does seem connected with secularity. The leading figures in this conversation have been the anthropologist, Talad Asad, and the philosopher, Charles Taylor.[2] Asad's primary concern is with the cultural reordering that results from worldwide diffusion of the West's secular/religious binary. Taylor's main focus is on modern agency, on what it feels like to live in a secular age. However, while Asad focuses on changes in culture and Taylor highlights shifts in agency, neither seriously attends to shifts in social structure. But others have done so, especially within sociology and political science.

In this chapter, I review these three literatures and put them in conversation with the morphogenic thesis. The global religious order is currently undergoing a fundamental transformation – that much is certain. Still, I conclude that it is too early to tell whether the result will be a new form of stability or one of ongoing morphogenesis.

Reflexive Secularity as Cultural Structure

The "anthropology of secularism" has become something of a growth industry in recent years (Cannell 2010). Talal Asad and his students did the seminal work in this field.[3] They draw heavily on the late Foucault and the late Wittgenstein. Specifically, they focus on the interrelationship between "discourses" and "practices." By "discourses" Asad roughly means networks of concepts that acquire their meaning in relationship to one another. By practices, he means ways of doing things that are part of a particular "form of life." He argues that discourses and practices support

[1]On global Pentecostalism, see: Donald E Miller and Tetsunao Yamamori, Global Pentecostalism: The New Face of Christian Social Engagement (Univ of California Press, 2007); David Martin, Pentecostalism: The World Their Parish (Blackwell Oxford, 2002). On the Qigong craze, see David A Palmer, Qigong Fever: Body, Science and Utopia in China (Cambridge Univ Press, 2007). On the Gulen movement, see: M Hakan Yavuz and John L Esposito, Turkish Islam and the Secular State: The Gèulen Movement (Syracuse University Press, 2003).

[2]The key works are: Talal Asad, Formations of the Secular: Christianity, Islam, Modernity (Stanford, Calif.: Stanford University Press, 2003); Charles Taylor, A Secular Age (Cambridge, Mass.: Belknap Press of Harvard University Press, 2007).

[3]In addition to Asad's own work, see especially: Saba Mahmood, Politics of Piety : The Islamic Revival and the Feminist Subject (Princeton, NJ: Princeton University Press, 2005); David Scott and Charles Hirschkind, Powers of the Secular Modern: Talal Asad and His Interlocutors (Stanford University Press, 2006).

one another. On the one hand, discourses help to organize and legitimate various domains of practices. For example, they tell us what is "religious" and what is "secular" and how and why the two must be bounded off from one another. On the other hand, practices help to stabilize and reproduce the meaning of discourses. Hiking through the Grand Canyon and taking Mass in the Reims Cathedral may inspire similar feelings of reverence and awe, Asad might argue, but we are taught that the first practice is "secular" while the second is "religious", at least in the form of life that now exists in the modern West.[4]

Where secularization theory treats religion and secularity as successive stages of historical development, Asad treats them as a conceptual binary that derives from Western Christianity. To see how, let us briefly examine the conceptual history of each term before reflecting on their interrelationship. Western scholars of religion have now been studying the genealogy of the "religion" concept for more than half a century (Smith 1998). The etymology of the word "religion" remains a subject of debate. Some argue that its root meaning is "to bind"; others suggest that it is "to go over again." In the Christian Middle Ages, the "religious" were the cloistered, those who had bound themselves to a monastic rule. By the Renaissance, "religion" had become a synonym for "Christianity." One could speak of "true" and "false" religion, but not of "religions" in the plural. That began to change after the Reformation. Some started to speak of the three major confessions – Catholic, Lutheran and Reformed – as distinct "religions." In the modern era, the category was expanded still further to include non-Christian "religions", as in "world religions." But it was also contracted to denote a particular sphere of life that was distinct from, say, politics and economics, as well as from "culture" and "civilization."

Now, consider the term "secular." It, too, has a long and complex genealogy. In pre-Christian Rome, a "saeculum" was an "age." In early Christian discourse, the saeculum was "this age" as opposed to the eschaton. In both periods, its primary meaning was temporal. In the Middle Ages, it acquired a spatial connotation as well. A monk who left the cloister became a member of the "secular" clergy. The term "secularization" was coined following the Reformation. Its meaning was legal. Church properties seized by the state were said to have been "secularized." The term "secularism" was first introduced over three centuries later. It had an ideological connotation. "Secularists" were "freethinkers" and "agnostics" who opposed traditional religion, put their faith in science and championed the "separation of church and state."

As should be clear, these conceptual histories are contingent, polyvalent and tightly linked. They are contingent insofar as the meaning of both concepts was shaped by historical events. They are polyvalent because each event deposited a new layer of meaning on top of the old. And they are linked insofar as the

[4]This example is inspired by Asad's insightful critique of Geertz's religion concept in Talal Asad, Genealogies of Religion : Discipline and Reasons of Power in Christianity and Islam (Baltimore, Md.: Johns Hopkins University Press, 1993). For Geertz's position, see Clifford Geertz, Interpretation of Cultures : Selected Essays (New York: Basic Books, 1973).

meaning of "religion" inflected the meaning of "the secular" and vice versa. Thus, secularism still retains the temporal, spatial, legal and ideological connotations it has accumulated over time. Indeed, these various connotations still inform scholarly discussions of the secular, though most often at a tacit level. The same holds for religion. It can still be used to denote devotion, truth, affiliation and belief, and so on, though scholars of religion are usually more conscious of this genealogy than are students of secularization. Finally, the meaning of secularity is linked to the meaning of religion. The secular demarcates the boundaries of the religious: there are secular times, secular spaces, secular institutions, secular ideologies and so on. The religious also denotes the limits of the secular. It pertains to the historical, the material, the worldly, the bodily and so on. In other words, the religious/secular divide is connected to a whole host of other conceptual binaries.

Now, let us now return to Asad's anthropology of secularism. It is closely modeled on Edward Said's theory of orientalism (Said 1979). Like orientalism, Asad argues, secularism is a Western construct that helps legitimate colonial domination.[5] How so? Let us start with the religion concept. It serves two interrelated purposes: commensuration and subordination. It commensurates by creating equivalencies. Certain discourses and practices of the colonized are categorized as "religions." For example, a certain set of Brahmanic traditions might be recorded as "Hinduism", while the classical learning of Chinese officialdom is rechristened as "Confucianism." It subordinates by ordering the world's religions into a multi-tiered hierarchy. At the bottom are "pagan" and "ethnic" religions that pertain only to a particular people and do not have a universal ethic. Then come the various "world religions" which aspire to universality but may still lack one or more features of a "fully developed" religion (e.g., written scriptures, a universal ethics, a learned priesthood and so on). At the apex is Christianity. It too is internally gradated. Catholicism is at the bottom because it still contains "pagan" remnants (e.g., sacramental magic and idolatrous rituals). Protestantism is fully "purified" of these elements. In short, "religion" is tacitly conceived in Protestant terms, and thereby placed on the top rung of the cultural ladder. Because the category of religion has been so deeply shaped by the history of Christianity, Asad argues, and especially of Protestant Christianity, non-Western and non-Christian discourses and practices are made deficient by definition.

Now consider the secularism concept. It also facilitates colonial rule. How so? For one thing, by authorizing a division between religious institutions, which are peopled by natives, and political institutions, which can be staffed by colonial officials. Secondly, by relegating religion to the private sphere, secularism defangs its political bite. Thirdly, by insisting that religion is a matter of individual belief, secularism undercuts ritual life and communal solidarity, which might serve as a

[5]On this point, see also: Tomoko Masuzawa, The Invention of World Religions: Or, How European Universalism Was Preserved in the Language of Pluralism (University of Chicago Press, 2005); Russell T McCutcheon, Manufacturing Religion: The Discourse on Sui Generis Religion and the Politics of Nostalgia (Oxford University Press New York, 1997) esp. Chapter 7.

basis of anti-colonial resistance. Finally, secularism reinforces Western claims of cultural superiority, insofar as Christianity, and especially Protestant Christianity is compatible with secularism in ways that other religions are not.

Asad's theory has been subjected to a number of critiques. Peter Van der Veer has challenged it on two fronts (Van der Veer 2009, 2014). First, he argues that there is a "missing third" which mediates between the religious and secular binary in modern societies, namely, "spirituality." Van der Veer persuasively shows that the "spirituality" concept emerges during the late nineteenth century in tandem with the modern meanings of "religion" and "secularism." On his reading, the spirituality concept is constituted by a double rejection. On the other hand, it eschews certain features of religion (e.g., institutions, rituals, hierarchies, and dogmas). And on the other, it refuses certain features of science (e.g., stringent materialism, empiricism, determinism and physicalism). In more positive terms, nineteenth century spirituality embraced the experimentalism and anti-traditionalism of the scientific ethos and combined them with the spiritualism and transcendentalism of a religious metaphysics.

Van der Veer also contests Asad's claim that these categories are purely a product of Western Christianity. In fact, he argues, they arose interactively out of "imperial encounters" between colonizers and colonized (Van Der Veer 2001). Western orientalists did not "invent" Hinduism and Confucianism all by themselves, he argues. They had a great deal of help from non-Western intellectuals who were anxious to reshape Indian and Chinese traditions in a more "Christian" or "Protestant" direction, by creating scriptural canons, identifying universal ethics or promoting "preaching." The same was true a fortiori of the concept of "spirituality." It entailed a double critique of Western culture, first for its excessive materiality and second for its excessive dogmatism. "Asia" was more "spiritual", some argued, and also more inclusive. If the "world religions" concept implied the cultural superiority of the West, the "spirituality" concept inverted the hierarchy. And that is part of what made it attractive, not only to some native elites but also to many Western intellectuals and freethinkers.

Prasenjit Duara's work on East Asia highlights a further difficulty with Asad's theory: the effects of translation (Duara 2008). When the categories of "religion", "secularism" and "spirituality" were introduced into East Asian languages, they were translated by means of neologisms. Interestingly, these neologisms were first coined in Japan, which was initially more open to Western ideas. The resulting characters were then introduced into Chinese. Subtle shifts in meaning occurred at each step, not because the translations were somehow faulty but because they evoked different linguistic connotations and historical associations. For example, the Chinese term for "religion" is associated with the term for "sectarianism" which evokes long-standing worries about millenarianism that go back to the White Lotus Rebellion. Meanwhile, the term for "spirituality" is closely associated with the language of "medicine" which evokes in turn certain forms of "self-cultivation." Thus, while the introduction of Western terminology into East Asian languages reordered the discursive field, it did not simply reproduce the Western discourse of secularism, as Asad is sometimes wont to imply.

There is at least one further difficulty with Asad's approach: it implies that social practices and human artifacts are like blank screens on which cultures project meanings. But this is too simple. Practices and artifacts often carry memories and codes when they are transplanted from one context to another. Consider the example of "mindfulness meditation" in the contemporary West.[6] In the United States, it has been incorporated into therapeutic regimes used to treat anxiety, depression and other psychological problems. It is taught in medical clinics and often covered by health insurance. The particular practice of "mindfulness" that is most often taught in such "stress reduction" programs is rooted in the Vipassana school of Hinduism. The principal proponents of mindfulness practice also operate a network of Buddhist retreat centers. While mindfulness is taught as a form of secular therapy, the transition to meditation qua spiritual practice is quite easy. All the more so, because it often deploys artifacts that are spiritually encoded, such as Tibetan prayer bells from Buddhist monasteries.

In their magisterial study of religion in modern China, Vincent Goosaert and David Palmer deliver a paradigmatic application of the new anthropology of secularism (Goossaert and Palmer 2011). Like Asad, they are attentive to how the introduction of Western categories such as "religion" and "secularism" reconfigured Chinese discourse and practice. Like Van der Veer, they locate these categories within a wider network of concepts that includes widely diffused notions like "spirituality", "magic", and "science" but also specifically Chinese ideas about "medicine", "self-cultivation" and "civilization." And like Duara, they are sensitive to how the connotations and associations of these terms shift when they are rendered into Chinese. More than any of these scholars, however, they provide detailed accounts of the ongoing struggles over the definitions of these terms and their relationship to practices. Tai-Chi and Qigong provide striking examples. Are they a form of traditional medicine? Asian spirituality? Sectarian religion? The answer is: all of the above in one context or another. Local ancestor cults provide another salient example. Are they a form of "popular superstition"? "Traditional religion"? Or "Chinese culture"? The answer is the same. Naturally, which account triumphed was not determined solely by intellectual debate. These were high-stakes struggles that often involved political conflict and sometimes also physical violence. Goosaert and Palmer are likewise attentive to the fact that such struggles concern, not just the definitions of particular categories but also jurisdiction over particular practices and artifacts.

What general lessons can we draw from the new anthropology of secularism? First, that the religious and the secular are "linked concepts." They are historically intertwined and mutually constitutive. Second, that the religious/secular binary has a "missing third" – spirituality – and that this conceptual triad is suspended within

[6]On the diffusion of mindfulness practice, see Jaime Kucinskas, "From Buddhist-Inspired Meditation to Mindfulness," (Bloomington, IN: Indiana University, 2013). On the diffusion of Buddhism more generally, see Wendy Cadge, Heartwood: The First Generation of Theravada Buddhism in America (University of Chicago Press, 2008).

a wider web of concepts that includes magic and science amongst other things. Third, that this discursive web is not solely the product of Western history; it was also shaped through "imperial encounters." Fourth, that the shape of this web is historically and culturally variable, insofar as it is influenced by processes of translation and conflict. Fifth, that practices and artifacts are ensnared in these webs and cannot simply be stripped of meaning and redeployed into a new context.

How does this new model of secularity differ from the old theory of secularization? In the old model, "magic", "religion" and "secularism" were like three buckets connected by a single hose. First magic drained into religion; then religion drained into secularism. In the new model, they are more like three faces on a Rubik's cube. You cannot move the squares on one plane around without simultaneously moving squares on the other five. Nor is there just one player. There are many hands busily struggling to rearrange the cube into one pattern or another. As a result, it is impossible to "solve" the puzzle without the application of considerable force. Nevertheless, we are impelled to try, at least for ourselves. Modern secularity is deeply reflexive. It confronts us with a variety of existential stances and compels us to choose. It is also deeply pluralistic. We can hardly help but be aware that our own stance is not the only possible one, and that others have chosen differently from us. How the Western world came to be secular and how secularity feels to modern Westerners is the subject of Taylor's magnum opus.

Reflexive Secularity and Human Agency

Like Asad, Taylor is more interested in understanding the varied and shifting meanings of "secularity" than in debating the historical and sociological dynamics of "secularization."[7] He opens his analysis by distinguishing three different senses of "secularity." "Secularity 1" refers to the differentiation between religious and secular spheres of life. "Secularity 2" refers to the decline in religious practice. And "Secularity 3" refers to changing "conditions of belief." Orthodox secularization theory is typically concerned with Secularity 1 and/or Secularity 2. Taylor's main focus is Secularity 3.

Having framed his argument in analytical terms, he then reframes it in more historical ones. In the year 1500, he asserts, irreligion was virtually unthinkable. Five hundred years later, however, it is not just thinkable; it has actually become the "default option" in many parts of the Western world. Why? What brought about this monumental shift in the "conditions of belief"?

---

[7]The fullest version of Taylor's argument may be found in Taylor, A Secular Age. The basic argument is first adumbrated in Charles Taylor and James Heft, A Catholic Modernity?, (New York: Oxford University Press, 1999). On the pivotal concept of social imaginaries, see also Charles Taylor, Modern Social Imaginaries (Duke University Press, 2004). For discussion and critique see also Michael Warner, Jonathan Van Antwerpen, and Craig J. Calhoun, Varieties of Secularism in a Secular Age (Cambridge, Mass.: Harvard University Press, 2010).

On one account, canonized in secularization theory, the rise of religion is attributed to force and fraud, and its decline is attributed to emancipation and science. Religion persists so long as priestly powers team up with secular rulers to propagate superstition and instill fear into the masses. It declines once natural science and human emancipation begin stripping away illusion and oppression. Taylor refers to such accounts as "subtraction stories." He argues that they are one-sided at best. There was no "war between science and religion" in the early modern era. And, he adds, religion provided as many arguments for democracy as against it (Toft 2011).

Taylor's own account is more of an addition story. The defining feature of our secular age, he says, is not the subtraction of traditional religion so much as the addition of other options. The most important of these options is "exclusive humanism." By "exclusive humanism", Taylor means a nontheistic humanism, as opposed to the theistic humanism of, say, Erasmus or Kierkegaard. In the modern West, he adds, we must now speak of exclusive humanism in the plural. There are Enlightenment versions and Romantic versions, Kantian ones and utilitarian ones, and so on and so forth. Nowadays, there are too many versions to transpose. There are also many anti-humanisms (e.g., Nietzschean and Sartrean) and now also various transhumanisms as well (Geroulanos 2010). Taylor refers to this rapid proliferation of competing worldviews as "the nova effect."

But isn't this just another kind of subtraction story? Isn't exclusive humanism just Christian humanism minus God? Not exactly, says Taylor. On his account, the genesis of exclusive humanism is also a transformation story. Specifically, it involves a fundamental transformation in what Taylor calls our "social imaginary." By "social imaginary", Taylor means a set of widely-shared, background assumptions about humanity, society and the cosmos, and their relationship to one another. The main purpose of Taylor's book, *A Secular Age*, is to narrate this transformation.

For purposes of the present discussion, the most important of these transformations concerns human agency. Until fairly recently, Taylor argues, the Western social imaginary presumed a "porous self." "[F]or the porous self", Taylor says, "the source of its most powerful and important emotions are outside the "mind"; or better put, the very notion that there is a clear boundary, allowing us to define an inner base area, grounded in which we can disengage from the rest, has no sense" (Taylor 2007: 38). A porous self can be permeated by outside forces and powers which may summon or even possess it. Since the early modern era, however, the porous self has been increasingly supplanted by a "buffered self." In this imaginary, the self has outer boundaries which seal off and protect its "inner depths." And these depths in turn underwrite the modern ideal of "autonomy" that originates with Kant.

The shift from the porous to the buffered self goes together with a corresponding shift in our understanding of society. Prior to the secular age, Taylor argues, the social order was widely understood as both natural and sacred. In the European Middle Ages, for example, the social imaginary was premised on a trifold division between "those who pray, those who fight and those who labor", that is, between the clergy, the nobility and the peasantry (Duby 1982). Indeed, the French anthropologist, Georges Dumezil argued that a trifold imaginary was an underlying feature of

"Indo-European" civilization more generally (Dumezil 1958). These arrangements were understood to enjoy divine sanction of some kind. Taylor refers to this as a system of "hierarchical complementarity." In the modern social imaginary, by contrast, this system gives way to "the order of mutual benefit." On this view, social orders are human artifacts created to secure individual wellbeing. Hobbes' version of social contract theory provides a particularly clear example. Individuals are presumed to be pre-social and, indeed, anti-social. They come together solely for purposes of self-preservation. They concede a portion of their natural rights to the sovereign in exchange for a guarantee of security; nothing more and nothing less.

The third shift in the modern social imaginary concerns nature. Here, the shift is from a purposive cosmos to what Taylor calls "the immanent frame." The pre-modern imaginary was an amalgam of Athens and Jerusalem. From Athens, it took the idea of purpose in nature. From Jerusalem it took the distinction between the mundane and the transcendent. The modern imaginary could be seen as an amalgam of Epicureanism and skepticism. From the former, it takes mechanism – a combination of monism and determinism. From the latter, it takes scientism, the view that reality is exhaustively described by science. The immanent frame doesn't completely close the door on transcendence. But it does suggest that there is probably nothing on the other side. The immanent frame has what Taylor calls a "closed spin."

In Taylor's view, there is an inevitable connection between our social imaginary and our moral imaginary, between how the world seems to be and what it seems we should do. Following Heidegger, Taylor describes this connection as "ontic." He argues that the there is an ontic link between the emergence of the immanent frame and what he calls "the affirmation of everyday life." By this, he means the view that the highest human good consists in ordinary human flourishing – in family ties, social relationships, meaningful work, physical wellbeing and so on. He contrasts this with the ethics of the world religions, all of which presume that the human good is not exhausted by everyday life and that achieving the good may involve the devaluation or even the renunciation of everyday life.

But Taylor also believes that there is an ineluctable tension between the modern moral imaginary and the phenomenology of everyday life. This tension arises out of the experience he calls "fullness." Fullness is the feeling, perhaps fleeting, that there might be something more than the fulfillments of everyday life. "These may be moments", says Taylor, quoting Robert Musil, "when 'ordinary reality is 'abolished' and something terrifyingly other shines through'" (Taylor 2007: 5). Such experiences needn't be understood as "religious." Some may interpret them as "spiritual" or aesthetic or epiphanic. However understood, such experiences are the root cause of the nova effect. For some, they give rise to an ethic of subjective experience (e.g., Romanticism). In others, they may inspire efforts to transcend "the all-too-human" (e.g., Nietzscheanism). And so on and so forth.

So, what does it feel like to live in a "secular age"? First, conflicted or, as Taylor puts it "cross-pressured." We may be avowed secularists, who occasionally feel a "spiritual" pull. Conversely, we may be devout theists, who experience episodes of piercing doubt. The sheer proliferation of competing worldviews means that reflective people will feel simultaneously pulled in multiple directions. Secondly, we are apt to feel uncertain or, in Taylor's phrase, "fragilized." Why? Because we cannot really help interacting with people who do not share our worldview. And this inevitably leads us to question its verities.

While Taylor's account surely captures some people's experience of secularity, it just as surely misses others. Even in the West, there are religious subcultures that have shielded themselves from the sorts of "cross-pressures" and "fragilization" that Taylor discusses. Imagine a conservative evangelical family living in a small midwestern town in the USA. They attend religious services several times a week. They also participate in various social and charitable activities at their church. One child is home-schooled by the mother. The others attend a local Christian high school. They hope to attend a nearby Christian college after graduation. The father works at the local Christian radio station. The mother and daughters volunteer at a local crisis pregnancy center. At home, the family listens to Christian music and reads Christian novels. Apart from a small clutch of Latino families who work at the local meatpacking plant, the town they live in is quite homogeneous. Most of its residents would characterize themselves as "Americans", without any ethnic or racial prefix. Virtually everyone would characterize themselves as a Christian of some sort. There is a vague awareness of the "secular humanist" culture that exists in the nearby state capital and the distant coastal metropolises, and a vague anxiety about the "permissive" values that permeate American popular culture. This family may not live under a "sacred canopy" encompassing the wider culture (Berger 1969). But it is sheltered by a "sacred umbrella" created by the evangelical subculture (Smith and Emerson 1998). A similar sort of story could be told about an atheist or agnostic living in a college town or a coastal metropolis. They would certainly be aware of the evangelical subculture of the American heartland. And they might feel vaguely threatened by it. But they might not feel the least bit "cross-pressured" or "fragilized."

Of course, religious subcultures are less common in the West than they used to be and humanist subcultures more common. Even in the American "heartland", mobility, immigration, and the media are increasing the level of pluralism that people contend with in their everyday lives. But such encounters need not lead to cognitive dissonance. In many cases, argues Peter Berger, they are managed via "compartmentalization." Most people inhabit "multiple realities", he contends, each with its own "relevance structures." The relevance of one reality to another may not be clear. For instance, a conservative evangelical may take an antibiotic without this impinging on his or her views of evolution. Or there they may have a reason for compartmentalizing the two. The person in question may accept the sort of "micro evolution" that occurs in microbes while rejecting the reality of "macro evolution" that gives rise to new species of mammals. Further, experiences of cognitive dissonance may also be mitigated by norms of "reasonableness." A recent study by Robert Wuthnow found that such norms usually lead American Christians to tone down their views when they interact with people outside of their faith community (Wuthnow 2012). This also serves to mitigate cognitive dissonance.

Modern Westerners may live in a secular age. About that, Taylor is quite right. But not everyone feels "cross-pressured" and "fragilized", at least not to the same degree. The experience of secularity is mediated by the existence of subcultures and by practices of compartmentalization. Taylor's account of pluralism is too one-dimensional. He is right to emphasize the pluralization of worldviews. To this, however, one must add the pluralization of social milieu and variations in individual reflexivity. A comprehensive theory of modern secularity must attend more closely to social structure.

Reflexive Secularity and Social Structure

For methodological purposes, Taylor's analysis brackets "secularity 1" (the differentiation of religious and non-religious value spheres) in order to focus on "secularity 3" ("conditions of belief"). Moreover, Taylor's analysis of secularity 3 focuses mainly on the interplay between culture and agency. In this section, I un-bracket and expand on his analysis. Specifically, I consider how the differentiation of value spheres influences conditions of belief. I also consider how secularity 3 is influenced by global capitalism. In a word, I put structure back into the equation. I suggest that the degree and form of optionality is influenced by both the local organization of secularity 1 and by the global networks of modern capitalism. Specifically, I argue that: (1) regimes of secularity 1 limit and channel experiences of secularity 3; and (2) the globalization of the economy leads to what I will call "dis/embedding" and "dis/assemblage processes."

Secularity 1 was long a central focus of secularization theory. In the orthodox theory, Secularity 1 was usually conceptualized in terms of "differentiation" and/or "privatization." The theory predicted that religious "spheres", "institutions", and "roles" were becoming more and more "differentiated" from non-religious ones and/or that religious "beliefs", "practices" and "symbols" were being more and more relegated to the "private" realm.[8] Proponents of the theory spent a great deal of time trying to "operationalize" differentiation and privatization and "measure" them in various societies. They interpreted these variations as indicators of the degree of secularization.

That is no longer true. Today, scholars are more interested in identifying and explaining different forms of secularity, not only in the West but in other parts of

[8]On the conceptualization of differentiation, see M. Chaves, "Secularization as Declining Religious Authority," Social Forces 72, no. 3 (1994); Mark Chaves, "Secularization: A Luhmannian Reflection," Soziale Systeme 3 (1997); D. Yamane, "Secularization on Trial: In Defense of a Neosecularization Paradigm," Journal for the Scientific Study of Religion 36, no. 1 (1997). For examples of operationalization and measurement, see Karel Dobbelaere, Secularization: An Analysis at Three Levels (Peter Lang, 2002); Steve Bruce, God Is Dead: Secularization in the West, Religion and Modern World (Oxford, UK ; Malden, Mass.: Blackwell Publishers, 2002).

the world as well.[9] Scholars working in this area no longer speak of secularity in the singular, as if there were just one model that originated in the West and then diffused to the rest of the world. More often, they speak of different regimes of secularity, which are the result of complex historical conjunctures and institutional path dependencies. And they try to understand the resulting variations – why American secularism is different from French secularism, say, or why Indian secularism is different from Chinese secularism.

The new scholarship on comparative secularity is still at an early stage of development. It would be premature to advance a comprehensive typology of the various types. Still, some of the dimensions of variation are slowly coming into view.

For example, we might begin by treating "privatization" and "differentiation" themselves as variables rather than as trends. Take "privatization." Just as "the religious" can only be defined in relation to "the secular", so "the private" can only be understood in terms of "the public." Amongst other things, "public" implies "visible", "shared", and "political", while "private" suggests "hidden", "individual" and "non-state." One could then distinguish various degrees of privatization in terms of which and how many of these meanings are mobilized. Recent debates about the various "headscarf affairs" provide an illustration (Bowen 2007). In France, the "privatization of religion" implies the public invisibility of a person's faith. The French version of secularity, known as "*laïcité*", requires that religious signs be confined to private spaces. Thus, the wearing of headscarves in "public spaces" is regarded as a violation of French secularity. In the United States, by contrast, the "privatization of religion" is not understood quite so expansively. Faith is generally understood to be "private", but mainly in the sense of "personal." Many also believe that it should be "private" in the sense of "non-political." But few if any would insist that religious signs be banished from public view. Personal attire is coded as "private" rather than "public." In short, we might say that the symbolic boundaries between public and private space are drawn differently in the two countries.

"Social differentiation" can also be turned into a variable. The most sophisticated theory of social differentiation is to be found in the systems theory of Niklas Luhmann. Luhmann distinguishes between four types of differentiation: "segmentary", "center/periphery", "hierarchical" and "functional." (Luhmann 1997, 2000) Drawing on Luhmann, we can distinguish four types religio-political differentiation. I will call them consociational (segmentary), imperial (center/periphery), confessional (hierarchical) and liberal (functional).

[9]Recent examples include Craig J. Calhoun, Mark Juergensmeyer, and Jonathan VanAntwerpen, Rethinking Secularism (New York: Oxford University Press, 2011); Nandini Chatterjee, The Making of Indian Secularism : Empire, Law and Christianity, 1830–1960, Cambridge Imperial and Post-Colonial Studies Series (Basingstoke, Hampshire; New York: Palgrave Macmillan, 2011); Christian Smith, The Secular Revolution : Power, Interests, and Conflict in the Secularization of American Public Life (Berkeley: University of California Press, 2003); Ahmet T. Kuru, Secularism and State Policies toward Religion : The United States, France, and Turkey, Cambridge Studies in Social Theory, Religion, and Politics (Cambridge; New York: Cambridge University Press, 2009).

Consociational secularity involves segmentary differentiation of religio-cultural groups. Each group has its own autonomous subculture, outfitted with autochthonous institutions (e.g., religious communities, educational institutions, media outlets, and political parties). Each subculture is formally represented within state institutions via its political wing. The concept of "consociationalism" was originally developed by political scientists to describe the power-sharing systems that emerged in small multi-confessional polities such as Belgium and Switzerland (Lijphart 1969). However, it also captures certain features of social organization in large, religiously diverse democracies such as India, Malaysia and Indonesia (Lijphart 1996; Lustick 1979).

Imperial secularity is premised on center/periphery differentiation between the unified high culture of court and capital on one hand and the various folk religions and cultures that are subject to it on the other. Pre-modern China is perhaps the paradigmatic example. However, similar structures may be found in many other historical empires as well (e.g., Roman, Mughal, Ottoman). In modern times, the imperial type was probably most closely approached by certain communist societies, such as Poland, which combined an official culture of state atheism with a folk culture of traditional religion.

The confessional type involves hierarchical differentiation in which an official, state religion is *primus inter pares* and other religions are either passively tolerated or actively repressed. Early modern Europe provides an excellent example (Schilling 1988). Confessional structures live on in modern Europe as well though, both in the official state churches (e.g., in the UK and parts of Scandinavia) and in the informal public cultures as well, which often have great difficulty incorporating non-Christian religions, particularly Islam and Judaism.

The liberal form of secularity, finally, corresponds to the principle of functional differentiation. It is premised on a clear distinction between public and private spheres and, within the private sphere, between religious and non-religious spheres (i.e., the economy, the culture), each of which has its own values and rules. It underlies the constitutional principle of "separation of church and state" and also generic accounts of "social differentiation."

If Luhmann's systems theory provides one useful set of conceptual tools, then Rodney Stark's "religious economies approach" furnishes another (Finke and Stark 1992; Stark 1999). Stark and his followers apply the basic principles of neoclassical economics to religious life. They speak of religious supply and demand, religious markets and firms, religious consumers and entrepreneurs, and so on. The theory generates "predictions" about "religious vitality" based on two "variables": the structure of the "religious market" and the degree of "state regulation."

While the predictions have not fared so well, some of the metaphors are still useful (Chaves and Gorski 2001; Voas et al. 2002). For example, we can distinguish between situations of "religious monopoly", "religious oligopoly" and "religious competition", based on the number of religious communities that are competing for influence in a given context. On this analysis, Iran would be an example of monopoly, Indonesia of oligopoly and the US of a "free market."

Similarly, we can distinguish between various forms of state regulation such as: (1) state financial subsidies directed towards a particular religious community or set of religious communities; (2) formal legal privileges enjoyed by members of some religious communities but not others; (3) barriers to entry such as the need to attain official recognition or approval; (4) various forms of repression directed at certain communities.

Discussions of "religious freedom" provide another vantage point on regimes of secularity. Religious freedom can be and has been thought about in very different ways that closely track earlier discussions about political freedom. For example, we can distinguish between individual and collective freedom and positive and negative freedom. Combining these two distinctions generates four types of religious freedom. The most common are: (1) liberal (individual and negative), meaning "liberty of conscience" and its "free exercise." This is how religious freedom is most commonly understood in the West. The United States comes very close to the "pure type." (2) communal (collective and positive), meaning state support for the social institutions of recognized religions (e.g., schools, charities, seminaries, media, etc.). This is how "secularism" has generally been understood in post-independence India. The multi-confessional polities of Northern Europe also incorporate elements of this model. (3) accommodationist (collective and negative): the state actively encourages "religion in general" without supporting any particular religious institutions. The Indonesian "pancasila" system closely approaches this type. (4) spiritualist (individual and positive): the state views individual spirituality as a public good and takes various steps to encourage it. I am not aware of any examples of this type in the contemporary world. However, some business enterprises have adopted a "spiritualist" form of human resource policy, which provides direct and indirect support for the spiritual formation of their employees, such as time out of the working day to practice 'mindfulness'.

As should be clear from the foregoing, there are many actual and possible regimes of secularity, which will differ greatly in the range, degree and form of "religious options" they permit or encourage. For example, Germany does not prohibit the Church of Scientology, but it does not recognize it as a religion either. Consequently, Scientologists do not enjoy the sorts of legal privileges and protections afforded to recognized religions such as Catholicism or Islam. Conversely, the Chinese state permitted Falun Gong so long as it was understood as a form of "traditional medicine" or a "spiritual exercise" (Chang 2008; Junker 2012). However, it was later reclassified as an "evil cult" and is now actively suppressed by the state. In countries which define religious freedom in collective terms, finally, individual freedoms are sometimes restricted – indeed, converting to another religion or marrying outside one's birth religion may be difficult or even impossible. Conversely, in countries that define religious freedom in individual terms, such as the US, religious communities do not enjoy any special protection or recognition qua communities. They are not permitted to establish separate courts or religious laws of any kind, nor may they engage in collective rituals that violate secular law (Sullivan 2005). As these examples show, a focus on cultural structures alone yields only a partial understanding of optionality. A full understanding of secularity requires more attention to social structures. Conditions of belief are channeled and constrained by local regimes of secularity.

If the diffusion of the nation-state form has generally tended to limit and channel religious optionality, the globalization of capitalist production and free markets mostly presses in the other direction. Why? Because it has enlarged and accelerated global flows of information, human beings and cultural artifacts. Take the modern history of the sacred scriptures of the world religions. The Bhagavad Gita was first translated into English in 1785 (Davis 2015). It was then translated from English into German in 1802. In 1843 portions of the Gita were published in The Dial, the main organ of the Transcendentalist Movement in the United States. This was one of the first attempts to bring the text to a lay audience. The first Penguin Classics edition appeared in 1962. Today, of course, various translations and interpretations may be easily accessed over the Internet as may high quality films and videos of memorable parts of it. Similar stories could be told about other major texts such as the Koran, the Analects, the Heart Sutra and so on. Once jealously guarded by priestly elites, sacred texts are now widely accessible to a global laity. One result of this availability, it should be noted, is a "textualization" or "creedalization" of religions that traditionally emphasized orality or ritual.

These accelerated flows of information have been paralleled by flows of human beings. One hundred and 50 years ago, "Hindus" and "Muslims" were still presented to Western audiences as if they were zoological curiosities. Today, Hindus and Muslims are a common sight on the streets of New York and London – more common, perhaps, than practicing Christians. Today, every religious community has its own global diaspora. And these diasporas now intersect with one another in urban centers through the world. To what effect? In the United States, where religious communities have long played a vital role in the assimilation process, there is often a trend towards Protestantization (Yang and Ebaugh 2001; Warner and Wittner 1998). By Protestantization, I do not mean conversion to Protestantism – though this also happens, of course. Rather, I mean the adoption of Protestant practices, forms and styles. For example, a Buddhist Temple in Oakland's Chinatown may hold weekly services on Sundays, sponsor a soup kitchen and a youth group, and encourage members to read certain sutras. The Protestantization of non-Protestant religious communities in the United States illustrates processes of disconnecting and embedding. By disconnecting and embedding, I mean the weakening of ties between the center and periphery of a religious community and a reshaping of the peripheral community that renders it more homologous with its new environment.

Global flows of information and people can also have the opposite effect, however. They can lead to disembedding and reconnecting. By this, I mean a process whereby religious communities are "purified" of their local "cultural" particularities and brought into tighter contact with a broader network of local communities sharing titular membership in the same world religion. The deep historical background for this development is the gradual formation of global religious diasporas. This process was driven by various mechanisms: missions, conquests, expulsions, colonization, trade and so on. All of the world religions have also experienced numerous episodes of disconnection, in which network ties have been severed. Disconnections can also be caused by a variety of mechanisms: the dissolution of empires, the secession of new nations, the collapse of trade networks, or the insertion of rival religions into a network node, to name just a few. Disconnection creates the preconditions for embedding – for local religious communities to absorb local cultural characteristics. The French anthropologist, Olivier Roy, has been patiently documenting a process of disembedding and reconnecting within the Islamic diaspora (Roy 2004). The tendency, he argues, is towards the formation of a "global umma." Muslim beliefs and practices become more homogeneous. Global centers of Muslim learning and culture (re)emerge as central nodes of cultural formation. Muslim identity "trumps" other markers ("ethnicity", "class" etc.) and shapes political concerns.

What will be the final result of this interaction between embedding and disembedding, disconnection and reconnection? At the moment, at least, disembedding and reconnection might seem to have the upper hand. If so, then the result may well be what José Casanova (2008) refers to as "global denominationalism." By this, he means the formation of globalized religious communities whose local relations are a mix of peaceful competition and ecumenical cooperation. The more pessimistic scenario is contained in Huntington's "clash of civilization" thesis. On this view, civilizations will replace nations as units of conflict in the international order.

Finally, let us now turn to the effects of the global circulation of cultural artifacts. In this context, I use the term "artifact" quite broadly to refer, not only to human-made material objects but also to cultural forms and practices that can be "exported" and "imported." Viewed from the vantage point of a process ontology, cultural artifacts are typically inserted into routine flows of human activity.[10] This is true in both religious and secular settings. For example, the striking of a prayer bell might normally occur at a particular moment in a monastic ritual. Likewise, the appearance of a team mascot might normally occur at a particular moment in a football match. To the degree that the artifact in question is regarded as "sacred" in the broadly Durkheimian sense, its deployment will typically be strictly controlled and narrowly circumscribed. In this way, the artifact in question remains tightly embedded within a particular activity flow. However, in an "age of mechanical reproduction" and global markets, these strategies are easily disrupted. Tibetan artisans begin to mass manufacture prayer bells – and prayer flags, prayer wheels and prayer rugs – for a global market. The same obtains a fortiori for replicas of a local football mascot. As a result, the Tibetan prayer might find its way into the sanctuary of an evangelical megachurch in the United States and a football jersey might be sighted during Friday prayers at an Anatolian mosque. In other words, the global flow of cultural artifacts qua capitalist commodities leads to the disassembly and reassembly of religious and secular activity flows and the creation of new and sometimes hybridized flows. We may regard this disruption of routine with delight or despair, but this much is certain: it disturbs local mechanisms of cultural reproduction.

[10] Here, I am drawing inspiration from "actor-network theory." For a succinct overview, see Bruno Latour, "On Actor-Network Theory: A Few Clarifications," Soziale welt (1996).

Which of these countervailing mechanisms will prevail? Disembedding and re-connecting? Or dis-connecting and re-embedding? Only time will tell.

Conclusion: 'Reflexive Secularity'?

Two decades ago, Beck et al. (1994) announced the arrival of a new era of "reflexive modernity." They argued that the globalization of the capitalist economy was undermining the power of the nation state and also of cultural traditions, thereby emancipating the individual and creating the potential for new solidarities. Reflexive modernity was a new era of modernity, insofar as it was systematically dispensing with traditional institutions and structures that had stabilized the first phase of modernization, such as religious belief, national identity and the nuclear family. It was reflexive, insofar as the ongoing process of detraditionalization was compelling individuals to consciously choose their life paths. The hope was that this sort of self-conscious choice might also be extended to the societal level.

The reflexive modernization thesis has not fared particularly well. Nationalism and religion are both alive and well. Neither shows any signs of disappearing. If anything, they are more vital now than they were two decades ago. Meanwhile, de-traditionalization has led, not just to individuation, but also to fundamentalism, religious fundamentalism in the first instance, but also to secular fundamentalisms as well, as in the cultural revolutions of the Communist era or, more benignly, the "new atheist" movement of the present day. And if there is a global threat to the power of the nation-state, it is not NGOs or international institutions so much as secession movements and armed insurgencies. While its forecasts of individuation and post-traditional identity may have some local validity within Northern Europe, the theory of reflexive modernization now seems like a projection of the hopes and fears of a certain group of Western intellectuals onto a global canvas since painted over with rather different images.

The failures of the reflexive modernization thesis – so clear in retrospect – should give us pause as we consider the future of reflexive secularity. Taylor's optionality thesis probably does accord fairly well with the experiences of a certain stratum of educated professionals living in metropolitan settings. Such people are aware of many different ways of believing and disbelieving. They are exposed to many different forms of human well-being and ill-being. Typically, they are also well insulated from external pressures to choose one set of beliefs and practices over another, so long as it is compatible with the competent performance of their professional responsibilities. What we should not do is confuse the way their lives feel – the way our lives feel – with the "conditions of belief" that others face. Nor should we be naïve about the ways in which a liberal democratic polity and a capitalistically organized economy shape our own conditions of belief. Are we really free to choose a life of ascetic self-flagellation such as some medieval monastics practiced? Or drug induced communal ecstasy that characterized some Native American religiosity? Would that not clash with the affirmation of everyday life and the ethic of vocational responsibility that constitute the modern social imaginary? The answer is clear.

Nor should we imagine that reflexive secularity evokes a uniform response even within our own milieu. In principle, one can easily imagine a wide range of possible responses to the "reflexive imperative" in the religious realm, just as wide as those which Margaret Archer discovered in the secular sphere. Based on her work, we would anticipate that these responses would minimally include: (1) neo-traditionalism, meaning the affirmation of a particular tradition as the embodiment of an exclusive truth. Note that neo-traditionalism comes in both religious and secular variants. The religious variant is "fundamentalism." The secular one is "scientism"; (2) syncretistic fideism, meaning a conscious choice to remain within one's "native" tradition because it is like one's native language, rather than because it is believed to contain an exclusive truth; (3) syncretistic seeking, meaning the pursuit of one's own individual "path" or "journey" based primarily on personal "experience" or "calling." This may lead to a hybrid worldview that combines elements of religion, spirituality, magic, science, therapy and so on. (4) aesthetic self-creation, meaning the conscious rejection of all forms of collective identity or received tradition and the embrace of choice as a good in itself and the pursuit of a wholly unique form of individual identity. The relative prevalence and conceptual exhaustiveness of these responses is of course a matter for empirical investigation.

Does reflexive secularity help to usher in a morphogenic society? The evidence is mixed. Since the Axial Age, religious communities have played a central role in the reproduction of normativity and, more generally, in the stabilization of social orders. Indeed, one might argue, as Robert Bellah recently did, that the Axial Age breakthrough created the cultural conditions for social cooperation on a hitherto unprecedented scale. But whether religious communities will continue to do so remains to be seen. It will depend, in part, on the interaction between the embedding and dis-embedding mechanisms discussed above and on their interactions with local cultural and political conflicts. In the optimistic scenario, a system of global denominationalism forms the basis for a period of global ecumenicism that could legitimate new forms of transnational cooperation. In the pessimistic scenario, conflicts within and between the various world religions become an enduring source of international instability preventing the human race from confronting deepening threats to its continued existence. At the moment, both scenarios seem equally plausible.

References

Acquaviva, S. S. (1979). *The decline of the sacred in industrial society*. Oxford: B. Blackwell.

Asad, T. (1993). *Genealogies of religion: Discipline and reasons of power in Christianity and Islam*. Baltimore: Johns Hopkins University Press.

Asad, T. (2003). *Formations of the secular: Christianity, Islam, modernity*. Stanford: Stanford University Press.

Beck, U., Giddens, A., & Lash, S. (1994). *Reflexive modernization*. Cambridge: Polity Press.

Berger, P. (1969). *The sacred canopy: Elements of a sociological theory of religion*. Garden City: Doubleday.

Bowen, J. R. (2007). *Why the French don't like headscarves: Islam, the state, and public space*. Princeton: Princeton University Press.
Bruce, S. (2002). *God is dead: Secularization in the West. Religion and modern world*. Oxford: Blackwell Publishers.
Cadge, W. (2008). *Heartwood: The first generation of Theravada Buddhism in America*. Chicago: University of Chicago Press.
Calhoun, C. J., Juergensmeyer, M., & VanAntwerpen, J. (2011). *Rethinking secularism*. New York: Oxford University Press.
Cannell, F. (2010). The anthropology of secularism. *Annual Review of Anthropology, 39*, 85–100.
Casanova, J. (1994). *Public religions in the modern world*. Chicago: University of Chicago Press.
Casanova, J. (2008). Balancing religious freedom and cultural preservation. *The Review of Faith & International Affairs, 6*(2), 13–15.
Chang, M. H. (2008). *Falun Gong: The end of days*. New Haven: Yale University Press.
Chatterjee, N. (2011). *The making of Indian secularism: Empire, law and Christianity, 1830–1960*. Basingstoke/New York: Palgrave Macmillan.
Chaves, M. (1994). Secularization as declining religious authority. *Social Forces, 72*(3), 749–774.
Chaves, M. (1997). Secularization: A Luhmannian reflection. *Soziale Systeme, 3*, 439–449.
Chaves, M., & Gorski, P. S. (2001). Religious pluralism and religious participation. *Annual Review of Sociology, 27*, 261–281.
Davis, R. H. (2015). *The Bhagavad Gita: A biography*. Princeton: Princeton University.
Dobbelaere, K. (1981). Theories of secularization. *Current Sociology, 29*(2), 15–30.
Dobbelaere, K. (2002). *Secularization: An analysis at three levels*. Brussels: Peter Lang.
Duara, P. (2008). Religion and citizenship in China and the diaspora. In M. M.-H. Yang (Ed.), *Chinese religiosities* (pp. 43–62). Berkeley: University of California.
Duby, G. (1982). *The three orders: Feudal society imagined*. Chicago: University of Chicago Press.
Dumézil, G. (1958). *L'idéologie Tripartite Des Indo-Européens*. Latomus (revue des études latines).
Finke, R., & Stark, R. (1992). *The churching of America, 1776–1990: Winners and losers in our religious economy*. New Brunswick: Rutgers University Press.
Geertz, C. (1973). *Interpretation of cultures: Selected essays*. New York: Basic Books.
Geroulanos, S. (2010). *An atheism that is not humanist emerges in French thought*. Stanford: Stanford University Press.
Goossaert, V., & Palmer, D. A. (2011). *The religious question in modern China*. Chicago: University of Chicago Press.
Junker, A. (2012). *Sacred and secular protest in Chinese Diaspora: Falun Gong and the Chinese democracy movement*. Dissertation, Yale University.
Kucinskas, J. (2013). *From Buddhist-inspired meditation to mindfulness*. Bloomington: Indiana University.
Kuru, A. T. (2009). *Secularism and state policies toward religion: The United States, France, and Turkey*. New York: Cambridge University Press.
Latour, B. (1996). On actor-network theory: A few clarifications. *Soziale, 47*, 369–381.
Lijphart, A. (1969). Consociational democracy. *World Politics, 21*(02), 207–225.
Lijphart, A. (1996). The puzzle of Indian democracy: A consociational interpretation. *American Political Science Review, 90*, 258–268.
Luhmann, N. (1997). *Die Gesellschaft Der Gesellschaft* (1st ed.). Frankfurt am Main: Suhrkamp.
Luhmann, N. (2000). *Die Religion der Gesellschaft*. Suhrkamp: Frankfurt am Main.
Lustick, I. (1979). Stability in deeply divided societies: Consociationalism versus control. *World Politics, 31*(3), 325–344.
Mahmood, S. (2005). *Politics of piety: The Islamic revival and the feminist subject*. Princeton: Princeton University Press.
Martin, D. (2002). *Pentecostalism: The world their parish*. Oxford: Blackwell.
Masuzawa, T. (2005). *The invention of world religions: Or, how European universalism was preserved in the language of pluralism*. Chicago: University of Chicago Press.

McCutcheon, R. T. (1997). *Manufacturing religion: The discourse on Sui Generis religion and the politics of Nostalgia*. Oxford: Oxford University Press.
Miller, D. E., & Yamamori, T. (2007). *Global Pentecostalism: The new face of Christian social engagement*. Berkeley: University of California Press.
Palmer, D. A. (2007). *Qigong fever: Body, science and utopia in China*. Cambridge: Cambridge University Press.
Roy, O. (2004). *Globalized Islam: The search for a New Ummah*. New York: Columbia University Press. In association with the Centre d'Etudes et de Recherches Internationales.
Said, E. (1979). *Orientalism*. New York: Vintage.
Schilling, H. (1988). Die Konfessionalisierung Im Reich: Religiöser Und Gesellschaftlicher Wandel in Deutschland Zwischen 1555 Und 1620. *Historische Zeitschrift, 246*(1), 1–45.
Scott, D., & Hirschkind, C. (2006). *Powers of the secular modern: Talal Asad and his interlocutors*. Stanford: Stanford University Press.
Smith, J. Z. (1998). Religion, religions, religious. *Critical Terms for Religious Studies, 1998*, 269–284.
Smith, S. (2003). *The secular revolution: Power, interests, and conflict in the secularization of American public life*. Berkeley: University of California Press.
Smith, C., & Emerson, M. (1998). *American evangelicalism: Embattled and thriving*. Chicago: University of Chicago Press.
Stark, R. (1999). Secularization, R.I.P. *Sociology of Religion, 60*(3), 249–273.
Sullivan, W. F. (2005). *The impossibility of religious freedom*. Princeton: Princeton University Press.
Taylor, C. (2004). *Modern social imaginaries*. Durham: Duke University Press.
Taylor, C. (2007). *A secular age*. Cambridge, MA: Belknap Press of Harvard University Press.
Taylor, C., & Heft, J. (1999). *A Catholic modernity?* New York: Oxford University Press.
Toft, M. D., Philpott, D., & Shah, T. S. (2011). *God's century: Resurgent religion and global politics*. New York: W.W. Norton.
Tschannen, O. (1991). The secularization paradigm: A systematization. *Journal for the Scientific Study of Religion, 30*(4), 395.
Van der Veer, P. (2001). *Imperial encounters: Religion and modernity in India and Britain*. Princeton: Princeton University Press.
Van der Veer, P. (2009). Spirituality in modern society. *Social Research: An International Quarterly, 76*(4), 1097–1120.
Voas, D., Crockett, A., & Olson, D. V. A. (2002). Religious pluralism and participation: Why previous research is wrong. *American Sociological Review, 67*(2), 202–230.
Warner, R. S., & Wittner, J. G. (1998). *Gatherings in diaspora: Religious communities and the new immigration*. Philadelphia: Temple University Press.
Warner, M., VanAntwerpen, J., & Calhoun, C. J. (2010). *Varieties of secularism in a secular age*. Cambridge, MA: Harvard University Press.
Wilson, B. R. (1985). Secularization: The inherited model. In P. E. Hammond (Ed.), *The sacred in a secular age* (pp. 9–20). Berkeley: University of California Press.
Wuthnow, R. (2012). *The God problem. Expressing faith and being reasonable*. Berkeley: University of California Press.
Yamane, D. (1997). Secularization on trial: In defense of a neosecularization paradigm. *Journal for the Scientific Study of Religion, 36*(1), 109–122.
Yang, F., & Ebaugh, H. R. (2001). Transformations in new immigrant religions and their global implications. *American Sociological Review, 66*, 269–288.
Yavuz, M. H., & Esposito, J. L. (2003). *Turkish Islam and the secular state: The Gèulen Movement*. Syracuse, NY: Syracuse University Press.

Chapter 4
Emergence, Development and Death: Norms in International Society

Colin Wight

Introduction

If we begin with the assumption that there is something called International Society (Bull 1977) then it should come as no surprise that that society operates under the influence of some norms. Indeed, the study of norms in International Relations (IR)[1] has become something of a cottage industry since the emergence of social constructivist theory (Kratochwil 1989; Onuf 1989; Wendt 1992, 1999). Prior to the emergence of constructivism, international relations typically turned to economics for its theoretical models (Waltz 1979). The incorporation of social theory, and the cultural turn in the Discipline, however, has now meant that sociological models of state interaction are themselves the norm (by which, for now I mean accepted standards of theoretical innovation).

However, even prior to the social turn, IR was already dealing with the concept of norms, although the effectiveness of how it did so was diminished due to the constraints of positivism, which had dominated the Discipline until the mid-1980s. Regime theory had already incorporated the idea of rules and norms as a central aspect of its definition of a regime. Regimes, according to Stephen D. Krasner are '[i]mplicit or explicit principles, norms, rules and decision-making procedures around which actors' expectations converge in a given area of international relations' (Krasner 1982: 185). In regime theory, norms are typically embedded within a

[1] I use the capitalised form to refer to the Discipline of International Relations, and the non-capitalised form to refer to the practices that the Discipline studies.

C. Wight (✉)
Department of Government and International Relations, The University of Sydney, Sydney, Australia
e-mail: colin.wight@sydney.edu.au

M.S. Archer (eds.), *Morphogenesis and the Crisis of Normativity*, Social Morphogenesis, DOI 10.1007/978-3-319-28439-2_4

framework indebted to rational choice theory, which means that they are effectively treated as intervening variables between self-interest and international political outcomes (King et al. 1994). Or, they were conceptualized as part of the context within which self-interest was framed. Rarely, however, were norm treated as casual factors in their own right.

With the emergence of constructivism in the late 1980s, however, more sociological approaches to norms were developed which attempted to demonstrate that norms were not merely intervening variables, but were causal mechanisms in their own right. Despite this theoretical development, much of the literature dealing with norms in IR remains confused about the status of them, about how they might be defined, about what role they play, about how they can function as explanatory variables, and about how their influence can be measured. Few doubt that norms play a significant role in structuring social practices, but methodologically, it is not clear how their impact can be assessed or demonstrated. We know norms affect behaviour, but isolating those effects is methodologically difficult, if not impossible (Mercer 2010; Sasley 2011). A particular problem in this respect is how to separate the influence of norms from that of self-interest.

In this chapter, I aim to outline the dominant approach to norms in IR, and on the basis of that analysis, demonstrate how morphogenesis (Archer 1995) can help illuminate how norms emerge, develop, change; and hence shape accepted modes of behaviour in the international political system. The chapter proceeds by first exploring the concept of norms. I argue that it is analytically important to differentiate norms from ideas, rules and laws. Second, I consider how the concept of a 'norm life cycle' is developed and used in IR. Third, I use this discussion to develop an account of norm emergence, development and death, consistent with morphogenesis. Essentially, my argument has two aspects. First, that the concept of a 'norm life cycle' is a useful way to consider how norms emerge, develop and die, but that it can be improved if placed within the context of morphogenesis. Second, that a fundamental aspect of late modernity, or the morphogenic society is the manner in which cultural and structural elaboration now operate in (almost) the same temporal dimension. Cultural elaboration has an almost instantaneous impact on structural elaboration and vice versa. What explains this is the compression of time and space, which is itself explained by the emergence of new modes of interaction, new technologies and the glimmers of an emergent global civil society. As a nascent, yet to be, society, however, its norms are highly dynamic, fragmented, malleable, constantly changing, and highly contested.

Defining Norms

There is substantial debate as to the definition of norms. Despite this, it is generally accepted that all societies have rules and norms that guide and affect social behaviour. These are often complex combinations of ethical, religious, and practical prescriptions. Some of these norms can be said to be functional in that they promote the preservation of society itself. Norms surrounding incest, for example, have been shown to have an important functional role in so far as they protect the genetic diversity of the population (Wolf and Durham 2005). Equally, norms limiting violent behaviour, and in particular murder, can be said to be functional in terms of the protection of the well-being of the society itself. These norms, and others like them, seem to be almost universal across all human societies and suggest that some norms have a biological or genetic origin rather than a cultural one (Brown 1991). In IR, it has been argued that the norms surrounding non-use of nuclear weapons has saved the human race from self-destruction (Rublee 2009; Tannenwald 2007). On the other hand, many norms seem to have no functional role and only specify accepted modes of behaviour within a given society.

Functional or not, few would disagree that an understanding of human behaviour requires a consideration of a society's norms. At the international level, where states and not individuals are typically viewed as the actors, and where anarchy is the organising principle, norms have been frequently ignored or marginalised as explanatory variables. Often those who explore the influence of norms on state behaviour are criticised as being naive or unrealistic. Edward Hallet Carr, for example, provided a damning critique of 'interwar idealism', arguing that the hope that new norms of conduct among states could lead to long term peace were the conditions of possibility for war (Carr 1946). Carr thought that any attempt to introduce new norms and institutions to govern state behaviour at the international level could only be reflective of great power interests.

Carr characterises this 'utopian idealism' as embodying a commitment to reason, confidence in the possibility of human progress, a sense of moral integrity, and, the belief that there exists an underlying harmony of interests. The inter-war idealists believed that war was an unnecessary and unwanted rupture in the course of ordinary human life. War could be prevented through the education of people so that they could come to recognise their harmony of interests and build international institutions able to promote norms of collective security such as the League of Nations (today the United Nations). These new norms, it was believed, would provide guides to behaviour no longer predicated on naked self-interest. According to the interwar idealists the 'harmony of interests' meant that global norms surrounding peace that all could agree with were possible; the only thing stopping their emergence was that the norms inherited from the past acted as a barrier to the development of new norms able to govern state behaviour. Carr challenged this moral universalism and its attendant commitment to an ill-defined 'harmony of interests'. He declared that "morality can only be relative, not universal" (Carr 1946: 19), and claimed that the dogma of the harmony of interests is invoked by privileged groups "to justify and maintain their dominant position" (Carr 1946: 75).

For Carr, state-leaders who refer to universal interests are, in fact, acting in their own interests (Carr 1946: 71). The harmony of interests, he argued, was a myth, and the world is characterised by the particular interests of different individuals and groups. In such a conflictual context, order can only be based on power, not morality. In fact, according to Carr, morality is the product of power (Carr 1946: 61).

Values and norms that idealists view as universal, such as peace, prosperity, social justice, and international order, serve to preserve the status quo. Moreover, the status quo powers regard the current arrangements as just and therefore preach peace to forestall attempts at revolution. "Just as the ruling class in a community prays for domestic peace, which guarantees its own security and predominance, ... so international peace becomes a special vested interest of predominant powers" (Carr 1946: 76).

This sceptical and pessimistic kind of thinking has been influential. Scholars and policymakers in the international realm stress the need for pragmatism (masquerading as realism[2]) when dealing with international relations. Moreover, the requirements of objectivity necessary for narrow accounts of science place an added premium on models that explain how states 'actually' behave rather than how they 'ought' to behave. In addition, the commitment to empiricism embedded in most positivist accounts of science makes the analysis of norms almost impossible given the difficulty of quantifying them and then discerning their influence (Goldstein and Keohane 1993: 8).

As such, IR has tended to privilege self-interest as the sole explanatory variable and this has led to many theories accepting the view that in an anarchic international environment the dominant logic is that of a Hobbesian war of all against all (Hobbes 1946). Yet, is international relations actually a form of social practice where the law of the jungle prevails? Clearly not, and international standards of behaviour exist, cooperation among states seems endemic, and peace is the norm rather than war. Moreover, even in war there are norms that govern behaviour and conduct.

Carr's sceptical realism, however, has to be placed in context. He was writing as the international system was beginning its descent into World War II. Since that time it is undeniable that some of the norms that govern interactions between states have fundamentally changed, and for the better. Decolonisation, human rights, the anti-apartheid movement, women's emancipation, the prohibition on first use of nuclear weapons, and increased sensitivity towards environmental catastrophe, are all areas that have witnessed significant normative change. Of course, many of these areas are still considered to represent the norms promoted by powerful states in pursuit of their self-interest. Humanitarian intervention, for example, is often criticized as a means through which powerful states continue to exert control over weaker states and interfere in their domestic affairs. Likewise, the promotion of democracy driven by norms surrounding political participation has been argued to be simply the means through which Empire is exercised today. There is something to these critiques, but the origin of a norm, or set of norms, cannot function as the sole critique of its value. Human rights may indeed be primarily a western discourse, but that does not lessen their value.

Although the role of norms in engendering and sustaining international cooperation has garnered much attention from IR scholars, the literature tends to confuse

---

[2]Realism here refers to political realism and bears no relationship to the philosophical realism that is embraced by morphogenesis.

them with ideas. The concept of 'ideas' is difficult to define; encompassing such diverse notions as world-views, cognitive paradigms, theories, norms, principled beliefs, policy programs, and frames (Campbell 2002: 21). Judith Goldstein and Robert Keohane argue that ideas may function as 'road maps,' 'focal points,' and/or 'glue' among actors making choices within groups (Goldstein and Keohane 1993: 13–25). Goldstein and Keohane also argue that ideas may become institutionalized, reflecting both the power of particular ideas and "the interests of the powerful" (Goldstein and Keohane 1993: 21) Likewise, Stephen Krasner argues that the origins of the nation-state system demonstrate that ideas, such as state sovereignty, are institutionalized because they serve the interests of the powerful (Krasner 1993). Krasner's approach illustrates that ideas and norms are not formulated or institutionalized in the absence of the power and interests of actors.

Although related, norms and ideas are distinct. Norms are a particular kind of idea. Norms are intersubjective and associated with appropriate action. They express expectations about certain behaviours. Norms 'simplify choices of actors with non-identical preferences facing each other in a world characterized by scarcity' and serve as justifications and models for ways in which specific tasks should be accomplished (Kratochwil 1989: 14). Norms also socialise state actors and are linked to actor identity in complex ways. The internalisation of norms can lead to the emergence of new identities. When this occurs, the norm no longer functions to simplify choices but becomes definitive of who we are; a 'good father', an 'honest person', a 'good international citizen' (Horner and Connor 2014). Norms are also fundamentally about power and control. This control is exercised in differing ways. Social norms can be formally enforced (sanctions) or informally (e.g., through body language and/or non-verbal communicative techniques). Norms create conformity. As social beings, individuals and groups learn appropriate behaviour through social interaction; when to say certain things; which words are appropriate in which contexts; whether to discuss certain topics at particular times; or, what to wear (when, why and how).

Norms are fundamental to foreign policy debates and constrain action by limiting the range of alternatives that elites are likely to perceive as acceptable and legitimate. Policy makers' values, norms, and principled beliefs may affect their position on policies by helping them decide which policies are the most appropriate – an important consideration when, as is commonly the case, there is no conclusive indication about which policy option is most likely to work best. When norms influence policy makers they do so by operating according to a logic of appropriateness, not a logic of consequences (March and Olsen 1989). In this sense norms often act as barriers to certain kinds of behaviour rather than producers of it.

However, the relationship between norms and policy outcomes is not easy to grasp. The most pressing issue is whether/how norms impact on political outcomes, and if so, under what conditions. Many approaches to norms assume a direct causal connection, but it is doubtful that norms can be treated in this way. In any policy discussion state-managers and other actors will generally have a range of possible outcomes that can be pursued. The role of norms in the decision-making process may be crucial but not decisive. In the immediate aftermath of 9/11, for example,

US politicians and CIA personnel not only ignored international laws relating to torture, but dismissed the norms relating to that practice as well (Wikipedia 2014). In complex decision-making situations, multiple norms may be in play, and epistemologically it is difficult to specify if the norm was directly causally implicated in the outcome.

In an influential paper, Martha Finnemore and Kathryn Sikkink define norms in a way that makes this link to identity explicit. According to Finnemore and Sikkink, norms are a 'standard of appropriate behaviour for actors with a given identity' (Finnemore and Sikkink 1998: 891). Whilst the relationship between identity and norms is important, it is not a necessary one, and it is not clear why identity should be included in the definition of norms. The imperative to follow a particular norm may, at times, be so strong that the following of the norm runs counter to one's identity. Indeed, if it is possible to conceive of norms as potentially leading to a change in identity, then tying norms and identity so firmly together in this way seems problematic. It would suggest that internalised norms are almost impossible to change without a concomitant change in identity. However, in many instances, behaviour that follows the norm is precisely that kind of behaviour that reaffirms the identity, and in this sense there is something to the notion of identity as being performative of the norm. On the other hand, it is also possible to conceive of someone following a norm that runs counter to their perceived self-identity.

Second, the linking of norms with behaviour betrays a latent empiricism. Norms involve an expectation of a particular kind of behaviour, but they are not themselves that behaviour. On a realist depth ontology, norms can be considered some of the micro mechanisms that govern social practices. Other writers argue that norms are non-causal. Thus, for example, Friedrich Kratochwil argues that 'norms and rules do not function like causes' (Kratochwil 1989: 98). It is clear that Kratochwil has embraced a Humean account of causation that privileges efficient causal determination rather than treating causes in the realist sense of tendencies. In addition, Kratochwil accepts the argument that reasons are not causes, whereas on a realist account of cause they are. If norms are not causal, in the sense of being productive of behaviour, or in the sense of blocking certain behaviours, it is hard to see what explanatory role they could play. Moreover, Kratochwil also treats norms, rules, and laws as one and the same thing. This is an error, and distinguishing between norms, rules, and laws seems essential if we are to understand the explanatory role that each plays in social practices.

There are two main reasons why it is important to differentiate between norms, rules and laws. First, ontologically, norms, rules and laws are different, and the influences and impact of each on social practices may vary. We need an analytical framework that can recognise and deal with these differences. Second, and perhaps more importantly, we need frameworks that allow the formulation of how norms become rules or laws. Here the context becomes important. The recent example of 'campus rape' illustrates the importance of this differentiated framework (MacDonald 2014). There are norms concerning sexual behaviour between men and women. Universities also have rules that govern that conduct, in relation to such interactions when both, or either, party is a registered student at a University.

However, there are also laws relating to sexual interactions among men and women, which if violated, can lead to potential prosecution and imprisonment. Student sexual interactions are subject to all three, but the implications of each differs and any explanation of 'campus rape' would have to take all three into account, and explore the relationship between them.[3]

What distinguishes norms from rules and laws is both the type of sanction that ensues if the norm, rule, or law is not followed and the degree to which each is formalised in an explicit sense. I treat norms as informal intersubjective structures of understanding that govern social practices. If a norm is not followed the sanction that is imposed is at the level of social opprobrium. Thus, for example, there is a norm in many social circles that if invited to attend a dinner one takes a bottle of wine, or some other gift (Mauss 1969). If the norm is not followed the sanction that may follow is that of failing to get a further invitation. A rule, on the other hand, is a formalised norm that if broken typically leads to a sanction that is not only social in form. The breaking of a rule usually leads to an institutional sanction. Thus, we have rules that govern student submission of essays in universities. If a student fails to follow the rule, the sanction may be a penalty imposed by the University. In this sense the sanction comes from the institutional or organisational body responsible for the rule, and not from the student cohort. In fact, there may be a norm that students on a particular course are always late with their essays and the rules relating to late submissions may not be enforced, which only serves to strengthen the norm. Finally, laws can be considered to be rules that have been formalised into a state structure. The sanctions that flow from the breaking of the law, if discovered, always involve state agents. Hence, to avoid confusion and maintain analytical clarity we should differentiate norms from both rules and laws.

According to Gary Goetz and Paul F Diehl, there are four central elements that should guide research into norms in international relations (Goertz and Diehl 1992). First, is that of regularity and consistency in terms of behaviour. If the same set of circumstances leads a state to act differently then, it could be reasonably questioned as to whether the behaviour is guided by norms. If norms are to play an explanatory role there must be some expectation of the kind of behavioural outcomes that can be expected if the norm is being followed. The identification of a norm should imply some element of predictive potential. Of course, in open systems where multiple mechanisms can play a causal role, this would not be deterministic, but tendential. Nonetheless, unless there is some expectation about observed behaviour

[3]This is an interesting example because, in many respects, the norms surrounding this issue have led to a situation where the rules are underpinned by a different standard of proof than that required by the law. Thus, for example, campus authorities in the USA have moved to a norm of 'more likely than not' when considering these claims, rather than the one adopted in criminal cases where the standard is 'beyond a reasonable doubt'. MacDonald N. (2014) Washington throws the book at 'campus rape culture'. *CBC News*. (accessed 20 December 2014). There is also no doubt that the weakness of the norms surrounding these interactions is playing a major role here. It is as if the men and the women involved in these interactions no longer know where the normative boundaries are.

then claims regarding norms would seem, as Wittgenstein might have put it, 'idling' (Wittgenstein 1972: Para. 132).

Second, we must be able to distinguish between norms and rationality. Rationality is about the efficient means of attaining a predetermined end; norms are typically concerned with the desirability of the means and goals themselves. Rational behaviour can appear to be similar to norm following behaviour depending on the situation. Norm like behaviour may also be driven by pure self-interest. A regularity in social practices can be norm influenced, or it may be dictated by self-interest. In addition, norms are often used as convenient justifications for self-interested behaviour. It should be possible to disentangle the two. In theory, one way to disentangle norms and self-interest would be to identify instances of norm governed behaviour that conflicts with perceived self-interest. If norms and self-interest are always coexistent then we have no way of knowing if the norms are explanatory or not.

The difficulty here is that a third central aspect of norms is their relationship to sanctions. Sanctions often follow when codes of behaviour governed by norms are violated. As Robert Axelrod has put it "A norm exists in the given social setting to the extent that individuals usually act in a certain way and are often punished when seen not to be acting in this way" (Axelrod 1986: 1097). This provides an additional problem when trying to differentiate behaviour governed by norms from that pursued for self-interest. It is always possible that the self-interested desire to avoid the sanction is what explains compliance with the norm.

The fourth aspect of norms that was largely overlooked prior to the emergence of Constructivism is the relationship between norms and the normative. Norms invoke issues of justice and rights in terms of moral or ethical character. This does not mean that all norms are subject to a positive moral evaluation. The norms surrounding empire and colonisation, for example, were clearly morally reprehensible, but they did specify how colonisers ought to behave towards the colonised. Racism provides another example and there are clearly norms governing how racists of any kind ought to behave to races they deem inferior. To say that norms are normative is not a positive comment on the behaviour they prescribe.

To these four aspects I suggest two further considerations. It is important to distinguish norms from institutions. In international relations, for example, it is common to find authors referring to sovereignty as a norm. Yet, sovereignty is best considered as an institution that is constituted by a complex array of norms, rules and laws. State sovereignty is often said to have only emerged post-Westphalia (1648), and although it is now codified in international law in the early years following the treaties of Westphalia it is clear that sovereignty would have been governed solely by norms relating to how state rulers interacted with one another. Today there are international laws that govern state sovereignty, and rules as well as norms. Finally, it is important to note that norms can be strong or weak; norms differ in terms of their intensity. Strong norms typically carry strong sanctions and provide few problems once identified. Weak norms, however, present an additional epistemological problem. If the norm is so weak that sometimes it is followed and sometimes it is not, then how do we know if it is exerting any influence on behaviour?

Norm Emergence, Development and Change in International Relations

A key aspect of Late Modernity is the extent to which morphogenetic mechanisms seem to overwhelm morphostatic ones. There is a widespread perception that the pace of social change is intensifying (Archer 2015). Even if quantitatively and qualitatively difficult to prove, this perception can be said to validate the idea of 'morphogenic' society; that is a society where people believe change is the norm. Norms can be considered both some of the mechanisms that produce this change, and also, mechanisms that themselves undergo change. In this respect, norms can be said to feature in all the phases of the morphogenetic cycles (T1, T2, T3 and T4). Typically, norms can be considered to be part of the cultural system. However, since the social and cultural spheres interact, we can follow Margaret Archer and examine the socio-cultural system as a totality (Archer 1995, 1996). Archer argues that the conjunction between cultural morphogenesis and structural morphogenesis is 'the prime configuration for the rapid shrinkage of the category of primary agents and their transformation into new, varied and more powerful promotive interest groups... in this social formation, compared with all others, more and more groups acquire the characteristics of corporate agency – namely organisation and articulation' (Archer 1995: 318). The contemporary global system seems to fit this description. What is the state but a powerful interest group? But also, many new social formations, interest groups and networks seem to have acquired the characteristics of corporate agency. In addition, new mechanisms of communicative exchange mean that the time-lag between the cultural elaboration and structural elaboration is now compressed.

This is not to say that cultural and social elaboration always take place within an identical timeframe. However, in the interconnected globalized and informationally rich world of late modernity the interaction between the two forms of elaboration is accelerated. Indeed, it may well be that one defining feature of the morphogenetic society is that the time between cultural elaboration and structural elaboration is decreasing. In terms of understanding how norms emerge, develop, and become embedded within social practices, it is important to realise that this process differs over historical time. Historically, at least when considered on a global level, the cultural and structural systems would undoubtedly have interacted at a slower pace in eras when time and space were not as truncated as they are under conditions of globalisation. Hence, the place, role and function of norms differs across different historical eras. In our contemporary world, cultural and structural elaboration may well be interacting in the same timeframe, or at least a very truncated one. This framework is particularly well-suited to generating a theoretical understanding of how new norms emerge and develop and become accepted modes of behaviour.

The dominant model within international relations of this process again comes from Finnemore and Sikkink (1998), and it is worth considering it in some detail before considering what a morphogenetic approach can add to this account. We will find that although there are some similarities, taking the morphogenetic approach seriously allows us to suggest some crucial amendments to this influential account. In particular, exploring this framework through the 'analytical dualism' of morphogenesis enables us to better understand how norms in the international system emerge, develop and die.

According to Finnemore and Sikkink norms have lifecycles (Finnemore and Sikkink 1998: 895): To understand how norms emerge, develop and die, requires that one must understand the lifecycle of the norm. Finnemore and Sikkink argue that this process has three distinct stages. First is 'norm emergence'. Norm emergence typically takes place through the influence of 'norm entrepreneurs'. Norm Entrepreneurs are important and influential individuals who use their influence to try and persuade, cajole and/or coerce a 'critical mass' of states and other actors to adopt the new norms. If enough of the target audience is convinced to adopt the new norm they then begin to try to persuade key stakeholders in the system to adopt the emerging norm. An example here might be Princess Diana who played an influential role in promoting norms relating to the comprehensive mine ban treaty signed in 1997 (Rutherford 2000). Other examples might be Martin Luther King, who challenged norms relating to race relations and civil rights, which had a direct impact on the anti-apartheid movement in South Africa. Likewise, Gandhi played a significant role in changing norms relating to colonization and not only in India. These examples all highlight how domestic actors can influence international practices, but the process goes both ways, and norms can diffuse at the international level and become accepted and adopted in domestic contexts.

Typically, norm entrepreneurs are agents who are dissatisfied with the prevailing social context, and who advocate different ideas about appropriate behaviour. In general, their views are taken seriously because they are positioned in organizational settings that give their ideas credence. In some respects, their positionality (Lawson 2016) gives them credence; they speak with some sense of authority. These norm entrepreneurs can be political leaders, religious leaders, media figures, scientists and so on. Russell Brand is an excellent example of a contemporary norm entrepreneur who is attempting to change the norms in relation to political interaction, finance, social welfare, and authority (Brand 2014). Norm entrepreneurs strive to convince other agents to modify their behaviour in accordance with the norm entrepreneur's ideas of what is appropriate behaviour. In effect, this means that in the first instance, the norm entrepreneur is attempting to highlight and modify other agents' perceptions of the prevailing social context. This is an important point. The norm entrepreneur is not merely trying to change behaviour – this could be achieved by force, for example – but to get actors reflexively to consider their conduct in the context of prevailing social circumstances, and to accept that other forms of behaviour are more appropriate. An emergent new norm has more chance of social success if actors become committed to the moral logic of the arguments that underpin the norm. If a sufficient mass of actors accept the new ideas as appropriate, then Finnemore and Sikkink claim that a norm has emerged (Finnemore and Sikkink 1998: 901). From a morphogenetic perspective, this could be viewed as the tipping point at which the positive feedback mechanism becomes irreversible (Archer 1995). When a sufficient number of agents accept the new ideas then a threshold, or tipping point, is crossed, and a norm cascade ensues. This is the second stage in the Finnimore and Sikkink 'norm life-cycle'.

During the cascade stage of the norm life cycle, social acceptance of the new practices rapidly increases; Finnemore and Sikkink refer to this as a contagion effect (Finnemore and Sikkink 1998: 902). New technologies provide powerful transmission mechanisms at this stage, which cross national, community, and social borders easily. Multiple agents, even those once outside of the 'critical mass' who initially promoted the norm, now begin to embrace the appropriateness of the behaviour, which is embedded in the new norm. Eventually, and if enough agents adopt the norm, this leads to the final stage, which Finnemore and Sikkink refer to as 'internalization'. In this phase, the norm is taken for granted, and compliance with the practices related to it is no longer, or rarely, questioned (Finnemore and Sikkink 1998: 904).

Three points need to be emphasized about this framework. First, although not explicitly defined as such, it is undoubtedly an evolutionary framework. A change in the practices of some agents modifies the environment, which drives other agents to adopt the new patterns of behaviour related to the norm. This change in other agents occurs as all endeavour to do well, by acting in appropriate manners as specified by the new norm. Second, the framework provides a mechanism that explains norm emergence; norm entrepreneurs supply the new ideas that will eventually become new norms. As ideas of a particular kind, norm transmission can only be explained through the notion of reflexive agency (Archer 1996, 2000, 2007, 2010, 2012). Finally, within this framework we can locate the possibility of norm change as well as emergence. Finnemore and Sikkink rightly insist that norm entrepreneurs can only propose norms within a social environment already characterized by existing sets of norms (Finnemore and Sikkink 1998: 897). Indeed, norm entrepreneurs are often only proposing a modification to pre-existing norms when they articulate new ideas, rather than new norms. At some point, however, established norms can be altered to such an extent that old patterns of behaviour disappear entirely. Thus the framework, although not explicitly aiming to do so, also incorporates the idea of norm death.

Fundamentally, this approach suggests that a logic of appropriateness, rather than one of consequences, guides actor behaviour. Actors choose which action is most appropriate based upon institutional, moral, or normative standards. In addition, preferences and interests are themselves shaped by what is considered appropriate, thus giving norms some independent casual power to shape outcomes. As March and Olsen argue, "Action is often based more on identifying the normatively appropriate behaviour than on calculating the return expected from alternative choices" (March and Olsen 1989: 22).

Norms demand a degree of intersubjective agreement to exist and survive. If agents no longer feel that the behaviour designated by the norm is appropriate, they will cease to act in manner consistent with the norm. If this happens the 'norm' no longer exerts any influence over agents' interests and thus no influence over agents' behaviours. In such instances, cultural elaboration has occurred, and agents now occupy different cultural contexts. In such cases, we can say that the norm has ceased to exist. Norms only exist insofar as actors follow them. Intersubjective agreement surrounding norms does not just materialize automatically; norms do not arrive fully articulated and formed. "Norms do not as a rule come into existence at a definite point in time, nor are they the result of a manageable number of identifiable acts. They are, rather, the resultant of complex patterns of behaviour of a large number of people over a protracted period of time" (Ullman-Margalit 1977: 8). When a group of agents accepts a new form of appropriate behaviour based on the norm, the resultant behavioural patterns transform the socio-cultural context for the other agents in the community thus, potentially at least, producing change in other agents, as they strive to adapt their practices to the new environment created by the new norm.

This can be described as positive feedback and it is, of course, a key aspect of the morphogenetic approach. The feedback mechanism is based on the principle of successful action in appropriate contexts. A "principle that what works well for a player is likely to be used again, whereas what turns out poorly is more likely to be discarded" (Axelrod 1997: 47). This evolutionary view is one where agents judge 'what works well' within the context of a logic of appropriateness and strive to match their behaviour with the dictates of a dynamic social structure. The socio-cultural system created and/or reproduced by actors' behaviours and interactions, influences the agent's perceptions of how they are supposed to behave. As such, agents are constantly adapting to an ever-changing environment that they have a hand in creating and/or reproducing, and their actions continuously reproduce or transform that same environment with new norms emerging, developing and dying in an evolutionary manner through their actions and interactions.

Finally, once established, norms elicit self-reinforcing behaviour and eventually can become institutionalized and taken for granted. As the practices of agents change to accommodate the dictates of the new, the norm gains strength and is accepted as the appropriate standard of behaviour in a particular context. Eventually, if reinforced, practiced and adopted by enough agents it will be no longer be necessary consciously to describe, defend, or decide upon the behaviour. As Finnemore and Sikkink argue, "norms may become so widely accepted that they are internalized by actors and achieve a 'taken-for-granted' quality that makes conformance with them almost automatic" (Finnemore and Sikkink 1998: 904). However, not all norms survive. If there is not a significant intersubjective consensus, the nascent norm will die out. The "life cycle" is effectively an account of the norm's pattern of influence. It is an account of how that influence changes over time and in what ways. What is important in this respect, is not only the "life cycle" itself, but the different mechanisms, motives, and actors, that determine how the norm functions at different points throughout the cycle. As Finnemore and Sikkink argue, "Change at each stage ... is characterized by different actors, motives, and mechanisms of influence. It is through these things that we gain an understanding of how norms function within the social environment" (Finnemore and Sikkink 1998: 895). Finnemore and Sikkink, summarise these actors, mechanisms and processes in Fig. 4.1.

	Stage 1 *Norm emergence*	*Stage 2* *Norm cascade*	*Stage 3* *Internalization*
Actors	Norm entrepreneurs with organizational platforms	States, international organizations, networks	Law, professions, bureaucracy
Motives	Altruism, empathy, ideational, commitment	Legitimacy, reputation, esteem	Conformity
Dominant mechanisms	Persuasion	Socialization, institutionalization, demonstration	Habit, institutionalization

Fig. 4.1 Explaining norm emergence, development and death in morphogenic society

Norm emergence, development and death, are dependent upon the social environment. Nuclear weapons and the nonproliferation regime are a good example of how the social environment can change norms and of how that same environment provides the conditions of possibility for norm change. In the early days of the development of the atomic bomb, Leo Szilard argued against their use, but no norm was established (Szilard et al. 1978). It was only after the dropping of the bombs on Hiroshima and Nagasaki that a new norm could gain traction. What had changed was the social context, and in particular, the material proof of the destructive power of the bomb.

The notion of human rights had also been raised centuries before it was finally adopted in the international system. In sixteenth century Spain, a group of thinkers knows as the School of Salamanca were confronted with the practical and theoretical problems raised by the European discovery of the Americas and the American peoples. Provoked both by the horrific accounts given by missionaries, and by the Roman Catholic Emperor Charles V who sought guidance about his rights and obligations in the New World, Francisco de Vitoria used the idea of "human nature" as the basis for a natural law common to all human beings. Natural law that allowed Vitoria to articulate fundamental human rights and, by reformulating a customary "law of nations" or "right of peoples", paved the way to modern norms relating to human rights and eventually international laws (Vitoria et al. 1991). However, again, human rights only became enshrined in international law after World War II and norms relating to them had a torturous developmental process despite having emerged centuries earlier. Context in this respect may not be all, but it determines the extent to which a system is receptive to a new norm. This points to an important set of insights that morphogenesis can bring to this issue.

First, in order to understand the influence of norms we need a theory of agency. Ideas, and norms are essentially ideas, but must have carriers (Blyth 1997). We need to consider how norms are transmitted through conversation, cooperation, behaviour and censure and then translated into different national contexts and back onto the international system. Norms are not agents, because they lack abilities to choose between the various courses of action (or to assess and learn from past experience), but they may have causal efficacy. Finnemore's concept of norm entrepreneurs focuses attention on a small set of heroic individuals and organisations who leverage ideational influence and persuade actors in the international system of the appropriateness of particular norms and ideas. Whilst norm entrepreneurs may be vital in promoting new norms, they do not elaborate the new norm ex-nihilo. At T1 norm entrepreneurs are already structurally located, and the new norms they propose are emergent from a set of prior socio-cultural conditions. In this sense, the emergence of new norms generally signals the death of older norms. This death may be slow and protracted, but as behaviour increasingly moves to embrace the new norm the old norm dies out.

Colonization, Empire, slavery and privacy all provide examples of this process. New norms regulating behaviour in relation to these institutions have all emerged, to the extent that some of these social institutions which previously enjoyed normative support have now died out; colonization for example. However, it is important to see how norms may also mutate rather than die. Slavery, for example, although no longer existing in prior forms, is undoubtedly still with us (Skinner 2008; Bales et al. 2009; Shilliam 2014). Slavery as a social institution has not disappeared, it is just that many of the norms surrounding it have changed. This demonstrates the importance of distinguishing between slavery as an institution and the norms that govern it. Slavery, as an institution continues, but the norms that govern it have changed. Again, social context becomes important here as norms relating to slavery have had to adapt to changing circumstances. Hence, it is no longer acceptable (the norm) forcibly to remove people from their families, transport and sell them across the globe, but it is, in particular communities acceptable (the norm) to traffic young women and treat them as sex slaves. Nor is this example confined to only certain parts of the globe and many men in the west frequenting brothels are aware of the issues relating to the trafficking of women but consider it 'normal' to ignore this information. These examples demonstrate how an understanding of norms in social practice can rarely, if ever, examine them in isolation from other norms.

Second, morphogenesis forces us to consider in greater detail how norms become accepted. The idea of norm acceptance and a norm cascade provide us with a limited answer to this process. Morphogenesis fills in the gaps here through its stress on reflexive agency (Archer 2000, 2003, 2007). Finnemore and Sikkink have no explanation for how the cascade happens; a norm is either adopted or it is not. Archer, on the other hand, provides a detailed account of how agents reflect on their situations. This helps explain how particular groups of people can come to accept certain norms. In particular, the concept of an 'internal conversation' (Archer 2003) provides a theoretical model that allows us to see how actors reflect on their practices and situations and arrive at new and innovative outcomes. The internal conversation enables us to see how the social conditions existing at T1 are reflected on at T2, and T3 and lead to new articulations at T4. The 'internal conversation' is needed to explain how norms are internalized. At every stage, agency and structures are required elements since agents do not conduct the internal conversation in a structural vacuum. In addition to such internal conversations, however, are conversations that span other actors in the social field. New norms do not just emerge and cascade; they are negotiated and sometimes changed in the process of adaptation. Norms mutate as well as die.

Third, morphogenesis can help explain how norms become internalised and globalised. As the negotiation of new norms develops, so cultural elaboration and structural elaboration begin to emerge. Time is intrinsic to morphogenesis, and although diagrammatically the phases of the morphogenetic cycles appear discrete, in reality, they are a dynamic flow. Both the internal conversations actors engage in, and the social conversations that follow from the consideration of new norms, change social circumstances in minute ways. This change may not be observable, but it may be influential. These changes provide new conditions of possibility for norm development. The Information Age offers new opportunities for such change, and new virtual spaces open up for conversations that cross borders and nation-state boundaries. Everywhere new norms are emerging, and not all of them are positive. New forms of communication both require new norms and facilitate the spread of norms, and it is not clear that a consensus is developing around them. In a sense, the new dynamic normative environment is less coherent, and leading to a more fragmented social existence.

Conclusion

Norms surrounding issues like slavery, race supremacy, child labour, empire, and colonization have clearly changed over time. But these institutions can still be considered normal in some places around the world. Not every state or international actor will agree on what the appropriate standards of behaviour are in this respect. The issue of human rights, for example, shows that international norms regulating this area are not always agreed upon by every state, and implemented, in the same way, at the domestic level. Moreover, even some of the people that reside in those states most committed to such norms feel differently about the status of them. In addition, in many African and Muslim countries norms surrounding female circumcision (or female genital mutilation) remain, whilst Western nations argue that this practice goes against humanitarian norms. But equally, the norms surrounding this practice confront norms relating to the respecting of differences, and norms relating to non-intervention in the affairs of others. Thus, even at the domestic level norm domains are contested spaces. So whilst there is reason to believe that something like a global culture is emerging there are clearly differences in norms at the international level.

However, over time norms may start to change or transform states' domestic capabilities and institutions, their interests/preferences, or their role, in the international system; thus producing the transformative capacity inherent in morphogenesis. Likewise, morphogenesis provides a better account of the temporal dimension of norm development, in particular, in relation to how agents can change cultural and social contexts and in terms of how those same cultural and social contexts can impact back on the practices of agents. No conflationary account can achieve this level of theoretical detail. Finally, cultural elaboration and structural elaboration may now be so tightly aligned that the temporal distinction between them may lack any meaningful influence in social outcomes. Changes in one may almost instantaneously impact on the other. This might be (part of) what we mean when we talk of the morphogenic society.

References

Archer, M. S. (1995). *Realist social theory: The morphogenetic approach*. Cambridge: Cambridge University Press.

Archer, M. S. (1996). *Culture and agency: The place of culture in social theory*. Cambridge: Cambridge University Press.

Archer, M. S. (2000). *Being human: The problem of agency*. Cambridge: Cambridge University Press.

Archer, M. S. (2003). *Structure, agency, and the internal conversation*. Cambridge: Cambridge University Press.

Archer, M. S. (2007). *Making our way through the world: Human reflexivity and social mobility*. Cambridge: Cambridge University Press.

Archer, M. S. (2010). *Conversations about reflexivity*. London: Routledge.

Archer, M. S. (2012). *The reflexive imperative in late modernity*. Cambridge: Cambridge University Press.

Archer, M. S. (2015). How social regulation becomes anormative with morphogenesis. In M. Archer (Ed.), *Morphogenesis and the crisis of normativity*. Dordrecht: Springer.

Axelrod, R. (1986). An evolutionary approach to norms. *American Political Science Review, 100*, 1095–1111.

Axelrod, R. (1997). *The complexity of cooperation: Agent-based models of competition and collaboration*. Princeton: Princeton University Press.

Bales, K., Trodd, Z., & Williamson, A. K. (2009). *Modern slavery: The secret world of 27 million people*. Richmond: Oneworld.

Blyth, M. (1997). Any more bright ideas? The ideational turn of comparative political economy. *Comparative Political Studies, 29*, 229–250.

Brand, R. (2014). *Revolution*. London: Random House.

Brown, D. E. (1991). *Human universals*. London: McGraw-Hill.

Bull, H. (1977). *The anarchical society: A study of order in world politics*. London: Macmillan.

Campbell, J. L. (2002). Ideas, politics, and public policy. *Annual Review of Sociology, 28*, 21–38.

Carr, E. H. (1946). *The twenty years' crisis, 1919–1939: An introduction to the study of international relations*. London: Macmillan Press.

Finnemore, M., & Sikkink, K. (1998). International norm dynamics and political change. *International Organization, 52*, 887–917.

Goertz, G., & Diehl, P. F. (1992). Toward a theory of international norms: Some conceptual and measurement issues. *The Journal of Conflict Resolution, 36*, 634–664.

Goldstein, J., & Keohane, R. O. (1993). *Ideas and foreign policy: Beliefs, institutions, and political change*. London: Cornell University Press.

Hobbes, T. (1946). *Leviathan: Or, the matter, forme and power of a commonwealth ecclesiasticall and civil*. Oxford: Blackwell.

Horner, D. M., & Connor, J. (2014). *The good international citizen: Australian peacekeeping in Asia, Africa and Europe, 1991–1993*. Cambridge: Cambridge University Press.

King, G., Keohane, R. O., & Verba, S. (1994). *Designing social inquiry: Scientific inference in qualitative research*. Princeton: Princeton University Press.

Krasner, S. D. (1982). Structural causes and regime consequences: Regimes as intervening variables. *International Organization, 36/2*(Spring). Reprinted in S. D. Krasner (Ed.), *International regimes*. Ithaca: Cornell University Press, 1983.

Krasner, S. D. (1993). Westphalia and all that. In J. Goldstein & R. O. Keohane (Eds.), *Ideas and foreign policy: Beliefs, institutions, and political change* (pp. 235–264). Ithaca: Cornell University Press.

Kratochwil, F. V. (1989). *Rules, norms and decisions: On the conditions of practical and legal reasoning in international relations and domestic affairs*. Cambridge: Cambridge University Press.

Lawson, T. (2016). Collective practices and norms. In M. S. Archer (Ed.), *Morphogenesis and the crisis of normativity*. Dordrecht: Springer.

MacDonald, N. (2014). Washington throws the book at 'campus rape culture'. *CBC News*. http://www.cbc.ca/news/world/washington-throws-thebook-at-campus-rape-culture-1.2680147. Accessed 20 Dec 2014.

March, J. G., & Olsen, J. P. (1989). *Rediscovering institutions: The organizational basis of politics*. New York: Free Press.

Mauss, M. (1969). *The gift: Forms and functions of exchange in Archaic Societies*. London: Cohen and West.

Mercer, J. (2010). Emotional beliefs. *International Organization, 64*, 1–31.

Onuf, N. G. (1989). *World of our making: Rules and rule in social theory and international relations*. Columbia: University of South Carolina Press.

Rublee, M. R. (2009). *Nonproliferation norms: Why states choose nuclear restraint*. London: University of Georgia Press.

Rutherford, K. R. (2000). Internet activism: NGOs and the mine ban treaty. *International Journal on Grey Literature, 1*, 99–106.

Sasley, B. E. (2011). Theorizing states' emotions. *International Studies Review, 13*, 452–476.

Shilliam, R. (2014). "Open the Gates Mek We Repatriate": Caribbean slavery, constructivism, and hermeneutic tensions. *International Theory, 6*, 349–372.

Skinner, E. B. (2008). *A crime so monstrous: Face-to-face with modern-day slavery*. New York: Free Press.

Szilard, L., Szilard, G. W., & Weart, S. R. (1978). *Leo Szilard: His version of the facts: Selected recollections and correspondence*. London: M.I.T. Press.

Tannenwald, N. (2007). *The nuclear taboo: The United States and the non-use of nuclear weapons since 1945*. Cambridge: Cambridge University Press.

Ullman-Margalit, E. (1977). *The emergence of norms*. London: Clarendon Press.

Vitoria, F. D., Pagden, A. R., & Lawrance, J. (1991). *Political writings*. Cambridge: Cambridge University Press.

Waltz, K. N. (1979). *Theory of international politics*. Reading: Addison-Wesley Pub. Co.

Wendt, A. (1992). Anarchy is what states make of it: The social construction of power politics. *International Organization, 46*, 391–425.

Wendt, A. (1999). *Social theory of international politics*. Cambridge: Cambridge University Press.

Wikipedia. (2014). http://en.wikipedia.org/wiki/Senate_Intelligence_Committee_report_on_CIA_torture.

Wittgenstein, L. (1972). *Philosophical investigations*. Oxford: Blackwell.

Wolf, A. P., & Durham, W. H. (2005). *Inbreeding, incest, and the incest taboo: The state of knowledge at the turn of the century*. Stanford: Stanford University Press.

Chapter 5
The Normative Texture of Morphogenic Society: Tensions, Challenges, and Strategies

Andrea M. Maccarini

Introduction: Social Norms and Social Morphogenesis

Any distinct civilization is constituted by the crystallization of a cultural program, comprising a social *imaginaire* and an ontological vision, and extending to a whole mode of interpretation of the world. This is combined with the development of compatible social structures including a distinct set of institutions (Eisenstadt 2003). As all these dimensions entail strong normative claims, it is not surprising that the quest to grasp the meaning of globalization for social normativity lies behind most contemporary efforts in the field of social theory. The hypothesis that a 'morphogenic society'[1] is possibly emerging – and its underpinning morphogenetic-relational approach[2] – provides a promising, original vantage point from which such an issue can be examined.

In this perspective, the fundamental research question examined in the present chapter concerns what norms and values are being destroyed, preserved, or generated anew in the emerging MS. What normative processes are at work in the context of the structural and cultural landscape of the new world? In other words, how 'unbound' is morphogenesis going to be from normativity itself, from its prompts and restraints?

More precisely, I would like to examine both the implications of intensified social morphogenesis for social normativity and, conversely, the role played by

[1]Hereafter MS.

[2]This formulation, which links a morphogenetic and relational approach, is my own responsibility. I tried to clarify its rationale in Maccarini (2013).

A.M. Maccarini (✉)
University of Padova, Padova, Italy
e-mail: andrea.maccarini@unipd.it

M.S. Archer (eds.), *Morphogenesis and the Crisis of Normativity*,
Social Morphogenesis, DOI 10.1007/978-3-319-28439-2_5

normativity in social morphogenesis. The former means how morphogenesis is affecting normativity, causing both its disruption (de-normativization, *anomie*) and its regeneration. The latter means that, depending on what normative processes and contents prevail, the MS will take on different forms and even diverging civilizational paths.

The idea that social change, indeed that transitions between different societal-historical formations, can be studied through the change in the prevailing kind of law and social norms represents a classical analytical strategy for social science. Besides Montesquieu's monumental work, Henry Sumner Maine famously described the passage 'from status to contract' (Maine 1972), and it is well-known that Émile Durkheim's theory of the division of labour in society was illustrated through the shift from penal to civil law as the prevailing form norms take in the societal context characterized, respectively, by mechanical versus organic solidarity. Leaving aside other possible examples, exploring the connection between the MS and social norms places our study within an important sociological tradition. Within this context, for all the virtues these classical works have, it seems hardly plausible to produce similarly sweeping generalizations to describe our contemporary 'world society' (Stichweh 2000). On the other hand, my *démarche* here will sidestep the meticulous analysis of single norms. An extremely long list of changing, rising or declining norms would immediately come to the fore, stretching from the idea of marriage and the couple to many other issues concerning technology, soft law, etc.[3] But I will not focus on any of them, and will instead try to pinpoint the main issues and trends.

This is clearly no easy task. In his famous work on social differentiation, Georg Simmel (1890: 6–11) noted that in sociological questions, as well as those in psychology and metaphysics, it is typical for opposite principles to display the same degree of plausibility. For example, it is possible to regard the world as ultimately unitary – every difference being nothing but a false appearance – but also to believe that every part of it is completely individualized, not even one tree's leaf being identical to another one – from which it would follow that any unification is nothing more than a subjective act of ours, the consequence of a psychological urge for unity, for which there is no real, objective justification. According to Simmel, the cause of this uncertain knowledge lies in the fact that the objects described are *in themselves* complex and ambivalent, comprising such a huge variety of single facts that any thesis or statement about them can find support, bearing sufficient psychological weight to obliterate our consciousness of opposite experiences and interpretations. This means that the number of elements, relations and mechanisms simultaneously present prevents any sweeping generalization. Therefore, the connections created and explored both conceptually and empirically are always somewhat unilateral, though not necessarily wrong.

This amazingly up-to-date insight into social ambivalence, even sounding close to a realist outlook, could be a fair description of the present situation. Global

[3] For a discussion of some relevant changes see Archer (2014: 10–11). See also Porpora's Chap. 2 in the present volume.

society simultaneously feeds opposite phenomena. To quote only a few instances: the decreasing relevance of distance involves trust and cooperation, but also more confrontational attitudes between communities; therefore, we experience more unity *and* more fragmentation. There are more moral scandals, but also there is more moral indifference.[4] A growing sensitivity for human rights co-exists with war and violence to a degree unmatched since the two world wars. We have de-normativization and new norms, de-regulation and a growing bureaucratic threat. We experience the Internet as a locus of ideational diffusion as well as the arena of unprecedented cyber-wars.[5]

To sum up, it is impossible to indicate one single, unifying trend. What I try to do instead is to identify and outline what I regard as the main *foci* of normative tension, the essential *challenges*, and a few *strategies* that appear to be central in the symbolic and institutional arenas of contemporary society. These strategies describe ways in which protagonists of normative systems try to cope with intensified morphogenesis, avoiding sheer collapse and a resulting state of *anomie*. This involves the notion that a characteristic *type of norms* is currently emerging. The latter point may be further elaborated through a distinction between:

(a) the *cultural content* of norms – the worldviews expressed through them and the way they mould social relations;
(b) the very *nature of normativity* – namely, the type of obligation involved;
(c) the *normogenetic processes*, i.e. the ways in which norms emerge, are institutionalized and enforced.

Attention is focused on all these dimensions. The following analysis must provide an interpretation of some current phenomena, establishing their meaningful connection with the overarching situational logic and/or some specific mechanisms characterizing the situation of intensified and (relatively) freewheeling morphogenesis.

As hinted above, in this chapter I set out to examine norms that are being *destroyed, preserved or generated afresh*. More precisely, I try to answer a crucial question, namely whether *new* normative processes are emerging that constitute the

[4]See Alexander (2012) and Porpora et al. (2013) for interesting arguments and examples on each side of this distinction in the political domain. Another impressive example concerns pedophilia – one of the last moral taboos in the secular West that is currently becoming a contested phenomenon. Here we witness a growing quest for transparency and media driven scandals, expressing a more refined moral sensitivity, paralleled by a tendency to downgrade such an inclination from 'illness' to 'disorder', and finally to mere 'orientation' – which clearly involves a consistent march towards its moral (and in the end, legal) neutralization. This evolution is apparent in the political activity of the related protest groups, and can be traced through the various editions of the Diagnostic and Statistical Manual of Mental Disorder, issued by the American Psychiatric Association. For the most recent edition see American Psychiatric Association (2013).

[5]The argument for diffusion has been effectively presented by Archer (2015). As regards cyber-wars, the recent actions of the hacker group called the 'Guardians of Peace' (*sic!*), which threatened Sony Inc. into cancelling the movie 'The Interview', is a good case in point, with a still unknown plot that possibly involves State and non-State actors and groups.

MS's own *endogenous* forms of stabilization. This wording raises a further issue. Following Archer (2014), we must distinguish stability from stabilization. In a nutshell, it must be emphasized that stability does not always depend on morphostasis (*Ibidem*, 7–8). Stability may result from morphostasis, thereby depending on 'the continuing defence of pre-established *vested* interests' (*Ibidem*, 8). But it can also be the outcome of brand new forms of stabilization, of new norms and institutions, responding to and supported by newly emerging *objective* interests.[6] My principal aim is to gain some purchase on these emergent forms and processes, not to figure out the ways old normative arrangements may endure the chill of global winds.

One last point needs clarification. I accept Archer's statement, according to which the *sources* of such stabilization are to be found in the notion of *concerns*, and among those subjects she calls the meta-reflexives.[7] To this she adds the concept of *relational goods*.[8] We might sum up her argument as follows:

(i) the endogenous process of stabilization typical of a MS is characterized by the emergence of relational goods;
(ii) the process begins from a cultural change of values grounded in contingent complementarities...
(iii) ... and prompted by the concerns endorsed by meta-reflexive subjects;
(iv) thus, stabilization results from the manifest benefits generated by relational initiatives that produce added social value in terms of trust, cooperation, reciprocity.

With this said, I think it is necessary to add that values change among 'active minorities' first, and spread through the success of their experiments. This calls into question the category of *experience* and that of *culture*. The latter is important, because its *contents* are relevant. Someone can be a meta-reflexive, but the cultural contents involved in his/her concerns may be totally different from those that may produce relational goods – e.g. extreme individualism. Such are many subjects who currently spearhead protest movements and qualify as 'normative entrepreneurs', i.e. the generators of new social norms. The former comes into the picture as a relevant criterion through which experiences must be judged in the absence of stable, pre-defined and already stabilized principles. Of course, experience and culture are mutually related, because experiences are not self-interpretative, but must be articulated within a multidimensional symbolic space of values, practices, and institutions. Through such dynamics experiments and innovations may eventually result in stabilized norms, insofar as they are perceived as 'beneficial' by some particular subjects on some given grounds.

[6] Among other things, this means stability is not necessarily the offspring of 'defensive' struggles.

[7] See again Archer (2014: 3–14 ff). A full illustration of the above concepts obviously needs more extensive reading. See above all Archer (2000, 2003).

[8] As regards this concept, Archer refers to Pierpaolo Donati's work. See for example Donati and Solci (2011).

Having clarified my approach to the issue, in the next section "Normative tensions in morphogenic society: foci, challenges and strategies" I will outline what I consider to be the main challenges and the related responses, characterizing the relationship between the MS and the normative sphere. In the section on "Morphogenic society, morphological rights: the logic of opportunity and its ontological (dis)contents", the argument will focus upon the specific problems concerning personal ontology, which are bound to be of crucial importance to the whole normative and symbolic landscape of the emerging MS.

Normative Tensions in Morphogenic Society: Foci, Challenges and Strategies

Foci and Challenges

What is the major influence of the MS on social normativity? What we know is that the new societal conditions make both the normative *control* of behaviour and the *justification* of social norms more and more challenging and extremely hard to effect. It is increasingly difficult to set effective constraints on global actors and their unchained powers, while it is also hard to establish a shared legitimation of values and norms, given the crisis of all subjects, rationales, and institutional settings which used to provide a foundational background throughout modernity. Broadly speaking, this depends on four factors, namely (i) the multiplying opportunities for action and experience, (ii) the spread of contextual incongruity, (iii) the globalization processes, with their related forms of differentiation of society, and (iv) the increasing cultural fragmentation of global society, which involves the decline of most symbolic resources that would allow their mutual translation among various discourses and communities.[9] These very general problems are well known. But what we see here is only crisis and de-normativization. Is this all there is to say about the transformation of social normativity under the pressure of such conditioning factors?

First, there are a few major *foci* of normative tension in the MS, involving structural and cultural strains between conflicting innovations – some of which later find their respective 'chains of compatibility' making them mutually supportive – as well as being the case for agential struggles. They could be summarized as follows:

[9]The increasingly confrontational attitude of non-Western civilizations and movements against the basic premises of Western modernity is a good illustration of this point. Secularization should also come into the picture as a relevant component. The full consideration of all these issues is obviously far beyond the scope of this essay. Points (i) and (ii) are aptly examined by Archer (2012, 2014, 2015), and constitute the core of what is meant by a 'reflexive' and 'morphogenic' turn of society.

(i) material goods, needs, and spaces. This involves the availability of food, water, natural resources, a healthy environment, work, land, and the related Commons for large parts of the world population;
(ii) knowledge, (social and personal) memory and oblivion, related to the new conditions prompted by the digital revolution and its possible consequences;
(iii) human ontology and a new anthropology evoked by machines, hybrids, the manipulation of human biology, etc.

Most constructive (innovative) as well as conflictual processes in the MS revolve around these areas, whose normative relevance is evident. As hinted above, in each of these domains global society is facing both a problem of control and one of justification.

My thesis is that specific normative dilemmas arise concerning those problem areas, and their complex relationships. Two of them are upfront in my argument, because I believe they are redefining all other issues. They also represent instructive fields in which to discuss problems of control and justification, and to test the emerging solutions. The former is a problem of ontology, the latter has to do with universalism. They are also mutually related, as can be clearly seen in the problem of generating normative universals in the domain of human dignity. It is possible to draw two distinctions to describe the perimeter of the coming scenario:

(a) as regards ontology, the problem is what personal and social ontology is embedded in the emerging social norms of a MS. It makes a huge difference if the prevailing culture will be centred on the notion of human *indisposability*, instead of individual self-determination remaining the (only) guiding value of late modern society;
(b) as to universalism, in the twilight of the nation-state and of 'vertical' sources of justification, a significant divide is separating different types of processes intended to generate 'universality'. One finds expression in the attempts to reconstruct some normatively thick rules and definitions of social objects within 'networks of communities', while others lean heavily on technical standard setting, with the explicit aim of social engineering. The main differences between the two lie in the participation of the subjects involved and in the openness of dialogue to multiple rationalities[10] (or not).

Throughout this chapter, I have been guided by a unifying insight: that the need for normative regulation increasingly emerges *on the boundaries* between the functionally differentiated subsystems of global society, and their human and natural environment, as well as between the ontological layers that constitute the very stuff of social and personal reality.[11] The logic underlying such normativity, and the

[10]Throughout the present chapter, this term (or its equivalent, 'form of rationality') refers to the different forms of argument, derived from different cognitive as well as normative presuppositions that social actors exhibit in connection with their diverse interests and identities.

[11]As regards the boundaries between functional systems and their environments as important sources of new global normativity, I share this insight with Riccardo Prandini (2012: 64). My own

relevant *kind* of obligation and relationality involved, qualifies the developmental path we can expect the MS to follow.

One last remark must deal with social differentiation. Its prevailing form is going to have a profound influence upon the way these normative tensions and challenges are faced. In global society, social relations and communications, institutional arenas, and cultural domains are developing beyond national borders, which are becoming less and less meaningful. This is usually taken to mean that *functional* differentiation is now the primary form of differentiation.[12] However, such a post-national constellation (Habermas 2001) can hardly be reduced to the functional principle of differentiation. Social and political movements, lifestyle communities, criminal organizations, continually cross national boundaries, and transnational diasporas assume increasing importance (Ben-Rafael 2003). What they all have in common is that they perform actions, enter relations, and express allegiances that cut across societies *and functional systems* throughout the world, tending to become the primary obligation in cases of conflicting loyalties (*obligatio ligia*). This prevents them from being downplayed as forms of *segmentary* differentiation *within* the primary functional principle.[13] In that sense, one could speak of a social differentiation along cultural, ethnic or religious lines. Finally, there are forms of differentiation that are still coupled with a territorial principle, but exceed the level of nation-states. This does not mean that states disappear, or that they cease to condition the lives of their populations. It means that most relevant processes and decisions come to depend on a *civilizational* dimension, referring to geo-cultural, geo-political, and geo-economic areas, which transcend national borders, characterized by a relatively common cultural program and common institutional arenas, with their typical features and tensions.[14]

Such a plurality is itself an expression of the MS in its capacity to produce 'variety', in the form of social entities organized around different selective principles and endowed with specific forms of inner rationality. The normative tensions which characterize world society are largely an expression of this plurality. Therefore, the normative texture of the coming MS will be an emergent effect of such a complex game.

---

version of it has a wider scope, including (i) the ontological dimension, (ii) the emphasis on the type of obligation, and (iii) the complex nature of the differentiation of global society (see below).

[12] I don't even try to provide references for the concept of functional differentiation. Its clearest and most systematic statement to me remains that offered by Niklas Luhmann (1997).

[13] As in the case of nation-states surviving within the functionally differentiated system of politics. For this interpretation see Luhmann (1997: 806–812).

[14] This point brings up a complex issue, which I cannot follow up here. A different way to put it would be that nation-states only display sufficient vitality when they assume the *dimension* of sub-continental units – such as the USA or China – while their 'classical' modern format becomes hopelessly inadequate – as is the case with old European states.

Normative strategy	Guiding value	Guiding emotion(s)
a) autoimmune syndrome	individual self-determination	individual desire
b) social closure (enclaves and vortexes)	identity, controllability	fear, nostalgy, indignation ('purity and danger')
c) networking for foundations	'safe and righteous innovation', shared rationality and common goods	Desire to share experiences and (relational) goods

Fig. 5.1 Normative strategies in the morphogenic society

Strategies

The challenges I have just mentioned are met by different strategies, through which law and social norms, as it were, adapt and react to the relevant dilemmas. Three of them are particularly important (Fig. 5.1).

All these strategies describe ways, as it were, in which normative systems try to cope with intensified morphogenesis, avoiding sheer collapse and a resulting state of *anomie*. They entail the orientation to a guiding value, but also a 'guiding emotion'. Such a formula may raise some eyebrows in many sociological quarters. I use it here to mean the basic *intuitions*, close to experience and still not (fully) articulated on a rational level, through which normative (e.g. moral) feelings find a first expression. As commentaries on experience, they initiate the process of emergence of concerns (Archer 2000: ch. 6). Insofar as they are socially shared, they may become a powerful drive for normative claims to develop and for new norms to emerge.

Let us now examine the various strategies indicated in Fig. 5.1. Strategy (a) indicates those processes through which law reacts to disruptions in a self-destructive manner[15] – its guiding value being individual self-determination, desire (the satisfaction of personal preferences) being its guiding emotion. This explains its self-problematizing nature, because both elements make it particularly hard to set limits to behavioural variety. Coping strategies come in two shapes:

(i) Laws which temporarily legalize illegal behaviour. As such, these remain generally illegal (and may even be regarded as immoral), but are not negatively sanctioned for a given period of time or for a particular category of subjects,

[15]The application of the term 'self-immune syndrome' to the dynamics of the legal system – in the way I use it here – must be traced back again to Riccardo Prandini (2012). The meaning he attributes to the formula is here summarized at point (i) below. I extend its meaning to point (ii).

or under other special conditions. Frequent laws that condone abuses – e.g. regarding fiscal or construction law – are a good case in point, producing the breakdown of normative expectations as a collateral effect. The autoimmune aspect comes into full light when one considers that the strategy in question is often employed (*and legitimated*) as a 'necessary' or even 'rational' way to escape the impossibility of control.[16] Here the two broad dimensions of the normative crisis – control and justification – interact closely. Because the impossibility of control is a paradoxical form of justification for a norm, the effect on justification is devastating.

(ii) Technical regulative standards, which set prerequisites for individual or collective entities (e.g. nation-states, functional systems, etc.) to respect, where the autoimmune effect is generated through a different mechanism. The point is that such regulations often lack any apparent normative content that may possibly be traced back to any principled premise or assumption. Further, their importance for a given collectivity may also be less than clear in terms of utility.[17] Sometimes they even prevent the pursuit of some legitimate good – as it happens in the case of many bureaucratic constraints on action. Therefore, their content is often perceived as either arbitrary or hiding the sheer power and the interest of the stronger party. If this is the case, such standards induce a cost benefit calculation on the part of the subjects, and their normative nature is denied. These days, the EU fiscal compact and the norms concerning the GDP/debt ratio risk are regarded as an example of this strategy. As is apparent, this represents a significant factor in the legitimation crisis of the whole European project.

It is still relevant to note that form (ii) indicates, and in turn fosters, a lack of trust among the members of a network or of a collectivity. More generally speaking, this strategy develops as a fully heteronomous form of legislation, which is connected with the spiraling dynamics of 'freedom vs. control', as the result of its radicalization.[18] My point here is that such a strategy itself becomes just one option in the MS, where it is paralleled by other, emergent developmental paths.

Strategy (b) in Fig. 5.1 has to do with social closure, thereby involving those social enclaves and vortexes I discussed in a previous chapter (Maccarini 2015). It represents the attempt to outface the dynamics of growing morphogenesis by creating enclosures where strong normative premises may still be shared. Once again, the driving force may be the urge to fly from complexity and openness. The flipside would be the capacity to reconstruct social distance and to simplify

[16]The ineffectiveness of control is often used to justify legislative change, even in the 'hard cases' of morally contested issues such as abortion, euthanasia, etc. Appeal to this 'principle' is quite common, e.g. when it is deemed 'irrational' or even 'unfair' to forbid behaviour that is allowed elsewhere.

[17]Without this clarification, traffic lights would fall into this category – which would be absurd.

[18]I cannot follow this line of thought in its far-reaching implications. The very crisis of late modern society has been read as an outcome of such a problem. For this thesis see Donati (1997).

social dynamics. The prevailing emotion, however, may also be indignation, and the scandal produced by compulsory contact with different lifestyles. In Western societies, the integration problems concerning some immigrant communities are a case in point. Both the closure against them and their own self-closure within their 'bonding social capital' are examples of the same strategy.

Finally, strategy (c) is driven by the 'wish to share', coupled with the idea that a new 'common world' and some contextual congruity must be reconstructed from the bottom up, through networks connecting various communities. This is the only strategy that still posits the possibility of a normatively meaningful (i.e., not neutral) universalism, although this can only result from a networking process, not from a 'vertical' or hierarchical form of rationality or politics.

It should be noted at this point that empirically observable cases may at times be rather ambivalent as to whether they belong to one or the other strategy, and such an ambivalence often reveals profound social contradictions. A good example is the Italian law n. 67, 04/28/2014, which establishes a particular type of 'probation' for adult people. I will use this case to illustrate the ambivalence often occurring on this level. On the one hand, the law treads an innovative path in criminal legal reasoning, in that it institutionalizes alternative forms of punishment that do not involve serving any time in jail. Further, the social control of the convicted seems to be entrusted to a 'civil' network including the court, social work offices,[19] third sector associations, and possibly the family of the convicted and the victim him/herself. The ideal would seem to involve reconstructing trust and reciprocity. It also entails the need for different subjects to converge on a common definition of a situation and to organize common action, which involves mutual understanding between different rationalities and a delicate balance between the material and ideal interests of all the stakeholders. If the whole enterprise is conducted effectively, it could be an illustration of strategy (c), generating the common goods: 'security', 'social control', and 'rehabilitation of the guilty' for a given local community through an intense networking process. The organizational routines, as well as the professional *habitus* and established practices of lawyers, judges, social workers, third sector leaders, etc. are clearly challenged by a *reflexive imperative*, imposed by the new empirical and normative conditions.

On the other hand, many features of the law reveal its 'deflationary' aim (Bartoli 2014; Marandola 2014). The law was solicited by a recent ruling of the European Court of Human Rights (2013), which found Italy guilty of overcrowded jails, and came as a further attempt to decrease the number of inmates, without looking like one more 'pardon' that would cancel any punishment for the sake of reducing overcrowding. If such an instrumental goal prevails, then the novelty of the norm might boil down to a cosmetic change, paying lip service to the principles outlined above while really reducing the new complex process to a few bureaucratic rules which would allow it to meet the maximum number of inmates recommended by

[19]More precisely, the UEPE (office for external implementation of criminal law). I thank Cristina Selmi, Ph.D., for discussing this case with me and providing useful first-hand information.

the Court and by international legal standards. The results of implementation will be crucial to disambiguate the issue. In the last instance, this new institute will prove 'successful' or not – regardless of the standards met – depending on the experience of personal and social security-and-justice it will be able to foster. If people feel and their everyday social environments are experienced as being 'safer' (or not); if the various stakeholders involved perceive the relevant process as producing a 'fair' outcome, this will influence the experiment of the new norm, determining its success or failure. The experience of judges, lawyers, social workers, convicts, victims, police forces, and wider 'public opinion' will all be important in this respect. Such a shared experience is of course not a foregone conclusion, in that it always raises issues – in this and in other cases – both in terms of universalistic processes and of the content of norms.

Each of the three strategies I have rather cursorily illustrated has its own way of facing the ontological and the universalistic challenge. The former must now be further examined, as it can highlight one very important way in which these developments may come to qualify the MS as more or less, and differently, 'bound' or 'unbound'.

Morphogenic Society, Morphological Rights: The Logic of Opportunity and Its Ontological (Dis)contents

The Ontological Challenge in a Society Without an Exterior

Personal and social ontology were an essential element of modern society. On the personal level, an idea of *agency* is still pivotal in most social processes and in all functional subsystems of global society. On the social level, the very stuff of the 'body politic' and its articulation has been a central theme of the scholarly debate and – more concretely – of institutional creativity. Both levels are currently under pressure from intensified morphogenesis, whose impact is probing deeper and deeper into the most basic premises of our once 'modern' historical formation. As a consequence, it is not surprising that social and legal norms concerning the ontological dimension are spearheading the present changes. Arguably, they represent a key distinguishing factor between what may be called 'bound' and 'unbound' morphogenesis – and the related future of our society.

My thesis is twofold. First, I argue that the decisive point for the culture of global society is whether it is human indisposability[20] or individual self-determination

[20]Simply put, the idea of indisposability implies the normative request to treat the natural constitution of human beings as indisposable (unavailable), and is directed against the attitude of having it at one's disposal, as it happens in cases where parts of the human body could be patented and become available for industrial production or commercial exchange. There is obviously an extended literature on this subject. See at least Lohmann (2014: 167 ss.). See also Joas (2008: 125–132, 2013).

that constitutes the guiding value. The problem, of course, is not simply to assert either principle, but to articulate its justification in such a way that is culturally adequate and compatible with the structure and dynamics of the MS. Second, I hold that the crucial difference between these two cultural contestants is the way in which the relations between the ontological layers comprising the human being are conceived of and protected by law *and* by socially shared norms. The situational logic of opportunity can be instantiated in different ways. The difference, which qualifies a civilizational turning point, lies in the way the relationships in question are interpreted, distorted or denied, both conceptually – within the Cultural System – and practically, in Socio-Cultural interactions.

In this section, I focus upon certain normative phenomena regarding the ontological status of the human person. In terms of the dimensions of normativity listed above in my section "Introduction: social norms and social morphogenesis", the argument here revolves mainly around the content of norms. Before getting to the core argument, let us quickly outline its overarching context. Global society seems to place a strong emphasis on the idea of the 'human'. This means that the notion is increasingly appealed to, in frequent attempts to articulate fears that deep social change undermines the conditions for the existence of society – among which figures humanity itself.[21] Thus, the symbol of the human (and his/her *dignity*) expresses what risks being destroyed, while simultaneously evoking a possible barrier against destruction. 'Humanity' is meant to stop contingency, reducing the arbitrariness of actions, experiences, decisions, and socially possible connections.[22] This appeal to 'the human' is based on the premise that something may be saved from the whirlpool of social change, and 'remain fixed'. However, in a highly morphogenetic context the idea that something may resist contingency, including the human being in his/her very nature, becomes increasingly unlikely.

This situation can be described as that of a society *without exterior*. In a nutshell, the notion in question indicates a social formation which loses all references external to its own dynamics. Granted, the notion of a 'world without exterior' (*Welt ohne Extern*) appears in Luhmann (1996), addressing both the self-referential closure of social systems and the transformation of social, political, and cosmological concepts in modern philosophy. I, however, use it as a complex concept with multiple meanings, which include both the material and the symbolic domain. It refers to the lack of projection, of a space to roam, in which one may throw something, anchor something, experiment, erase or forget something, from which something may be received, in which one may mirror or transcend oneself. As it applies to society and its culture, one consequence is that providing permanent definitions of objects becomes a hard task. The way people live and 'change their lives' (Sloterdijk 2013) is also affected. It is important to note that I do not use 'loss of external references' as just another way to define the MS, or as a property that *necessarily* comes with it. On the contrary, it is meant to indicate a structural and cultural feature of contemporary

[21]Fuchs and Göbel (1994: 8). See also Donati (2009).

[22]Fuchs and Göbel (1994: 9, 14).

society that happens to *intersect* with its current morphogenic 'long cycle'. And such an interaction has a conditioning effect on the way social norms will construe personal ontology.

In this context, norms are directly involved. The emphasis on humanity is paralleled by growing attention and concern for human *rights*. This connection even promises to become the bearer of deep transformations in our legal systems. Starting with those mobilizations following the end of the cold war, and with the democratization processes in various regions of world society – from Eastern Europe to Latin America – new times and spaces opened up for law, which may prompt a revolution: "If the 'revolution of equality' was the hallmark of modernity, the 'revolution of dignity' signals a new time, as the offspring of the tragic 1900s, and opens the age of the relationship between the person, science and technology".[23] The path that once led from *homo hierarchicus* to *homo aequalis* would now extend to generate *homo dignus*, characterized by the emergence of new rights connected with a new anthropology.

All this entails a tremendous set of problems. If it is to be taken for granted that all 'external' references to reason, nature, and religion are gone, and cannot limit or constrain contingency, then how are intangible and indispensable norms to be produced? Given the present 'clash of civilizations' *within* the West, what could still serve as a foundation for human rights? The contours of the constitutionalization of the person (Rodotà 2012), that should contrast with the dehumanization of society, become ever more uncertain. What is its relationship with the transformations of the human that are prompted by science and technology? Will it still be possible to produce a shared culture of human rights and dignity within global society? What 'sources of the self' are still available to do this job?

Towards Morphological Freedom

The idea and value of human rights and dignity can be usefully conceived of as a process of *sacralization*, whose specific object is the human *person* (Joas 2013). The latter is not the only conceivable 'sacred object'. In fact, other concurrent, indeed rival processes of sacralization have been going on throughout modernity, centred on race, nation, socio-economic class, and more. Such processes are a way for societies to define their own identity. One implication of this is the misleading view that 'sacredness' only characterizes pre-modern societies and should be abandoned. What we deal with is rather a difference in objects and cultural contents.[24]

[23]Rodotà (2012: 184) (my translation).

[24]An impressive (irritating) demonstration of this came some time ago from one of the most distinguished representatives of Islamist terrorism. His fierce accusation to the West was *not* that it has de-sacralized everything. He did not go with the Weberian *motif* of disenchantment, which would supposedly scandalize a 'fundamentalist' person. On the contrary, his point was that Western societies were sanctifying *different* – and allegedly *wrong* – things and causes. The mistake

Now, the emergence and the relative 'success story' of human rights would seem to indicate that the sacralization *of the person* prevailed over other rival themes, at least in the European and Western society and in international institutions. The core of law comes to deal with the very root of humanity. But this is exactly the point. Given the intense multiplication of opportunities for action and experience, and the loss of external symbolic references, where is this root, how is the 'person' understood, and how is his/her value asserted and justified? On these issues, we must deal with sheer lack of consensus within the West – let alone between the West and 'the rest'. In fact, the contestation is getting to fundamentals. With the rising technical opportunity for humans to become neuro-bio-info-nano entities, the sharp alternative between being either human or 'anything else' (e.g. machines) will soon be unable to grasp the complexity of our coming ontology.

Law, and social norms in general, are caught in a potentially contradictory 'double mission', namely to safeguard the deep ontology of the human species and to foster, or at least not hinder the emergence of new, 'post-human' anthropologies.[25] Here two normative cultures part company, their guiding values leading social normativity in diverging directions. A culture of indisposability involves two principal tenets. First, the idea that every human being has an *untouchable* core,[26] which was not self-produced and does not depend on one's performance and capabilities. Therefore, such an 'inner core' cannot be lost or destroyed, and ultimately i*s not at one's disposal*. The second tenet entails the belief that human existence is no *mere fact*. The fact that human beings *are actually there* is not just a random event, but happens within a set of relationships with various layers of reality that gives it meaning and value. Such a relational bundle also generates obligations. The two aspects converge on the idea that human dignity means first and foremost the indisposability of the human. Now, it is certainly possible to leave foundational matters in the background, and admit that the above tenets may be supported by different conceptual tools. However, at the end of the day, the problem remains as to whether the symbolic resources to produce such a culture are still with us or not, and how indisposability could become a valid and motivating force, in the characteristic conditions of an emerging MS.

---

would be one of 'misplaced sacredness'. This, in his opinion, is the big divide between the two civilizations. The example comes from a video message issued by Al Zawahiri, broadcast by Al Jazeera in March, 2006. In that message he said the decline of the 'false' and 'dying' Western civilization depends on its making 'zionism, the Holocaust, and sexual perversity' its sacred objects. Thus, the notorious 'clash of civilizations' would amount to the confrontation between two ideas of the sacred, not between theocracy and secularism.

[25]The formula bears the obvious weight of a paradox. On the posthuman, the literature is now so extended that I give up quotations. I'll refer to a few important authors in the text below.

[26]About the relevance of *untouchability*, as related to other companion concepts like dignity, see Lohmann and other contributions in Albers et al. (2014).

The culture that holds individual self-determination as the main (indeed, absolute) value kicks off from very different premises. In this sense, systems theory has articulated an instructive interpretation, conceiving of human rights as essentially an emergent effect of functional differentiation (Luhmann 1993). Conceptually they correspond to the principled, mandatory openness of modern society, where every individual must be able to access every social subsystem. This excludes the validity of any limit imposed by 'rigid' classification. Human rights, therefore, appear as a particular way to assert freedom and equality, which comes into the picture when society gives up the forms of life that were typical of *Ancien Régime* stratification to adapt to the ongoing individualization of individuals.[27] The interesting point here is that in such a perspective human dignity is *opposed* to 'nature', which is the source of essential, indisposable distinctions.[28] Luhmann's intriguing argument is that the idea of 'nature' typically served the discriminatory purpose of positing ontological distinctions between different 'kinds' of people – i.e. *within* humanity – and enforcing practices of social exclusion. This has been culturally represented in terms of race, caste, or of any other symbol which could work as a possible ground for a 'naturalized' notion of social stratification. Therefore, in this context the notion of *indisposability* really means something like 'unfair rigidity', limiting access to given social spheres, and thereby stifling human freedom. My aim is not to follow the whole Luhmannian argument, but to highlight its connection with the legal doctrines which emphasize individual self-determination. The latter see nature only as chance and necessity, devoid of any normative meaning. Normative meaning should emerge from the human historical condition, in the particular sense that the person is his/her will and praxis, extended over the life course and applied to the ever varying situations and spheres of life encountered on the individual's biographical trajectory. In this game, the individual should be free to construct his / her personality, using all opportunities that are socially available. Accordingly, human rights may emerge, and their list be extended through protest and struggles in these various spheres and concrete situations.

As a result, what this culture has to offer in the face of the post-human challenge is a basic idea: innovation must go on, and no predetermined direction may be fixed. The only norm that is still perceived as valid says that equality of opportunities should be guaranteed for all (adult) individuals. In other words, equality and freedom are still the only categories that are expected to manage the technological revolution. The problem is that choice remains free, including access to self-enhancing technologies (Hughes 2004). Dignity appears at first as a *third* principle, beyond freedom and equality, but ends up being nothing more than an additive effect of 'freedom plus equality'. This does not come as a surprise, given the absence of an ontological dimension.

In this structural and cultural context, the symbolic vector of innovation is epitomized by the concept of *morphological freedom*, and its corresponding *rights*

[27]Luhmann N. (1993: 484, 515 ss).

[28]*Ibidem*, pp. 191–192; 233 ss.; 575.

(Bostrom 2005). These are the rights to enhance oneself by technical means. More precisely, it means to legitimate the will to give oneself a form that matches one's (self-)imagery, as well as to escape the limits of one's present (human) form. They apply to many crucial domains where human biology is involved, from procreation to human/machine relationships.

The carrier groups of these ideational and material interests are:

(i) the protest movements and advocacy groups which stand for morphological rights – everyone who claims his/her self-perception should bear normative meaning for society;
(ii) technoscience labs;
(iii) biotech corporations.

These actors and movements are currently riding on the Western mainstream. If this 'struggle for rights' is successful, technological liberation from nature will be accomplished.

To sum up, if dignity is understood *exclusively* as equally possible forms of self-determination, then the new challenges are met with the conceptual tools which served to fight the cultural-and-structural wars of classical modernity, when equality was the main problem *in principle*. I am perfectly aware that it still is *in practice*. Indeed, global society is currently producing less, not more equality. However, technological divides (the 'enhanced' versus the 'unenhanced') will surely add to the burden. My point is obviously not that freedom and equality should be dismissed as irrelevant. On the contrary, I deem it very hard to imagine an effective protection for such goods in the absence of an explicit ontology of indisposability. But this will be impossible, if the latter is mistaken as the comfortable soul mate of pre-modern hierarchical societies.

This point becomes clear if one considers what I call the 'ontological backlash'. By this I mean that the ontological changes prompted by the various 'anthropotechnics'[29] will feed back onto the very normative structures which try to make themselves indifferent to it. Such an attempt entails the bizarre illusion that ontological change will be inconsequential, but who can really imagine what meaning and value any 'indispensable norm' – indeed, any constraint – could still have for the post-human beings who will emerge from the (egalitarian) exercise of their morphological freedom? This means that science and technology intensify, and so to speak 'transfigure' the themes of freedom and equality, in that heteronomy and inequality can come to be rooted in our very personal ontology. This is exactly why it is hard to demonstrate that the exclusive value of self-determination can be a robust bulwark of human dignity. It seems much more realistic to accept

[29]I take the term 'anthropotechnics' from Peter Sloterdijk (2013). Using it in the present context, I change – or better, restrict – its meaning to *technologically assisted* manipulations of the human person.

that radical individualism and anthropotechnics stand in a relation of (contingent) complementarity. As with every contingent relationship, its outcome is – by definition – not a necessary one!

The human person in her indisposability versus pure self-producing individuality are the two 'sacred objects' that are posed to define the latent identity pattern of the MS. In the last instance, the issue at stake can be understood through the concept of 'transcendence', as applied to both individual and collective life.[30] Human enhancement techniques point explicitly to such an aim. The problem is whether humanity will preserve some sense of its transcendence – i.e. a relationship with some 'exterior'[31] – or it will try to produce (re-enter) it within an enhanced immanence. In a nutshell, the coming civilizational distinction is between conceiving of humans – indeed, of the whole world – as a material platform from which resources may be drawn and upon which powers and capacities may be implanted, and a non-utilitarian, relationally articulated recognition of their ontological integrity.

The enhanced society would confront us with a tough decision, namely whether the re-identification and protection of all that is human will depend on *recognition* or rather on a brand new *construction*. If human experience on the planet makes sense as self-transcendence within an immanent sphere, this involves *grasping-and-letting go* of our roots. In other words, the point is whether the human species still conceives of itself as not only *creating* meaning, but as an entity that is inherently *endowed with* meaning. Such meaning may only be discovered in and through social relationships, provided that humans still think of themselves as related to a world that is not totally of its own production, and is not merely the product of chance. Many ways may be opened for this recognition, but options should be made explicit in the culture and in the social norms advanced societies want to enforce. A choice will happen anyway, and will be crucial for the sense of human experience as a whole, for the quality of human life and the meaning attributable to its accomplishment. Needless to add, this is also a fundamental watershed for the profile of the coming MS.

Stepwise Post-Humanism?

The second part of my thesis connects the guiding values I have been discussing to a specific *type* of norms, values whose cultural content and underlying logic of obligation share a common denominator. In my view, a key feature of emerging

---

[30] This problem has triggered a renewed interest within sociology (not just history) for concepts such as the 'Axial Age' (Bellah and Joas 2012). For an interesting discussion of a strictly related topic see also Donati (2010). The issue is obviously far beyond the scope of this paper, but it would represent a way to 're-code' the whole argument I am presenting here.

[31] By this formulation I indicate that transcendence and 'exterior' are also strictly connected with relationality.

social norms concerns the way they conceive of and safeguard the relationships obtaining between the different layers comprising human ontology.[32] It looks as if our normative culture is currently running a particular experiment, which consists of separating the various dimensions of the human – material, biological, psychological, and social. The idea is to regulate social and individual opportunities of action *as if* each of these dimensions made no difference and were of no consequence for the rest. For example, norms would allow us to act as if our biological being would and should mean nothing to society, or as if social structures meant nothing to individual psychic systems. Even when such differences can be detected, they are normatively disregarded. Therefore, the human body becomes a platform that can be used to enhance its powers and virtual properties. The morphogenic thrust lies in the attempt to make all games, permutations, and combinations possible, through the *dissolution of the relationships* between ontological layers. Such a dissolution, making relationships invisible or at least totally contingent, and bereft of any reality status, serves the purpose of making all games possible, thereby increasing the opportunities for individual choice, action and experience. The rationale is that norms should *forbid constraining* individual creativity in its various possible forms – including technically assisted ones.

An example concerns so-called 'procreation rights', where the very definitions of a couple, of intra- and inter-generational relationships are becoming shaky, and where specific goals of actions and interventions tend to focus on one aspect of things, regardless of the possible impact on other dimensions – as if 'all other things remain equal'. Embryo selection for the enhancement of cognitive abilities is a similar case in point (Shulman and Bostrom 2014). Advocates of such (future) practices invoke the relevance of 'human capital'; genetic means are allegedly just another way to increase it. Their impact on society is usually predicted without any consideration about the social relations involved, or the symmetries and a-symmetries that would obtain within personal ontological layers. In some cases, the norm-creating strategy involved may be that of sheer 'openness', setting provisional standards that show no clear connection with any principled constraint. When this is the case, the role of 'regulators' is merely that they can speed or slow advance through rules on stem cell research and the private consumer genomics market.

A different example is that of a recent court ruling. On December, 2014, the European court of justice ruled upon unfertilised human ova.[33] The court overturned its own previous judgement, maintaining that an organism which is incapable of developing into a human being does not constitute a human embryo within the meaning of the European Biotech Directive. Accordingly, uses of such an organism for industrial or commercial purposes may, as a rule, be patented. In the judgment in question, the Court holds that, in order to be classified as a

[32] I use the formula 'social norms' here in its most general meaning, to include law and other norms. The reason is that the problem does not lie in law alone, but in the whole gamut of normative symbols shared at the socio-cultural level, playing a regulative *and* constitutive role for behaviour.

[33] European Court of Justice (2014).

'human embryo', a non-fertilised human ovum must necessarily have the inherent capacity of developing into a human being. Consequently, the mere fact that a parthenogenetically-activated human ovum commences a process of development is not sufficient for it to be regarded as a 'human embryo'. By contrast, where such an ovum does have the inherent capacity of developing into a human being, it should be treated in the same way as a fertilised human ovum, at all stages of its development. In that respect, it is for the High Court of Justice to determine whether or not, in the light of knowledge which is sufficiently tried and tested by international medical science, the organisms which are the subject of ISCO's[34] applications for registration have the inherent capacity of developing into a human being. In the previously cited Biotech Directive is EU Directive 98/44, article 6 is worded as follows:

1. Inventions shall be considered unpatentable where their commercial exploitation would be contrary to *ordre public* or morality.

This is the same principle used by the American Supreme Court in 2013 to deny Myriad Genetics Inc. the right to patent and copyright human genes Brca1 and Brca2, which the corporation labs had isolated. Therefore, this might well be – in an ironically strong sense – a case of 'cross-fertilization' between courts – one of the key principles in the soft law fostered by the 'global community of courts' (see above, section "Morphogenic society, morphological rights: the logic of opportunity and its ontological (dis)contents").

However, further study allowed the European Court of Justice to come to the conclusion of December 2014 mentioned above. Moreover, ISCO amended its application before the Hearing Officer, promising to avoid any further genetic manipulation aiming at making the parthenote able to develop into a human being.

Such a decision appears to be reasonable at first sight. However, these rulings are ambivalent enough to leave space for different interpretations. Indeed, this very ambivalence is an inherent feature of soft law. Further, the importance of interpretation as a basic way for soft law to evolve should not be underestimated. Nobody seems to be asking a few elementary questions.

First, where did the original ovum come from? It must have been taken from some human at some point. The procedure in question is not mentioned, and is definitely outside the Court's purview.

Second, the relevant parthenote will not be able to develop into a full blown human being, but it may become some part of a human body (tissue, cornea, etc.). Indeed, this was the medical (and economic) point of the whole operation.

Third, ISCO might keep its word, but we may not even need to apply *further* techniques. There are cases in which the same technologies used for a given purpose later turn out to lead to unexpected applications. For example, the same techniques

---

[34]ISCO stands for 'International Stem Cell Corporation' – a publicly traded biotechnology company based in California.

now used to avert disease – such as Tay-Sachs genetic disease – also seem likely to enable embryo selection for more complex heritable traits that involve many genes and environmental influences, such as height or cognitive ability (Shulman and Bostrom 2014).

Overall, this is a good example of the way law advances. Be it through unprincipled regulations or by cross-checked (criss-crossing) court rulings.[35] Change usually happens stepwise, not through severe 'cultural shocks', but by means of little steps which gradually and incrementally come to gain momentum and finally cross a morphological/ontological threshold.

Conclusion

My provisional conclusion will recapitulate the main points of this chapter, and to pave the way for further study.

I have focused attention upon two normative tensions characterizing the rising constellation of the MS, and upon three coping strategies that were identified as empirically relevant among social actors, intended to meet these challenges. The main tensions are those revolving respectively around personal ontology and normative universalism. As to the strategies, the former is the attempt to close social spheres against the threat of intensified morphogenesis. Although the resulting enclaves were seen (in a previous essay; see Maccarini 2015) to represent an empirically possible outcome in some regions of global society, the effectiveness of this strategy in meeting the challenges in question is very poor. The second strategy consists of a deep de-normativization of law, which becomes a merely adaptive device. Finally, there is the development of networks which incorporate and generate their own normativity – not as a predefined legacy of the past, but as a need and simultaneously a performance that is made possible by the inner relational structure of the network itself. We have also seen that empirical cases often stand in an ambivalent connection with some of these strategies.

My following point was to show that the current situational logic of opportunity is in itself consistent with all these strategies, and with different and even opposed approaches to the relevant normative tensions. Therefore, the emergent properties of

[35]The strategy of 'social closure' is bound to fail in the long run, should it try to create 'safe havens' where such experiments cannot enter. This goes for Western societies. The often confrontational attitude other civilizations may have as regards some of the behaviour in question is far from irrelevant, but its full consideration is beyond the scope of this chapter. The notion of 'cross-checked court rulings' refers to the new forms of network universalism that lean on technical deliberative or adjudicating bodies, typically courts and international arbitration boards. These courts and boards perform sort of a legal *bricolage*, deciding what laws are applicable and combining them so as to create a relatively consistent corpus of transnational law. The validity of a norm would then be left to the cross-check and cross-validation between these actors, constituting a 'global community of courts' through continuous mutual observation and adaptation (Burke-White 2002; Slaugther 2003; Teubner 2000, 2002).

our society will differ, according to the developmental path social normativity will take with respect to the challenges in question.

Finally, a cautionary note must be added as regards the prospective role of the courts of justice in this context. Their tremendously enhanced role assumes that their decisions can be grounded on a 'strong' legal rationality rooted in social reality, especially in the pattern of relationships. But what if legal arguments decide to break such a pattern, as happened in the case illustrated in section "Morphogenic society, morphological rights: the logic of opportunity and its ontological (dis)contents"? What guarantees that legal reason has the capacity to 'read' social reality and preserve the goods it generates? This task would involve a legal reasoning that is sensitive to ontology. But law is now also promoting a new anthropology, not only safeguarding the old. Law may well be actively promoting a 'big bang' of social relationships. To put it in a more sociological language, it could be facilitating the breakdown of the stability of some fundamental relational patterns. Both developmental paths are possible.

The concluding point is that justice (and indeed all normativity) can be neither constructed nor deduced. In the MS, neither social closure nor mere neutralization (i.e. the autoimmune denormativization of law) can generate shared norms or values. These can only be the emergent effect of complex social networks, insofar as they can also tap into symbolic resources endowed with adequate potentials for 'universalization'. In other words, this can only be the outcome of a generative encounter, through which the potential of a culture to read and evaluate social reality is newly elaborated to articulate individual and collective experience, by cultural elites who discover how this operation can lead to 'give order' to a new social world. Whether this will be human or inhuman depends on (i) the goals and interests (material and ideational) of such symbolic entrepreneurs, (ii) their cultural orientation, and (iii) the cultural repertoire they draw upon, with its ontological and universalizing potential.

This leaves us with a further task to accomplish. At the end of the day, the watershed between what can still identify 'the human' and what encourages its change beyond the boundaries of 'old humanism' ultimately lies in the symbolic resources that can still be mobilized for this task. Although it is hard to speak of cultural *contents*, and may be even harder to shape the argument in such a way that may remain firmly within the discourse of social science, the notion of human flourishing (versus enhancement) is the logical step ahead of the present work.

References

Albers, M., Hoffmann, T., & Reinhardt, J. (Eds.). (2014). *Human rights and human nature*. Dordrecht: Springer.

Alexander, J. C. (2012). *Trauma. A social theory*. Cambridge: Polity Press.

American Psychiatric Association. (2013). *Diagnostic and statistical manual of mental disorders, 5th edition: DSM-5*. Washington, DC: American Psychiatric Publishing.

Archer, M. S. (2000). *Being human. The problem of agency*. Cambridge: Cambridge University Press.

Archer, M. S. (2003). *Structure, agency, and the internal conversation*. Cambridge: Cambridge University Press.
Archer, M. S. (2012). *The reflexive imperative in late modernity*. Cambridge: Cambridge University Press.
Archer, M. S. (2014). Introduction: 'Stability' or 'Stabilization' – On which would morphogenic society depend? In M. S. Archer (Ed.), *Late modernity. Trajectories towards morphogenic society* (pp. 1–20). Dordrecht: Springer.
Archer, M. S. (2015). How agency is transformed in the course of social transformation: don't forget the double morphogenesis. In M. S. Archer (Ed.), *Social mechanisms transforming late modernity* (pp. 129–150). Dordrecht: Springer.
Bartoli, R. (2014). La sospensione del processo con messa alla prova: una goccia deflattiva nel mare del sovraffollamento? *Diritto penale e processo, 20*(6), 661–674.
Bellah, R. N., & Joas, H. (Eds.). (2012). *The axial age and its consequences*. Cambridge, MA: The Belknap Press of Harvard University Press.
Ben-Rafael, E. (2003). The de-civilizing process. In G. Skąpska, & A. Orla-Bukowska (Eds.), with the collaboration of K. Kowalski, *The moral fabric of contemporary societies* (pp. 283–289). Leiden: Brill.
Bostrom, N. (2005). In defense of posthuman dignity. *Bioethics, 19*(3), 202–214.
Burke-White, W. W. (2002). A community of courts: Toward a system of international criminal law enforcement. *Michigan Journal of International Law, 24*, 1–101.
Donati, P. (1997). La relazione libertà/controllo sociale nella società globalizzante. *Studi di Sociologia, XXXV*(4), 285–315.
Donati, P. (2009). *La società dell'umano*. Genova: Marietti.
Donati, P. (2010). *La matrice teologica della società*. Soveria Mannelli: Rubbettino.
Donati, P., & Solci, R. (2011). *I beni relazionali. Che cosa sono e quali effetti producono*. Torino: Bollati Boringhieri.
Eisenstadt, S. N. (2003). The moral dimensions and tensions of modernity. In G. Skąpska, & A. Orla-Bukowska (Eds.), with the collaboration of K. Kowalski, *The moral fabric of contemporary societies* (pp. 203–217). Leiden: Brill.
European Court of Human Rights (2013). *Chamber judgment 08/01/2013, applications nr. 43517/09, 46882/09, 55400/09, 57875/09, 35315/10 and 37818/10 – Torreggiani et al. vs. Italy*.
European Court of Justice (2014). *Judgment in case C-364/13, International Stem Cell Corporation v Comptroller General of Patents, Designs and Trade Marks.*
Fuchs, P., & Göbel, A. (Hg.). (1994). *Der Mensch – das Medium der Gesellschaft?* Frankfurt: Suhrkamp.
Habermas, J. (2001). *The post-national constellation. Political essays*. Cambridge: MIT Press.
Hughes, J. (2004). *Citizen Cyborg: Why democratic societies must respond to the redesigned human of the future*. Cambridge: Westview.
Joas, H. (2008). *Do we need religion? On the experience of self-transcendence*. Boulder: Paradigm Publishers.
Joas, H. (2013). *The sacredness of the person: A new genealogy of human rights*. Washington, DC: Georgetown University Press.
Lohmann, G. (2014). How to protect "Human Nature" – By human dignity, human rights or by "Species-Ethics" argumentations? In M. Albers, T. Hoffmann, & J. Reinhardt (Eds.), *Human rights and human nature* (pp. 161–172). Dordrecht: Springer.
Luhmann, N. (1993). *Das Recht der Gesellschaft*. Frankfurt: Suhrkamp.
Luhmann, N. (1996). Jenseits von Barbarei. In M. Miller, & H. G. Soeffner (Hg.), *Modernität und Barbarei* (pp. 219–230). Frankfurt am Main: Suhrkamp.
Luhmann, N. (1997). *Die Gesellschaft der Gesellschaft*. Frankfurt: Suhrkamp.
Maccarini, A. (2013). A morphogenetic-relational account of social emergence: Processes and forms. In M. S. Archer & A. Maccarini (Eds.), *Engaging with the world etc* (pp. 22–49). London: Routledge.

Maccarini, A. (2015). Turbulence and relational conjunctures: The emergence of morphogenic environments. In M. S. Archer (Ed.), *Social mechanisms transforming late modernity* (pp. 151–170). Dordrecht: Springer.
Maine, H. S. (1972) [1861]. *Ancient law. Its connection with the early history of society and its relation to modern ideas*. London: Dent.
Marandola, A. (2014). La messa alla prova dell'imputato adulto: ombre e luci di un nuovo rito speciale per una diversa politica criminale. *Diritto penale e processo, 20*(6), 674–685.
Porpora, D. V., Nikolaev, A. G., Hagemann May, J., & Jenkins, A. (2013). *Post-ethical society. The Iraq war, Abu Ghraib, and the moral failure of the secular*. Chicago: Chicago University Press.
Prandini, R. (2012). Complessità sociale e diritto riflessivo. Dall'auto-regolazione "regolata" fino alle costituzioni societarie. In R. Prandini (Ed.), *Culture e processi "costituenti" della società riflessiva. Globalizzazione, accelerazione e auto-regolazione sociale* (pp. 33–68). Bologna: Bononia University Press.
Rodotà, S. (2012). *Il diritto di avere diritti*. Laterza: Roma-Bari.
Shulman, C., & Bostrom, N. (2014). Embryo selection for cognitive enhancement: Curiosity or game-changer? *Global Policy, 5*(1), 85–92.
Simmel, G. (1890). *Über sociale Differenzierung. Sociologische und psychologische Untersuchungen*. Leipzig: Duncker & Humblot.
Slaugther, A. M. (2003). A global community of courts. *Harvard International Law Journal, 44*, 191–219.
Sloterdijk, P. (2013). *You must change your life. On anthropotechnics*. Cambridge: Polity Press.
Stichweh, R. (2000). *Die Weltgesellschaft. Soziologische Analysen.*. Frankfurt: Suhrkamp.
Teubner, G. (2000). Globale Privatregimes: Neo-spontanes Recht und duale Sozialverfassungen in der Weltgesellschaft. In G. Teubner (Hg.), *Zur Autonomie des Individuums. Liber Amicorum Spiros Simitis* (pp. 437–453). Baden Baden: Nomos.
Teubner, G. (2002). Hybrid laws: Constitutionalizing private governance networks. In R. Kagan & K. Winston (Eds.), *Legality and community: On the intellectual legacy of Philip Selznick* (pp. 311–331). Berkeley: Berkeley Public Policy Press.

Part II
Morphogenesis and the Decline of Normative Consensus

Chapter 6
In Letter and in Spirit: Social Morphogenesis and the Interpretation of Codified Social Rules

Ismael Al-Amoudi

Introduction

The extension and ramification of codified rules in most areas of social life has been understudied since Weber (1978) analysed the rise of modern bureaucracies and the development of formal rationality at the start of the twentieth century. Yet, the increasing reliance on codified rules constituted a crucial evolution of normativity since Weber's death. As I write these lines, in the twenty-first century's opening decades, participation in social life is conditioned by the adherence, explicit or implicit, to innumerable codified rules. In the USA, for instance, the Mercatus think tank measured the length of the Code of Federal Regulations at about 103 million words. This length corresponds to about 130 times the length of the Bible or the collected works of Shakespeare.[1] Furthermore, analysts at Mercatus remark that it would take over 5000 hours for a fast-reading person to read through the whole Code of Federal Regulation.

Yet, US Federal or European supranational laws are just the tip of an immense paper iceberg that governs, or ought to govern, everyday life. As workers, most of us are subject to our employer organisation's internal regulations and codes of practices in addition to national and international laws. As consumers, almost every product we use is subject to codified industrial and safety rules, from the carrots we eat to the houses we live in and from the clothes we wear to the electronic equipment we regularly throw away and replace.

[1] http://mercatus.org/publication/code-federal-regulations-ultimate-longread-game-thrones-hunger-games (checked 18 Apr 2015).

I. Al-Amoudi (✉)
Cardiff Business School, University of Cardiff, Cardiff CF10 3EU, UK
e-mail: al-amoudii@cardiff.ac.uk

M.S. Archer (eds.), *Morphogenesis and the Crisis of Normativity*,
Social Morphogenesis, DOI 10.1007/978-3-319-28439-2_6

Not only are we subjected to myriad codified rules, but these rules also present problems of interpretation. Firstly, these rules are typically codified in such ways as to restrict attempts at reinterpreting their spirit. Secondly, normativity is either ambiguous or non-existent and it remains dubious whether the agents issuing these rules are concerned with the common good or whether they are merely guided by their organisation's self-serving interests. But problems of interpretation persist even if we accept to set aside the questionable normativity of these codified rules and attempt instead to interpret them according to their letter. The vast majority of people, indeed, lack the time and juridical background to decipher, let alone contest in court, the letter of these codified rules. And only a handful of wealthy individuals and powerful organisations enjoy the actual capacity for deciphering, using and contesting the codified rules they are expected to respect.

The wide development of the Internet over the past decades illustrates this phenomenon spectacularly. A lengthy End User License Agreement must first be accepted whenever the user downloads a software application and, increasingly often, whenever she consults a webpage. These user agreements require users to abandon significant rights such as their right to a fair trial (superseded by arbitration clauses) or their control over any information they disclose about themselves while using the application or webpage. Anecdotal evidence suggests, however, that most users accept the agreement and end-up legally bound by it without having read it in full. As a case in point, the website Gamestation added (1st April 2010) an unusual clause to its End User Licence Agreement: users placing an order on that day were irrevocably giving their souls to the company. About 7500 users (88 % of the total) agreed to the contract without ticking the checkbox allowing them to opt-out of the 'immortal soul' clause. If the prank generated strong emotional responses and was widely mentioned in the press, this might be because it revealed a widespread, yet inconvenient and perhaps taboo, social phenomenon for which there are no ready-made solutions. It seems that, on the one hand, few agents are in a position to refuse to use internet services, while on the other, even fewer agents have the power to understand fully, let alone challenge and transform, the rules of utilisation imposed by the providers of these services.

In the current volume, Archer (2016) takes stock of the proliferation of bureaucratic regulation and explains this phenomenon by pointing to the fragmentation of normativity.[2] Moreover, she describes convincingly the manifold faces of anormative regulation: societies have been increasingly governed through political tactics rather than through normative strategic policy; anormative performance indicators have gradually replaced the once powerfully normative *esprit de corps*; and, finally, we have witnessed a flourishing of bureaucratic regulation that is both disconnected from and dismissive of citizens who are too fragmented to articulate and engage in meaningful resistance.

[2]For a reflection on the effects of morphogenesis on normativity in Late Modern societies, see also the contribution of Al-Amoudi (2014) to the second volume of the *Social Morphogenesis* series.

The present chapter addresses the general phenomenon of the proliferation of codified rules, though from a slightly different perspective than Archer. Instead of asking 'how does social regulation become anormative with morphogenesis?' it asks instead: 'what difficulties does morphogenesis make to the interpretation of codified rules?' This slight change of angle leads to an argument that is sympathetic and complementary, yet different in a number of ways. Firstly, the focus on 'codified rules' is larger than a focus on legislation or on anormative bureaucratic regulation. It encompasses these but also the deeply normative (Kunda 1992) and even neo-normative (Fleming 2009; Fleming and Sturdy 2009, 2011) forms of control operating in a number of firms and expressed through local codes of practice. Think for instance of the guidelines circulated among employees of large accountancy firms and investment banks regulating their body hair, their make-up or the length of their dresses in the names of professionalism and client orientation. More pervasively, employees are regularly subjected to formal appraisal procedures that evaluate their productivity (in terms defined by management) but also how satisfactorily they adhere to the organisation's managerially imposed culture (Alvesson and Willmott 2002) in terms of such appraisal categories as 'client orientation' and 'team play'.[3] Although moral considerations have been marginalised and even eliminated from public debate and the formulation of state laws (Porpora 2001, 2015), this has not necessarily been the case for the codes of private organisations. The latter typically include clauses punishing members whose behaviour may have brought 'bad repute'. How these clauses are invoked and enforced seems in many instances dependent on the decisions of those members with the organisational power to make such decisions.

Secondly, because Archer is anything but a determinist, a focus on difficulties (rather than say on evolutions) seeks to protect the argument from any perverse reinterpretation as an ineluctable historical development.[4] Difficulties are indeed adversarial *tendencies*; identifying them is often the first step before finding ways to overcome them. Thirdly, and more substantially, the present chapter develops an argument that is explanatory rather than descriptive. It seeks to identify the generative mechanisms that account for the difficulties encountered by people when they interpret codified rules in a morphogenic social configuration.

My argument starts from the ontological observation that the codification of rules is always fundamentally incomplete as codifications never fully specify the range of actions subject to them or the contexts in which they ought to apply (see my "Introduction"). A number of realist concepts are introduced in this section to account for how agents manage nonetheless to reach some form of consensus when interpreting codified rules. The second section mobilises these concepts to examine

---

[3]For disquieting accounts of compulsory fun at work see Fleming and Sturdy (2009, 2011).

[4]See for instance King (1999) who interprets Archer's framework as entailing a backdoor reification of social structure that 'consciously insists on the autonomy of the people and the parts, at certain moments in the social process' (King 1999: 201). Against King, my approach in this chapter assumes that structure, culture and agency depend on one another at every moment.

the import of *social integration* for rule interpretation in morphogenetic settings. The third and last section examines the import of *systemic integration* for rule coherence, first in a situation of predominant morphostasis and then in a situation of overwhelming morphogenesis. An example of contemporary relevance – tax optimisation – illustrates the argument.

How Do Agents Cope with Rules' Fundamental Incompleteness?

The interpretation of codified rules creates problems for agents in every form of society, morphogenic or otherwise. This section seeks to step back and appreciate the general philosophical problems relative to the interpretation of codified rules before analysing, in the rest of the paper, the specific form that these problems take in Late Modernity.

Letter vs Spirit: Two Modes of Interpretation

We might start our discussion by clarifying the idiomatic distinction that opposes interpretations according to the spirit against interpretations according to the letter. Interpretation according to the letter refers to a mode of interpretation that seeks to take into account exclusively the written code while ignoring the intentions of those who issued it. Conversely, interpretation according to the spirit seeks to complement, and in certain cases even overwhelm, the written code by taking into account the intention of those who promulgated it.

According to Wikipedia,[5] the earliest mention of this distinction appears in the Bible: 'But he is a Jew who is one inwardly; and circumcision is that which is of the heart, by the Spirit, not by the letter; and his praise is not from men, but from God.' (Romans 2:29). It is noteworthy that this biblical text establishes a clear, though implicit, link between the spirit of the law, normativity, inwardness and a person's authentic religious identity. Interpretations of the divine law that follow the letter but not the spirit may generate actions that might outwardly obtain some form of approval from other people. However, they fail to generate actions coming from the heart and that are pleasing to God. Being a Jew (i.e. in this context, a true believer) is internally related to seeking to understand, and taking to heart, the intentions of God rather than unreflexively following His written rules.

The opposition between the literal interpretation of rules and their spirit also forms a central aspect in the plot of many a work of literature. In *The Merchant of Venice*, to take a well-known example, Portia saves Antonio from Shylock's

[5]https://en.wikipedia.org/wiki/Letter_and_spirit_of_the_law (checked 22 Apr 2015).

inflexible rule 'you shall give me a pound of your flesh' precisely by invoking the letter of another well-established rule: that no blood may be shed. An exhilarating effect is produced when Shylock is entrapped through the same legalistic devices he had tried to use against Antonio who is now free.

Yet, while the religious and theatrical examples above favour interpretations according to the spirit over interpretations according to the letter, thinkers such as Montesquieu and Weber have also convincingly identified significant benefits of interpreting codified rules according to the letter rather than the spirit. To their analyses we now turn.

Montesquieu: Modes of Interpretation and Types of Government

Montesquieu's *De l'Esprit des Lois* (1748) is credited with offering both an early reflection on the links between the letter and the spirit of the law and for establishing the first bases upon which the sociology of law could subsequently develop (Durkheim 1892/1953). Montesquieu characterises interpretation according to the letter as an automatic process necessitating no thinking and no judgement. As he has it:

> In Rome, the judges would only state whether the accused was guilty of a certain crime, and the penalty was [already] in the law... *and for this all one needs are eyes.*' (Montesquieu 1748, Book VI, Chap. III, my translation).

Leaving aside for now whether literal interpretation is as automatic as Montesquieu suggests, or whether it always necessitates a modicum of social integration to be operational, let us notice how Montesquieu recognises the merits of both forms of interpretation. As he has it:

> In despotic states, there is no law: the judge is himself (sic) his own rule. In monarchic states, there is a law: and where it is precise, the judge follows it; where it is not [precise] he seeks its spirit. In a republican government, the nature of the constitution is such that judges follow the letter of the law. There is no citizen against whom it is possible to interpret a law, when his goods, his honour, or his life are at stake. (Montesquieu 1748, Book VI, Chap. III, my translation)

While Montesquieu is often critical of tyranny, he keeps a neutral attitude that does not judge political systems for their own worth but only relatively to (what we would call today) the sociological features of the people thus governed. These features are influenced by a number of factors, including the climate, religion, maxims, past examples and manners. For Montesquieu, modes of political organisation should first and foremost be congruent with the human passions that animate the people thus governed. While the passion central to despotism is fear, the passion central to the republic is virtue (i.e. love of the homeland) and the passion animating monarchy is honour. Thus, the exclusive recourse to literal interpretation is desirable for a people animated by the love of the homeland but not necessarily for a people principally motivated by honour. At this point, the myth of cultural integration (Archer 1985) seems to affect Montesquieu's reasoning: can we assume, indeed, that society exhibits the normative homogeneity he presupposes? While this supposition is arguably problematic regarding Ancient Rome and eighteenth century

France, it becomes almost indefensible in Late Modern societies characterised by a varying level of social integration across differing, yet connected, communities. I shall discuss in section "The Social Conditions of Rule Interpretation in Late Modernity" (below) what difficulties are raised by fragmentary social integration for the interpretation of the spirit of codified rules.

Weber: Substantive Justice vs Calculability

Max Weber offers an insightful analysis of the literal interpretation of codified rules in his reflections on formal, as opposed to substantive, justice. The formal rationalisation of law is exemplified in Germany by Pandectist law that provides

> a "logically formal law", characterised by abstract legal propositions constituting a "gapless system" that results in the legal ordering of all social conduct (Ewing 1987: 488, see also Weber 1978: vol. 2, pp. 657–8)

In England, the English case law system, while not displaying the characteristics of formal rationality of the German Pandectist law, operates nonetheless through a 'formal rational administration of justice' (Weber 1978: vol. 2, 813). Both systems are contrasted with 'khadi justice' that relies on the judge's interpretation of the law (according to its spirit) rather than on more formalised procedures of judgement.

Weber argues, convincingly, that formalised systems of justice (reliant on literal interpretations) provide guarantees of *calculability* and *stability* that are lacking in alternative approaches that rely further on the judge's own attempt to reach substantive justice, be it at the expense of formal justice. As he puts it

> Among those groups who favour formal justice we must include all those political and economic interest groups to whom the stability and predictability of legal procedure are of very great importance, i.e., particularly rational, economic, and political organizations intended to have a permanent character. (Weber 1978: 813)

At this stage, it is worth noting that neither Montesquieu nor Weber take fully into account the fundamental incompleteness of rules. Yet, this ontological feature of rules is of import for their commentaries. In particular, calculability or consensus can never be guaranteed as ambiguities persist and loopholes are sought and found. What problems does the rules' fundamental incompleteness create for agents? How do agents attempt to overcome, and sometimes benefit from, rules' incompleteness? And what are the consequences for the social and cultural systems through which they act?

The Fundamental Incompleteness of Rules

The incompleteness of social rules constitutes one of the significant philosophical discoveries of the twentieth century (Kripke 1982; Kusch 2006; Wittgenstein 1958). The following problem lies at the root of these investigations on rules, language, mind and society: no set of codified social rules, however carefully they are expressed, can account for the totality of the specific situations in which they ought to apply and for the specific modalities of their application. In other words, while rules can in principle be codified under the form 'do X rather than Y in context C' (Al-Amoudi 2010), logic alone does not guarantee that agents will agree on which actions count as acceptable or on which situations constitute a relevant context in which the rule applies. And yet, most social agents are capable of navigating through the social world and engaging in practices that respect most rules, or at least avoid breaking them too blatantly. How is consensus achieved over whether a given specific situation calls for an exception? And how do agents manage, in spite of rules' fundamental incompleteness, to engage in practices that accommodate the various rules to which they are subjected?

In a previous ontological study of social rules (Al-Amoudi 2010), I responded to the above questions by borrowing ideas from ethnomethodology (especially Sudnow's reflexive narrative on jazz improvisation) and post-structuralist literature (especially Laclau and Mouffe's reflections on hegemony and discourse). The recourse to conceptions borrowed from ethnomethodology and post-structuralist political philosophy was prompted by a perceived void in the sociological literature that relied on a mechanistic conception of socialisation inherited from Parsons. Under mechanistic conceptions of socialisation, the acquisition of rules is taken for granted and the incompleteness of rules is ignored. Equally neglected are the constant, fallible, efforts made by agents to act in ways that are congruent with the social rules respected by their community.

To my knowledge, Archer's works to date have not addressed directly the problems encountered, and the solutions found by agents, when interpreting rules. But I believe that her theorisation of social structure, agency and culture can offer an elegant way out of the conundrums of rule-following raised above. Moreover, her social theory is written in the same language as the *Social Morphogenesis* project, which spares us perilous translations between the vocabularies of critical realism and those of ethnomethodology or post-structuralism. The next sub-section provides the key elements that I borrow from Archer's social philosophy to address the question of how intensified morphogenesis affects the interpretation of codified rules.

Archer's Conception of Socialisation: A Refresher

Archer's morphogenetic approach breaks with the mechanistic functionalism of Parsons' social theory by vindicating the coexistence of existentially inter-dependent yet ontologically different kinds of entities: persons; social relations and ideas. In Archer's perspective, persons have reflexive powers of their own and are therefore irreducible to social relations or ideas. Two consequences follow. Firstly, social integration is heavily dependent on how people reflect on their social circumstances and cannot be viewed as an automatic process. Secondly, as Lockwood (1964) noticed, normative functionalists, such as Parsons, conflate two distinct mechanisms that influence whether social stability is maintained or disrupted. One is the mechanism of *systemic integration* through which the various parts of society communicate harmoniously and another is the mechanism of *social integration* through which the persons living in relation to one another come to share a similar cultural system.

The section on "The social conditions of rule interpretation in Late Modernity" (below) examines in further detail how the forms of social integration at play in Late Modernity influence people's ability to form consensual interpretations of codified rules. However, before focusing on specific contemporary configurations, we can provide the following general considerations: when confronted with the codified expression of a rule formalised as 'you should do X', social agents are capable of taking for granted alternatives Y and context C to the precise extent that they share elements of a common cultural system, defined by Archer (1995) as the ensemble of ideas accessible to members of a given society. Contrary to Mead (1967), and before him Montesquieu (1748), Archer avoids the assumption that agents face a homogeneous or non-conflicting system of rules and symbols.

The diametrically opposite picture *à la* Beck of individuals perpetually re-inventing themselves – as well as their concerns and the meanings they ascribe to things – in a social or cultural void is unconvincing. My general position, which I endorse alongside realist social theorists, consists in viewing cultural systems (ideas, including norms) as necessary requisites for human action while recognising that the former need not be consistent to be real. Indeed, because members of a given society have access to contradictory ideas, it does not follow that these ideas are less real.

The section on "Systemic integration and rule coherence" (below) examines how the forms of systemic integration at play in Late Modernity influence people's abilities to respect the letter of increasingly complex codified rules. Before discussing contemporary systemic configurations, it may be useful to reflect more generally on the relation between morphogenesis and complexity. This relation is best grasped by distinguishing two dimensions of morphogenesis (Al-Amoudi 2014). The first dimension could be termed *sequential morphogenesis* and consists in the accelerating displacement of one institution by the next. In situations of sequential morphogenesis an ever shorter time-lapse separates one institution from the following one. The novel institution may either replace the previous one (see Al-Amoudi and Latsis 2015 for a discussion of morphonecrosis) or it may exist alongside it. The multiplication of coexisting social forms constitutes the second dimension of morphogenesis and was identified as *concurrent morphogenesis* (Al-Amoudi 2014). While morphonecrotic sequential morphogenesis is typically at play in situations marked by the logics of elimination, concurrent morphogenesis mechanisms are typically at play in social contexts marked by the logics of opportunity in which people cherry pick those institutions that they believe suit their needs best (see Archer 1995 on situational logics).

Three Types of Conflicts Between Codified Rules

The elements above allow us to distinguish and discuss three types of conflicts between rules in the rest of the paper. First, conflict may arise between *differing interpretations of a rule*. This form of conflict typically arises when agents are faced with novel contexts that were unforeseen at the time of codifying the rules. A particular but significant case is provided when the cultural system has evolved so as to displace the meaning of a symbolic category. Think for instance of the meaning of 'adultery' as a threat to a house's bloodline. In the UK where I live, this evolution was confirmed in 1995 when the courts did not prosecute for high treason the lover of a British princess (married to the Crown's heir) who admitted adulterous practices.[6] The sentence that then consisting in hanging, drawing and quartering was therefore not applied.

The interpretation of codified rules raises problems that can be tempered, though never entirely resolved, through social and systems integration. The vocabulary in which the rule is codified must be shared between those expressing the rule and those seeking to interpret it. Thus, a rule codified in a forgotten language can be neither interpreted nor invoked. Moreover, the actions and objects whose legitimacy is scrutinised must be identifiable in terms of the codified rule. Hence, a rule regulating the circulation of boats is unlikely to be convincing for regulating the circulation of cars. Finally, the context in which the actions take place must be identifiable with the context, explicit or implicit, presupposed by the codified rule. This issue is perhaps more salient for sacred or traditional statutes that are scarcely amended than for civil laws subject to continuous amendment (see Weber 1978: 809–39). Indeed, the judicial *non sequitur* of the Princess's extra-marital affair owes both to the fact that punishment for religious sins is not acceptable in liberal democracies (Rawls 2001: 11) and to the fact that royal adultery no longer represents the threat to the British political system it once did. The whole story may have been embarrassing for some family members, but is hardly identifiable as a context qualifying as high treason or as a sin deserving capital punishment.

Second, conflict over rules can also take the form of *ideal conflicts between rules*. That is, when a rule contradicts another in such a way that the formulation of one rule logically contradicts the formulation of another. In practice, these tensions are minimised through a number of mechanisms. Codes of rules are typically stratified in such a way that the rules expressed in 'higher codes' (think of European law or the constitution) trump rules expressed in 'lower codes' (think of the internal regulations of a University). Moreover, an ongoing harmonisation is performed, both at the level of states (think, in European countries, of the efforts to harmonise national laws with the over-ruling EU law) and at the level of private organisations, think of the role of Human Resources departments which continuously adapt their organisation's internal regulations to the requirements of the legal system, especially when the latter are advantageous to owners and senior managers.

Third, and finally, conflict can take the form of *material conflicts between rules*. This form of conflict occurs whenever a set of rules affects the material means of functioning of other institutions (see Porpora 1993 on the reality and distinctiveness of material relations). In the section on "The social conditions of rule interpretation in late modernity" we will examine two rather well-known examples of this form

[6]"Editor defends Mirror over Diana letters". *BBC News*. 31 August 2000. Retrieved 29 Apr 2015.

of rule conflict: Weber's analysis of tensions between the bureaucratic and tax-levying systems in subsistence economies, and current problems created by the unprecedented opportunities for tax evasion for powerful actors.

The meta-theoretical clarification of the links between social integration and the first type of rule conflict; and between systems integration and the third type of rule conflict provide the central contribution of this chapter.

The Social Conditions of Rule Interpretation in Late Modernity

Once the myth of social integration is revealed as the convenient fiction that it is, then belonging to a particular society provides no guarantee that our interpretations will be in agreement with those of other members of the same society, especially if the latter have been socialised through different socio-cultural interactions. Yet, while Archer provides a very convincing critique of attempts to justify law in relation to consensually understood and accepted norms, the specific mechanisms linking socialisation and people's ability to reach a consensual interpretation of codified rules deserves additional unpacking. What are the general mechanisms through which social and systemic integration bear on people's ability to reach consensual interpretations and harmonious codified rules? And how much agreement can be expected in societies, such as late modern ones, characterised by low levels of social integration, salient contextual discontinuity and steep differences of power among persons and among organisations?

This section seeks to address these questions by examining how social integration enables people to reach consensual interpretations of codified rules. It first discusses the import of social integration for interpretations according to the letter. Then it examines how social integration facilitates interpretation according to the spirit. Finally, it examines the import of morphogenesis unbound.

The Social Conditions of Consensual Interpretations of Codified Rules

In the "Introduction" above, I have expressed a doubt about Montesquieu's claim that judging according to the letter required so little interpretation that for the literal interpretation of codified rules, 'all one needs is eyes'. Indeed, consensus on the letter of the law presupposes a minimal level of social integration. This minimal level of social integration is prompted by the need for agents to possess a common language and knowledge of the basic interactions presupposed by the clarification of the letter of the law such as rules of turn-taking, rules relative to the use of violence, or the payment of officials and so on.

Consensus on the letter of the law presupposes a relatively high level of systemic integration. If anything, there must exist institutions endowed with the authority to interpret the letter of codified rules over and above agents' private interpretations. Moreover, at least one of the parties must have an interest in entering a formalistic procedure rather than resolving the conflict through alternative means such as duels, coin-tossing or private arbitration. Finally, too wide a disconnection between formal justice and substantive justice (Weber 1978: 809–38) might threaten consensus on formal law. The major advantages of the literal interpretation of rules stem both from the calculability and predictability of judgements (favoured by entrepreneurs, investors and innovators) and by the dissociation of ethical conceptions from legal decisions, favoured in liberal societies in which multiple conceptions of the good life co-exist (Rawls 2001).

While consensus about the letter of the law necessitates strong systemic integration coupled with only minimal social integration, consensus on the spirit of the law can be satisfied with a *minimal level of systemic integration* but it requires, however, a *relatively high level of social integration*. The minimal level of systemic integration is prompted by the need for agents to be able to survive with at least minimal conditions of military peace and economic wealth. The relatively high level of social integration is prompted by agents' need to be able to reach satisfactory consensus when engaging in the interpretation of the intentions of legislators and of the purposes of codified rules. However, while social integration facilitates consensus, socialisation (as articulated by Archer 2003, 2007, 2012) guarantees neither social integration nor, *a fortiori*, consensus. Indeed, socialisation operates both through the adoption of pre-existing cultural forms, but also through their critical evaluation and, in some cases, rejection. Moreover, in the absence of censoring mechanisms, sub-communities that are relatively different from one another and whose members refer in their reflections and discussions to rather specific elements of the overall cultural system, can emerge and coexist within the same society. Finally, the resulting picture is complicated by intersectionality as each agent may be a member of several cultural sub-communities at once. The same person can be a mother, an employee, a practising Moslem and a fan of Metallica.

In sum, the normative fragmentation identified in Late Modern societies (Al-Amoudi 2014; Porpora 2015; Archer 2016 forthcoming) is problematic for consensual interpretations of the spirit of codified rules. Yet, Late Modernity is characterised neither by a complete dissolution nor by a hegemonic unity of social integration. The picture is ambivalent and deserves further description to understand the contemporary problems faced by agents attempting to interpret the spirit of codified rules.

Late Modernity's Ambivalent Social Integration

The above considerations provide us with elements to account for how Late Modernity's intensified morphogenesis affects people's ability to interpret and comply with the spirit of codified rules. The picture I would like to draw is characterised by ambivalence. On one hand, we seem to be witnessing the *fragmentation of social integration* referred to above. Different communities are formed, each sharing its own cultural referents which others do not access easily. The coexisting groups of *entrepreneurs* and *diffusionists* at the origin of the information systems revolution (Archer 2014) provide us with a case in point. Each group has its heroes (e.g. Bill Gates and Steve Jobs versus Julian Assage and Jimmy Wales); its rites (e.g. launching a successful Initial Public Offer versus gathering a high number of supporters); its modes of valuation (e.g. profitability vs fame) and their associated tests of value (Boltanski and Thévenot 2006).

On the other hand, we also seem to be witnessing the *extension of minimal social integration over unprecedently large geographical and social space*. The generalisation and standardisation of compulsory schooling has certainly equipped a whole generation of humans with a basic common discipline (Foucault 1977; Dean 2010; Prakash 1999) and basic common skills. Not only can the majority of people across the globe read and write but increasing numbers can also communicate in basic English. They also share basic common norms of hygiene (e.g. they wash their hands with soap) and cultural knowledge: many around the globe have heard about the Bible or even Shakespeare. The minimal social integration provided by compulsory education is reinforced both by the institutional isomorphisms resulting from the colonial era (most countries have a police force, tribunals, leaders claiming some form of legitimacy however shaky) and by the instruments of mass culture. Indeed, it is nowadays possible to talk about the latest mobile phone or the latest blockbuster Hollywood movie or the football World Cup with people around the globe. In the case of interlocutors who were exposed to a longer education, it is also possible to discuss international news.

How does this massive diffusion of basic culture affect people's ability to reach some form of workable consensus on the spirit of codified rules? It can be conjectured that a broader consensual basis than ever can be gathered around simple cases that involve non-contradictory norms that are broadly shared. Thus, increasing numbers of people around the planet understand firms' concerns with profitability and can interpret the codified rules of private organisations in these terms. And thus customers around the world do not need to read the small print to know that their line will be cut if they do not pay their phone bill.

On the other hand, complex cases involving conflicting norms or norms that are less widely shared are likely to generate particularly difficult conflicts in Late Modernity. The copyright wars offer a timely example. While the 'entrepreneurs' mentioned above interpret current laws as rightful extensions of the laws safeguarding private property, the 'diffusionists' recognise that private property ought to be respected as long as one's actions do not deprive the owner, but they also insist that actions that do not harm (and even contribute to enhancing) the property of others should be accepted. This conflict can be read as a conflict between two interpretations of the property laws on material cultural objects that preceded copyright laws. For entrepreneurs, the preceding law on material cultural objects sought to safeguard the profitable economic innovations of the creative industries; for the diffusionists the same law sought to safeguard individual purchasers from losing their property.

The quarrel between entrepreneurs and diffusionists is complicated both because the groups have opposing material interests in copyright law but also because they privilege different norms and have different representations of the preceding law. In the context of illustrating this section's broad argument, it can, however, be said that: before the information systems revolution, both groups complied with the same property law while they either interpreted its spirit differently or simply did not need to bother about its spirit at all. The information systems revolution dissociated the cultural object from its material support. It prompted people to interrogate the spirit of the laws of property and revealed two incompatible, yet coexisting, interpretations.

Global Village or Global Archipelago?

The resulting picture of the global cultural system, and of the conflicts of interpretation that traverse a globalising society, is neither that of the global village dear to the gurus and groupies of globalisation nor that of hermetically fragmented cultural systems. If a metaphor were sought, the image of an archipelago of interconnected villages might better capture a situation characterised by a layer of very thin, but widely shared, culture coexisting with thicker cultural systems that are more fragmented.

Yet, even this metaphor fails to grasp the fact of intersectionality as every person would be a member of several villages at once. The metaphor also fails to account for the arbitrariness of clear-cut boundaries: where does one village end and where does the other start? Finally, and most importantly, it would fail to account for their differential powers. Yet, some persons are able to navigate more easily than others. Even more significantly, some persons have the social power to obtain help from others who may act as translators, thus helping them to take full advantage of the globalisation *in principle* of culture.

Whenever concurrent morphogenesis is at play, it tends to generate a multiplication of cultural entities (including norms) accessible in principle to agents. The *in principle* clause signals, however, a power differential between those agents better equipped to understand and manipulate a multiplicity of cultural entities and those less equipped to do so. Indeed, particularly privileged agents may enjoy forms of training that allow them to understand and manipulate codified rules better than others (think of Bourdieu's works on 'cultural capital'). Thus, although Archer (2012) makes a convincing point regarding the obsolescence of familial habitus in working class families in situations of contextual discontinuity, my experience as a business school academic indicates that some (privileged) young persons are still particularly well equipped by their natal social environment to decipher and manipulate those codified rules at play in bureaucracies (including their own university) and in commercial enterprises (including their first employer). Quite often the same persons benefiting from enhanced understanding are also those who can count on an acquaintance or even a hired professional to help them understand, or at least guess, the spirit of the codified rules with which they have to deal.

To recap, the forms of social and cultural integration characteristic of Late Modernity create a two-tiered configuration in which some agents are better equipped than others to interpret the spirit of codified rules. In situations of differing interpretations of a rule, these privileged agents are better equipped than others to provide convincing interpretations that allow them to defend their vested interests. But how do the current morphogenetic processes affect the ideal and material contradictions between rules? And what are the consequences for social agents? To these questions we now turn.

Systemic Integration and Rule Coherence

The type of rule conflict that interests us here is not so much conflict of interpretation as much as conflicts of ideational contradiction (resulting in logical incompatibility) and conflicts of material contradiction resulting in the rules operating in certain institutions acting against the interests of other institutions structured by their own codified rules. For exposition's sake, I start from a familiar case of tensions operating within a morphostatic society before considering the case of morphogenesis unbound.

In a Morphostatic Situation

While social integration is a necessary condition for the possibility of consensual interpretation, systemic integration is constitutive of and constituted by a reduction in conflicts between different parts of society, that is, between different institutional complexes. Tensions between institutions are often though not necessarily expressed and realised through contradictory systems of codified rules. And conversely, even when a society is morphostatic, deficiencies in systemic integration generate conflicts between codified rules considered as essential to the functioning of the respective parts of society which they govern.

Weber's analysis of the necessary yet inherently conflictual relations between state bureaucracies and fiscal systems can be rehearsed to illustrate the relation between systemic malintegration and conflicts of material contradiction between rules. In near-subsistence economies, the rules organising fiscal systems are subject to conflicts of interest between ruler, officials, local landlords and peasants. This conflict of interests generates a tension between the rules governing bureaucracy and the rules governing taxation. In a context of peace and technological stability, when the rules of bureaucracy improve officials' pay or increase their numbers, the rules of taxation become unfit to cover bureaucracy's growing expenses unless they are amended so as to raise increased tax, thus adding to the burden of the peasants and eroding landlords' profits. Conversely, should the rules of taxation lighten the peasants' burden, the bureaucracy's ability to function is eroded, unless its system of rules is amended so as to allow it to cost less or employ fewer officials or seek payment from some of its users.

The mechanism of material contradiction between the codified rules of tax systems and the codified rules of bureaucracy is not confined to subsistence economies. Indeed, the current crises of the Welfare state in European countries can be interpreted through the same lens. Weber's analysis remains insightful today if we replace peasants with workers; landlords with rich investors; officials with civil-servants (and all those employees, including professors, dependent on public budgets); and the king with the elected government. Lockwood (1964) and Archer (1995) seem right therefore to remark that Weber's cases prove that systemic contradiction is not necessarily incompatible with a situation of overall social morphostasis. The characterisations of Late Modernity developed by the contributors to the *Social Morphogenesis* series point, however, at important aspects of contemporary societies which Weber could not address at the start of the twentieth century. First, what happens when some parts of society are more sequentially morphogenetic and undergo faster and more intense change than others? More precisely, what unprecedented normative tensions are generated in a society in which some corporate agents are capable of changing the codified rules of the institutions through which they operate faster than the state can promulgate new laws? Second, what happens when some corporate agents are better placed than others, including the state, to benefit from the multiplicity of institutional arrangements provided by concurrent morphogenesis?

In a Morphogenetic Situation

Let us now examine the tensions operating on systems of codified rules in social configurations characterised by intense concurrent and sequential morphogenesis. Since morphogenesis does not happen above agents' heads but rather through their socio-cultural interactions (Archer 1995), it is important to take into account the differences in power between agents. The powers that interest us here are those allowing an agent (corporate or otherwise), to make the best use of the multiple opportunities engendered by concurrent morphogenesis so as to take the best advantage of the literal application of the codified rules.

For clarity's sake, I present my argument by distinguishing three types of agents. First, administrative authorities that produce codified rules that are mandatory for other agents. Second, relatively powerful individuals (or organisations) who are sufficiently equipped in terms of human and intellectual resources, and in terms of access to competent advice, to be able to change their practices and statuses so as to make the best use of the existing codified rules in play at a certain time and to adapt promptly to changes in the rules. Third, are agents who lack the power to adapt their practices and statuses so as to take advantage of the existing codified rules at a certain time or adapt promptly to transformations in the rules.

Archer's (1995: 157) diagram representing social elaboration (or reproduction) over time is helpful to represent the dynamics and the transitions at play. She represents the diachronic re/production of social structure and culture by distinguishing several general temporal phases. The initial phase of the analysis is conventionally represented as T1 and corresponds to the structural conditioning of agents before cultural transformation proper takes place. In the context of our analysis of the morphogenesis of codified rules, T1 corresponds to the period during which an initial set of codified rules is at play. The next period distinguished on Archer's diagram (T2/T3) corresponds to a period of socio-cultural interaction during which agents interact so as to transform the structures in play at T1. Logically, the T2–T3 period starts before codified rules are transformed and ends up afterwards.[7] Thus, T2 is located before the end of T1 and T3 is located after, once the elaboration is completed. In cases of morphogenesis, T4 represents the period of time during which the novel (social or cultural) structure emerges, and typically replaces or complements significantly, the structure at play in T1.

Like any contribution to meta-theory, the morphogenetic diagram explains nothing on its own. The determination of the phases T1, T2, T3 and T4 is contingent on the observer's research questions and theoretical presuppositions. Thus, the diagram provides an explanatory framework for specific explanations rather than an explanation itself. It offers a useful template for locating the temporal steps of the emergence of a novel structure through agents' socio-cultural interactions. I also believe that this diagram can be usefully extended to trace parallel morphogenetic processes operating in different organisations or in different areas of society.

I therefore employ a (slightly) extended version of Archer's diagram to represent visually and systematically the parallel emergence, and interactions, of codified rules across three significant kinds of social agents. Thus, Fig. 6.1 juxtaposes the morphogenesis of codified rules by an ensemble of administrative authorities with the morphogenetic transformations introduced by other agents over the internal codified rules regulating their own social practices and statuses. This juxtaposition allows one to follow agents' responses to those changes initiated by the administrative authorities. A distinction is made between those agents most capable of swift adaptations fit to their own purposes (designated as 'powerful agents') and those agents who are not able to adapt fittingly (designated as 'less powerful agents'). The time sequences relative to the activities of more powerful actors are notated with a star symbol while those relative to the activities of less powerful agents are notated with a prime symbol.[8]

[7]This is not a logical implication *strictu sensu* as it relies on a metaphysical assumption about the nature of time, i.e. that efficient causes are chronologically posterior to material causes and anterior or concomitant to the effects they produce.

[8]In a strict sense, the administrative authorities are also social (corporate) agents. The codified rules they produce may or may not apply to themselves.

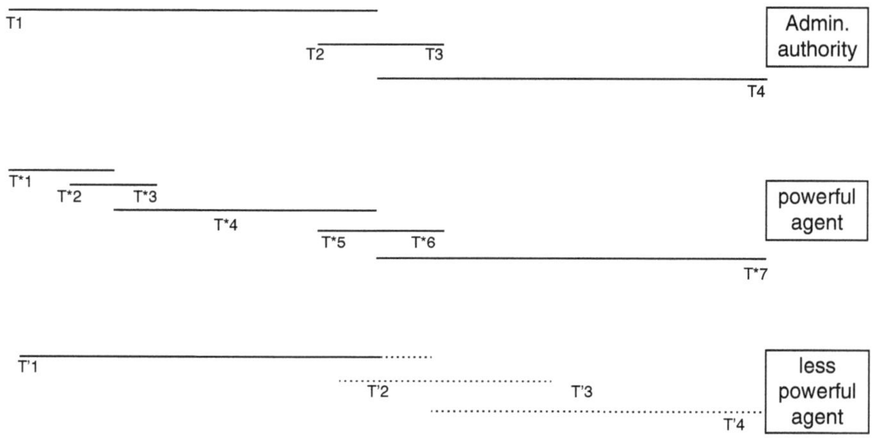

Fig. 6.1 Power differences and the morphogenesis of codified rules

Figure 6.1 allows us to follow the sequences of social elaboration as they unfold in parallel through the activities of the three types of agents. More significantly, the figure is helpful to trace agents' successful (or unsuccessful) mobilisation of ideal and social resources to take advantage of codified rules. The sequence starts for all agents at the same point in time T1, T*1 and T′1. At that time, there exist certain codified rules which are imposed in a certain way on all types of agents be they powerful or not. However, relatively shortly after the start of this sequence, the powerful agents initiate a cycle of socio-cultural interaction (T*2–T*3) through which they transform their practices and statuses in order to take the best advantage of the rules operating in T1. The greater the agent's self-transforming powers, the shorter they can keep the T*2–T*3 phase. As a result of these interactions, the powerful agents have completed the reorganisation of their statuses and activities by the start of T*4. Over the period T*4, they benefit from a privileged situation relative to less powerful agents who have not been capable of reorganising their activities and statuses.

At some point, represented as T2 on the diagram, the administrative authorities notice the disparities of treatment between the more flexible and the less flexible agents. They thus initiate a transformation of the codified rules through several socio-cultural interactions (T2–T3). These interactions result in a novel set of codified rules starting in T4. The rules in T4 are typically more stringent and more complex than at T1 as they seek to close the loopholes identified in the former set of codified rules.

The transformation of the codified rules operating between T1 and T4 is not an insuperable problem for the more powerful agents as they can promptly initiate a phase of socio-cultural interaction (represented as T*5–T*6) through which they once more transform their own practices and statuses. Thus, from T*7 on, these agents are, again, subjected to the codified rules in a way that is more advantageous for them than the administrative authorities had expected.

The picture is not complete, however, unless we also consider the activities of less powerful agents. Although in T′1 their activities and statuses are not optimised so as to take the best advantage of the codified rules, the situation gets worse for them at T4. Because of their lack of flexibility they may not be compliant with the novel structure by the deadlines set by the administrative authorities (thus T1* is prolonged beyond T1). In that case, they are likely to incur penalties for their non-compliance. Their difficulties do not stop here though as the codified rules seeking to limit the number of loopholes and to keep a limit on the number of cases of non-compliance are more complicated and more demanding in T4 than in T1. The fact that less powerful agents struggle to satisfy the new requirements of T4 is represented through the use of dotted lines to represent the T′2–T′3 and T′4 periods.

A Concrete Case: Tax Optimisation and Evasion

Figure 6.1 is helpful in representing one of the major problems plaguing Late Modernity, that is, the ability of multinational firms and high net worth individuals to escape much of the tax they owe in the countries where they reside (for individuals) or operate (for firms). The diagram also allows us to trace some of the significant side-effects of the morphogenetic processes at play.

In the context of tax legislation, new measures are introduced regularly by the government and tax administration to ensure both a fair treatment of economic actors and sufficient revenues to cover the costs of basic regalian functions (i.e. territorial defence, justice, police and money production), of welfare state institutions and of state bureaucracy. A number of agents such as banks, accountancy firms, law firms and legal departments offer, for those willing and able to afford their services, advice on how to proceed through the T*2–T*3 phase and become a fiscally optimal organisation in T*4. Moreover, these powerful agents are capable of lobbying the administrative authorities to ensure that the novel codes coming into play in T4 are not excessively adversarial to their interests or, at least, that they are informed sufficiently in advance of reforms to take appropriate action in T*5–T*6. In particular, major accountancy firms (Price Waterhouse Coopers, Deloitte, KPMG, Ernst & Young) help the authorities writing the new laws and then advise their clients on how to exploit loopholes. The abilities of clients to know about and exploit loopholes in the national tax system is in part owing to their intrinsic powers as agents but also to some of the characteristics of the international legal environment. As Morgan (2011) remarks, the corporate ethos holds that 'whatever is not formally prevented is allowed' rather than the equally plausible 'whatever is not formally allowed is prevented'. Moreover, different nations operate with different, and constantly evolving, tax systems. And finally, it is in each nation's own (narrowly defined) interest to attract and tax, even lightly, capital that would otherwise be taxed in another nation. As a result, Late Modernity has witnessed intensified fiscal competition between states.[9] Although a distinction is made between tax optimisation which is legal and tax evasion which is illegal, there exists in practice a grey zone that covers many a 'fiscally aggressive' practice. Moreover, the financial opacity guaranteed by some countries facilitates illegal practices of tax evasion that include:

> money laundering, income tax evasion, round tripping (taking money offshore, dressing up in secrecy structures then pretending to be foreign investors in order to take advantage of tax breaks and exchange rates only available to foreigners); back to back lending games; export subsidy fraud; avoidance of import duties; corruption. (Henry 2012)

It is not so surprising, therefore, that in 2006 the US Internal Revenue Service estimated the amount of unreported income at about $2 trillion per year, thus generating a net gap of $385 billion (IRS).[10] In a similar vein, the tax Justice Network estimated the overall amount of capital having escaped some form of taxation (overall offshore assets) at between $21 and $32 trillions.

While concurrent morphogenesis is advantageous for the most powerful agents, this is not necessarily the case for less powerful agents (mainly Small and Medium Enterprises and individuals falling below the threshold of High Net Worth). Not only are the latter affected by the tax bill left unpaid by the former, and not only do they have to compete with agents who pay taxes on a lower rate, but they also have to navigate in an increasingly complex environment without necessarily having the resources to do so. Thus, a recent report from the British House of Commons' Committee of Public Accounts laments that HM Treasury's Office of Tax Simplification was established to provide the government with independent advice on how to simplify the UK tax system. Deloitte and PWC told us that they have seconded staff to work at the Office of Tax Simplification. The Office, however, is under-resourced and employs fewer than six full time staff. So far it has focused on the deletion of tax reliefs which are not used. To make headway it needs sufficient resources to take a more radical approach to simplifying UK tax law (House of Commons 2013, p. 12).

The above statement points to a cruel and widening power imbalance between tax authorities and the most powerful corporations. While the State has been, from the Late Middle Ages to the mid-twentieth century, the most powerful corporate agent and a guarantor of equality in relation to the law, the situation is dramatically different in Late Modernity. The largest accountancy firms, but also their clients and numerous financial agents are comparatively much better resourced than the state. Even more worryingly, the fact that Deloitte and PWC seconded staff to help the Tax Office indicates that the relation of dependency and domination has now been

---

[9]See for instance the Competitiveness of the UK Tax Administration Review. Accessible on https://www.gov.uk/government/publications/competitiveness-of-uk-tax-administration-review (checked 29 Apr 2015).

[10]http://www.irs.gov/pub/irs-soi/06rastg12overvw.pdf (checked 29 Apr 2015).

reversed. It is now the state that needs the support of powerful private corporate agents to maintain codified tax rules that are operational for the majority of less powerful agents.

In sum, the preceding analysis is presented mainly for illustrative purposes. It offers but an extremely sketchy picture of the situation and issues of tax evasion in Late Modernity. It indicates, however, that the combination of unbound morphogenesis with literally interpreted codified rules tends to generate perverse spirals, which are at once overly beneficial for those already powerful and detrimental for the majority. What remedies are currently proposed? To this question I now dedicate this section's last part.

Remedies Currently Under Consideration

The general analysis above of the perverse effects of morphogenesis unbound on the fairness of codified rules also indicates areas where remedial action can be sought. For clarity's sake, I focus the analysis on the case of tax evasion and base much of the argument on the enquiry conducted by the British House of Commons' Public Accounting Committee with the heads of tax operations in the UK's top four accountancy firms. The core of this enquiry is constituted by the examination as witnesses of the heads of tax operations of the four major global accountancy firms (Ernst, KPMG, Deloitte and PWC).

Most of the mechanisms I identify, however, are generalizable or relevant to other cases combining literally interpreted codified rules and unbound social morphogenesis. They can be roughly categorised into three different types of measures: legal reform at the national level, international collaborations, and the encouragement of interpretations according to the spirit, rather than the letter, of the law. The report and interviews can be consulted on http://tinyurl.com/bwjc7ge.[11]

The National Level: An Obsolete Unit of Analysis?

We can observe several actions initiated at the national level by the legal authorities against fiscally aggressive activities. First, a permanent chase to close those loopholes revealed by the (relatively few) schemes uncovered and the prosecution of their users. However, this chase is limited by two mechanisms. First, to be operative, they suppose international multilateral agreements that are likely to take, in the estimates of the Committee of Public Accounts, a decade at least to negotiate, while in the meantime leaving free-rein to multinational corporations. National legislative amendment alone is insufficient even to bring about laws as obvious as those requiring that corporations operating over the internet (e.g. Amazon.co.uk and

[11]Last accessed on 29 Apr 2015.

google.co.uk) be taxed where they generate profits, employ people and sell goods rather than where their servers are located.

Second, while calls for 'simplification' and 'transparency' are ritualistically reiterated by all actors (including the big accountancy firms), the national tax authorities of all countries – except perhaps the USA – lack the human resources needed to analyse detailed information from corporations operating on their territory.[12] Furthermore, a broader look indicates that the imbalance of human and financial means between tax collector and tax payer may be even harsher than the report suggests. Indeed, the latter focuses on the firms of accountants and ignores their clients' considerable internal resources.[13]

In this configuration, it is not surprising that most suggestions presented by the Public Accounts Committee to the big four accountancy firms were dismissed as overly complicated by the latter who proposed instead to collect aggregated information. When firms of accountants and their clients are far better resourced than the state, the latter is unable to analyse, and determine when it is appropriate to challenge non-aggregated information from the former. How information should be aggregated, and whether the aggregation would create new loopholes was not clarified, however, by the public enquiry.

International Conventions: The Problem of the Weakest Link?

Most solutions considered against tax evasion or aggressive optimisation involve international collaboration at some point. Yet, although all the governments on the Globe seem to agree that tax evasion *from* their country should be fought, the opposition of interests between nations slows down attempts at multilateral or even bilateral initiative. The USA opened the way through the Foreign Accounts Tax Compliance Act (FATCA), a series of bi-lateral agreements through which non-US

[12]In the words of the Public Accounts Committee:

> HMRC is not able to defend the public interest effectively when its resources are more limited than those enjoyed by the big four firms. The four firms employ almost 9000 people as part of their UK tax practice. For instance HMRC has 65 transfer pricing specialists whereas the big four firms alone have around 250. In our report on tackling marketed avoidance schemes we found that HMRC does not know what level of resource it commits to tackling tax avoidance. Government must ensure that HMRC is properly resourced to challenge the advice given by the four firms and others to companies and individuals seeking to aggressively avoid tax (House of Commons 2013, p.6).

[13]So considerable are the internal resources of multinational corporate clients that, in the words of one of the senior auditors.

> '**Q232 Ian Swales:** Would you personally accompany the client to discussions at HMRC at that point? Is that a thing a tax partner would do?
>
> ***Jane McCormick:*** If my client asked me to, but actually, most of my clients do not. They are big organisations and do not feel they need an adviser if they have to talk to HMRC' (House of Commons 2013, p.44).

countries agree to share financial information with the US tax authorities about US citizens holding a bank account on their territory.

At the time of writing this paper, about 50 countries have ratified FATCA and it has entered into force in 9 of these countries (including such tax havens as the UK and Switzerland). Moreover, a similar initiative was launched by OECD (the Common Reporting Standard) in 2014. At the time of writing, 47 countries have agreed to implement it, starting in 2017.

While such initiatives are likely to contribute towards a reduction of tax evasion, and while their fast growth is promising, they are unlikely to be truly effective unless all countries on the planet participate in them. Moreover, the greater the number of countries signing such conventions, the higher become the financial opportunities for the remaining countries who did not sign them. Thus, tensions can be expected at some point between signatories and non-signatories or, among signatories, between those complying scrupulously and those who are less scrupulous.

Further Regulating the Experts?

The British House of Commons' Committee of Public Accounts' 44th report hints that improvement might be obtained by regulating further the activities of large accountancy firms. For instance, many senior auditors keep close ties with the government and engage in 'revolving doors tactics' consisting in spending periods of time working for the government before going back to private activities and advising tax payers.[14]

Another mechanism identified by the same Committee consists in regulating the type of services that may be offered by firms of accountants and which currently continue to sell schemes 'with as little as 50 % chance of succeeding if challenged in court'. Yet, the same report does not address or clarify whether or not the clients could continue to benefit from advice provided by offshore branches of the same consultancies.

Finally, the chair of the PAC mentions a number of regulations for accountants in her oral examination of witnesses, for instance, separating their auditing and tax advice activities or banning tax advisers from participating in public markets.

The lengthy hearings of the auditors also reveal attempts from the Panel's Chair to appeal to the accountants' sense of substantive normativity. Thus, on several occasions, she insists that lost cases indicate wrong (rather than merely mistaken) judgements or that their practices in giving tax advice are not conducive

[14]As the House of Commons' Committee of Public Accounts' report puts it.

> 'we have seen what look like cases of poacher, turned gamekeeper, turned poacher again, whereby individuals who advise government go back to their firms and advise their clients on how they can use those laws to reduce the amount of tax they pay' (House of Commons 2013: 4).

to the greater good.[15] The response of the accountants is, however, depressing for anyone hoping for a reaction indicating sophisticated normative reflexivity. They unanimously repeat, as a mantra, that they are 'incredibly proud' of their firm and that they make a 'fantastic contribution to society'. Moreover, it takes a long, and almost surrealistic, exchange before the head of one of the accountancy firms admitted (very reluctantly) that court judgements indicate not only that 'the interpretation of the law proved to be wrong' but also that the actions performed were unlawful.

The resulting impression is that of accountants who combine remarkable intellectual faculties of instrumentally and formally rational analysis coupled with a weak and almost childish substantive reflexivity based on simplistic notions. In their morally impoverished discourse: 'helping clients' is good and legal judgements indicate that 'the interpretation of the law proved wrong'. Little room is left for critique or ethical reflection proper. This is interesting since, while the literature on business ethics criticises the simplistic equation of the legal and the legitimate often performed by corporate managers (and management students), it seems that these professionals dealing with law displace the denial of ethical reflection one step further by considering that even negative legal judgements are not indicative of unethical behaviour. However, such scepticism towards the legal order is less troubling than the absence of normative questioning it seems to signal.

Encouraging Interpretations According to the Spirit?

Since the Inland Revenue Commissioner versus Duke of Westminster case in 1936, it has been a guiding principle in British tax law that individuals were free to arrange their affairs in such way as to optimise or avoid tax. Thus, until recently, tax law has been interpreted in the most literal sense possible. Since the end of the twentieth century, however, a more purposive approach to tax law seems to have been increasingly advocated. Braithwaite (2002) encouraged such a transformation as a development necessary to break the vicious circle of tax avoidance, legislative response and renewed tax avoidance through novel loopholes. The interpretive approach to law combines intentionally loosely drafted legislation with enhanced powers of interpretation attributed to judges. Thus, the judge is not merely expected to analyse the congruence of each legally recognisable action with the code of law. S/he is also expected to take a position on the combination of acts as a whole, especially when the individual actions seem to have no commercial purpose.

While countries such as Canada have effectively implemented General Anti Avoidance Rules (GAAR) that allow judges to ignore corporate arrangements

[15]At one moment, the House of Commons' Panel's chair even exclaims:

Q225 Chair: I think you are a bunch of really clever people. You are clever, well remunerated and very experienced, I have no doubt of that. What depresses me is that you could contribute so much to society and the public good and you all choose to focus on an area that reduces the resources available for us to build schools, hospitals and transport infrastructure. You choose that, and I do not get it. I do not know why you do it (House of Commons 2013, Ev. 23).

which are motivated by tax-optimising rather than business purposes, these are still under scrutiny and debate in others such as the UK. Norton (2012) for instance offers a critical and philosophically informed interpretation of the debate and of its stakes. He identifies a move away from what he identifies as a liberal Kantian approach towards a 'communitarian' or 'Hegelian' approach which pictures state and individual in dialectical struggle. Norton remarks insightfully that General Anti Avoidance Rules bear on the role and practices of accountants. As he puts it:

> Professional advisors are no longer able to give guidance in a tax optimal manner with absolute certainty that, provided there is literal compliance with the relevant statutory provision, there is no risk of them being 'unravelled' or disaggregated by the judiciary at a future time. In this regard accountants must become more nuanced in their advice, and less absolute or certain in their recommendations (Sikka and Willmott 1995). As knowledge experts they are required to be significantly more adaptive or 'fleet of foot' in an environment in which legal parameters are more susceptible to extra-parliamentary change in the future and, of greater concern, in the past through the use of retrospective legislation. Instead, in the new context of principles-based interpretation, accountants must strive to justify purpose rather than exclusively form in multi-component tax structures. (Norton 2012: 118, see also Alexander and Jermakowicz 2006)

Moreover, Norton's position is critical of GAAR requiring from judges interpretation of the spirit of the law as it was intended by parliament. His arguments are firstly that judges tend to respond through a cautious and self-limiting approach through which they also tend to interpret cases in favour of the tax-payer rather than in favour of the state. And secondly, GAAR constitutes a de facto delegation of legislative power to the judiciary and therefore violates the principle of the separation of powers, which could lead to a slippage similar to the Enabling Law of 1933 that freed the executive from parliamentary oversight in Nazi Germany.

The imbalances of power theorised in this section run against Norton's argument that relies on judges' self-limiting tendencies, unless one expects GAAR to open the door for ample practices of magistrate corruption by powerful corporate agents. Yet, while such corruption is not implausible, it is not clear how the result would generate less tax avoidance than is presently the case.

Moreover, Norton's worry about the authoritarian slippages seems exaggerated and he provides very little detail of the processes through which encouraging judges to use their common sense in tax questions could lead to a *coup d'Etat*. If anything, Hitler's coup was secured through the physical intimidation of members of parliament rather than through a purely ideological slippage of legislation. Norton's worries might be symptomatic of a TINA (there is no alternative) conservative ideology that favours the status quo, the rich and the powerful. His more general point, however, deserves consideration. As we have seen in the section on "How do agents cope with rules' fundamental incompleteness?" above, interpretations according to the spirit of the law are likely to be particularly contested in societies characterised by relatively ambivalent social integration in which consensus can only be expected over broadly defined values.

Conclusion

This chapter sought to provide a theoretical complement to Archer's contribution in the same volume. While she provides a clear historical thread and many empirical examples that are missing from my paper, I seek to provide as much clarification as I can on how the (ontological) natures of morphogenesis and codified rules make the latter more difficult to interpret when the former is at play.

Morphogenesis unbound presents novel problems for the interpretation of codified social rules. The problems identified in this paper are explicable in terms of the modalities of social and systemic integration in Late Modernity. On the one hand, reliable interpretation according to the spirit presupposes homogeneous social integration across society. Yet this social integration is missing as soon as we are dealing with non-trivial issues (see the section "How do agents cope with rules' fundamental incompleteness?"). In the absence of social integration it is not surprising to witness a multiplication of codified rules where agreements based on trust and honour would have sufficed in a not-so-distant past.

On the other hand, interpretation according to the letter of the law is sustainable only if contextual continuity is assured, or at least if the speed of the authorities issuing rules exceeds that of free-riders. And yet, we have seen in the section on "The social conditions of rule interpretation in late modernity" that the contemporary configuration falls short of fulfilling this condition. A minority of actors seem capable of moving faster than the law and can draw a competitive advantage from fast-changing, complex, codes of legislation. The vast majority of actors – including the state, SMEs and most individuals – are burdened, however, with ever longer codes of legislation.

References

Al-Amoudi, I. (2010). Immanent non-algorithmic rules: An ontological study of social rules. *Journal for the Theory of Social Behaviour, 40*(3), 289–313.

Al-Amoudi, I. (2014). Morphogenesis and normativity: Problems the former creates for the latter. In M. S. Archer (Ed.), *Late modernity: Trajectories towards morphogenic society*. Cham, New York: Springer.

Al-Amoudi, I., & Latsis, J. (2015). Death contested: Morphonecrosis and conflicts of interpretation. In M. S. Archer (Ed.), *Generative mechanisms transforming late modernity*. New York: Springer.

Alexander, D., & Jermakowicz, E. (2006). A true and fair view of the principles/rules debate. *Abacus, 42*(2), 132–164.

Alvesson, M., & Willmott, H. (2002). Identity regulation as organizational control: Producing the appropriate individual. *Journal of Management Studies, 39*(5), 619–644.

Archer, M. S. (1985). The myth of cultural integration. *The British Journal of Sociology, 36*(3), 333–353.

Archer, M. S. (1995). *Realist social theory: The morphogenetic approach*. Cambridge: Cambridge University Press.

Archer, M. S. (2003). *Structure, agency and the internal conversation*. Cambridge: Cambridge University Press.
Archer, M. S. (2007). *Making our way through the world*. Cambridge: Cambridge University Press.
Archer, M. S. (2012). *The reflexive imperative in late modernity*. Cambridge: Cambridge University Press.
Archer, M. S. (2014). The generative mechanism reconfiguring late modernity. In M. S. Archer (Ed.), *Late modernity: Trajectories towards morphogenic society*. Cham, New York: Springer.
Archer, M. S. (2016). A normative social regulation: the attempt to cope with social morphogenesis. In M. S. Archer (Ed.), *Normativity and the crisis of social morphogenesis*. New York: Springer.
Boltanski, L., & Thévenot, L. (2006). *On justification: Economies of worth*. Princeton: Princeton University Press.
Braithwaite, J. (2002). Rules and principles: A theory of legal certainty. *Australian Journal of Legal Philosophy, 27*, 47–82.
Dean, M. (2010). *Governmentality: Power and rule in modern society*. London: Sage.
Durkheim, E. (1892/1953). *Montesquieu et Rousseau, précurseurs de la sociologie. Note introductive de Georges Davy*. Paris: M. Rivière.
Ewing, S. (1987). Formal justice and the spirit of capitalism: Max Weber's sociology of law. *Law and Society Review, 21*(3), 487–512.
Fleming, P. (2009). *Authenticity and the cultural politics of work. New forms of informal control*. Oxford: Oxford University Press.
Fleming, P., & Sturdy, A. (2009). "Just be yourself!": Towards neo-normative control in organisations? *Employee Relations, 31*(6), 569–583.
Fleming, P., & Sturdy, A. (2011). Being yourself in the electronic sweatshop: New forms of normative control. *Human Relations, 64*, 177–200.
Foucault, M. (1977). *Discipline and punish: The birth of the prison*. New York: Random House LLC.
Henry, J. S. (2012). *The price of offshore revisited*. Document prepared for the Tax Justice Network.http://www.taxjustice.net/cms/upload/pdf/Price_of_Offshore_Revisited_120722.pdf. Last accessed 29 Apr 2015.
House of Commons. (2013). *Tax avoidance: The role of large accountancy firms*. http://www.publications.parliament.uk/pa/cm201213/cmselect/cmpubacc/870/87002.htm. Accessed 29 Apr 2015.
King, A. (1999). Against structure: A critique of morphogenetic social theory. *The Sociological Review, 47*(2), 199–227.
Kripke, S. A. (1982). *Wittgenstein on rules and private language: An elementary exposition*. Oxford: Blackwell.
Kunda, G. (1992). *Engineering culture: Control and commitment in a high-tech corporation*. Philadlephia: Temple University Press.
Kusch, M. (2006). *A sceptical guide to meaning and rules: Defending Kripke's Wittgenstein*. Chesham: Acumen.
Lockwood, D. (1964). Social integration and system integration. In G. K. Zollschan & W. Hirsch (Eds.), *Explorations in social change* (pp. 244–258). London: Routledge & Paul Kegan.
Mead, G. H. (1967). *Mind, self and society from the standpoint of a social behaviourist*. Chicago: University of Chicago Press.
Montesquieu. (1748). *De l'esprit des lois*. Available on http://classiques.uqac.ca/classiques/montesquieu/de_esprit_des_lois/de_esprit_des_lois_tdm.html (checked 29 Apr 2015).
Morgan, J. (2011). Ethos and reform of the finance systems, a tentative argument. *Real-World Economic Review, 58*, 89–94.
Norton, S. D. (2012). Judicial interpretation of the will of the state: A Hegelian perspective in the context of taxation. *Critical Perspectives on Accounting, 23*(2), 117–133.
Porpora, D. V. (1993). Cultural rules and material relations. *Sociological Theory, 11*(2), 212–229.
Porpora, D. V. (2001). *Landscapes of the soul: The loss of moral meaning in American life*. New York: Oxford University Press.

Porpora, D. V. (2015). Why don't things change? The matter of morphostasis. In M. S. Archer (Ed.), *Generative mechanisms transforming the social order*. New York: Springer.

Prakash, G. (1999). *Another reason: Science and the modern imagination of India*. Princeton: Princeton University Press.

Rawls, J. (2001). *Justice as fairness, a restatement*. Cambridge, MA/London: The Belknap Press of Harvard University Press.

Sikka, P., & Willmott, H. (1995). Illuminating the state-profession relationship: Accountants acting as department of trade and industry's investigators. *Critical Perspectives on Accounting, 6*(4), 341–369.

Weber, M. (1978). *Economy and society: An outline of interpretive sociology*. Berkeley: University of California Press.

Wittgenstein, L. (1958). *Philosophical investigations*. Oxford: Oxford University Press.

Chapter 7
Anormative Social Regulation: The Attempt to Cope with Social Morphogenesis

Margaret S. Archer

Introduction

Social morphogenesis is intensifying in late Modernity and is currently transforming the contours of social stratification, altering the workings of all major social institutions, and impacting negatively upon societal integration. In turn, these changes pose novel problems for legal regulation in general and for its justification. Traditionally, the philosophy of law has treated legal justifiability in two ways and both are dependent upon morphostasis: either upon the stability of societal structuring or on the durability of socio-cultural conventions and most frequently on some combination of the two. Neither morphostatic source can continue to operate as once was held because social structures and social conventions also become changeable once intense morphogenesis has engaged societally. In other words, they cannot be regarded as fixed points around which other morphogenetic transformations swirl.

Radical social change accompanied by changes in the law has always been problematic in legal philosophy since it challenges the presumed grounding of lasting legal *validity* in lasting *social normativity*. French Revolutionary law, itself swiftly displaced by the Napoleonic Code, proved exercising in practice for other independent States (when or whether to recognize either) and still more so in the philosophy of law (what validated one or the other, since both broke with previous social norms but were at variance with each other). Yet if legitimacy was denied to them, then validity was also withheld from these novel laws. Consequently, each new legal corpus would have had to be deemed a matter of coercion alone. Conversely, if legality was granted to either (and it became more difficult to withhold as the Imperial Code was quickly spread to Napoleon's European conquests where

M.S. Archer (✉)
Centre for Social Ontology, University of Warwick, Coventry, UK
e-mail: margaret.archer@warwick.ac.uk

M.S. Archer (eds.), *Morphogenesis and the Crisis of Normativity*,
Social Morphogenesis, DOI 10.1007/978-3-319-28439-2_7

it was not ephemeral), then legal validity did not seem reliant upon its grounding in the normativity particular to every nation state.

Already, various problems have clustered around the generic notion of *social regulation being based upon lasting social normativity*: from the implications of morphostasis versus morphogenesis for legal stability or change to the *actuality* of law (considered valid by some when actually in force in a particular social setting) versus the *legitimacy* of law (whose validity, to others, could only derive from conventional morality). These are central to the 'problem of normativity'. At its most *general, normativity concerns the role that society's moral or value system, norms and conventions play in social regulation.*

Traditionally, both legal and social theorists had made recourse to such forms of normativity to account for the 'bindingness' or crucial sense of obligation held to inhere in the law.[1] Fundamentally, it was shared normativity that put the 'ought' into social action and accounted for legal conformity. But which way round did it work? Was it shared normativity that orchestrated social change, or did social transformation engender changes in norms and values? This remained the central problem for legal and social theorists alike, as was argued in the Introductory Chapter.

The morphogenetic approach does not treat this central problem in either/or terms, siding neither with Durkheim's conviction that changes in the 'collective conscience' *followed* the transformation in the division of labour from early segmented societies to modern functionally differentiated ones,[2] nor with Kelsen (in the bulk of his work), to whom legal regulation *derived* from its rooting in a foundational 'groundnorm' that underwrote its normative validity (Kelsen 1945). The reason for not taking sides is principled: the explanation of any social phenomenon whatsoever always comes in a SAC because it must incorporate the interplay between Structure, Culture and Agency, rather than causal primacy automatically being accorded to one of them, as was assumed by Durkheim and Kelsen in opposed ways. Given the complexities of this inter-disciplinary debate, it seems best if I now spell out the three main propositions that will be advanced and defended in this chapter.

(a) To most legal philosophers the connection between Law and normativity is fundamentally morphostatic and works in terms of negative feedback between them. To philosophers of social science – at least to nearly all the present contributors – the relationship today is morphogenetic, with positive feedback amplifying both legal and normative changes, without assuring their compatibility.

[1]Since Pufendorf (1964 [1688]), the obligation attaching to or the binding character of the law was the key element to be understood.

[2]Durkheim's position was nuanced by his concern that the Third Republic in France required substantial increases in civic morals and moral education as essential normative reinforcements in order to produce a stable and just society. See the last chapter of *The Division of Labour* dealing with remedies for its pathologies.

(b) The generative mechanism that I ventured and developed in the last two Volumes[3] also accounts for the rapid demise of any shared normative system, resulting in tensions within Cultural Systems and the heterogeneity of Socio-Cultural influences from different sections of the (global) population in conflict with one another.[4] Amongst the consequences of this mechanism are reductions in social integration, an increasing deficit in social solidarity, a growing 'macro-moral disconnect'[5] between religious/ethical systems and members of society, all of which have negative repercussions upon the traditional normative components of the legal order: the law, norms/rules, conventions, customs and etiquette.

(c) All five elements above are held to be giving way to the 'Anormative Regulation' of the contemporary social order or, if preferred, its 'Bureaucratic Regulation' – replete with Weber's 'iron bars'. In other words, normativity plays a much reduced role in furnishing guidelines for social action because the law and social custom diminish proportionately in relation to non-normative forms of regulative social control.

The processes and consequences of such Anormative Regulation in its various guises will be traced for different levels and activities in the social order before asking, in conclusion, if these are *necessarily* the case for any society that is undoubtedly undergoing intense morphogenesis.

As social change has intensified over the last three decades as a consequence of the synergy between digital science and economic financialization, novel opportunities for crime have created a novel problem for legislative regulation, namely 'how to keep up?' This inverts the traditional relationship between the legal order and the social order. Increasingly, the law lags behind innovative malfeasance and, since variety generates more variety in ways that are unpredictable, it outdistances the possibility of jurisprudence ever catching up. There are two legal alternatives. Either the law can try to 'run faster', but this inflates the quantity of legislation and still remains a retrospective tidying up operation. This has been attempted and abandoned. For example, between 1983 and 2009 the British Parliament approved over 100 criminal justice bills and over 4,000 new criminal offences were created. In response to that trend, the Ministry of Justice established a procedure to limit the designation of new crimes (Cabinet Office 2013). In fact, the volume of Government primary legislation diminished between 1979 and 2009, whilst the quantity of Statutory Instruments augmented (House of Lords 2011). The latter is the alternative to futile legislative frenzy. It consists in an increasing cascade of regulations, passing

---

[3]This is the synergy developing around 1980 between digital science and multinational/financialized capitalism and its consequences for late modernity. (See Archer 2014a, 2015).

[4]For the distinction between the C.S. (which concerns the type of logical relations between the corpus of ideas available) and the S-C (which concerns the relations of power and influence between protagonists of each set of ideas upon others) see Archer (1988) and the Introduction to this Volume.

[5]Douglas V. Porpora coined this term in Porpora et al. (2013) and he uses it in this Volume.

downwards through a plethora of Agencies, culminating in increased bureaucratic rather than legal regulation. The next section is devoted to the growth and role of administrative regulation[6] in late modernity, focusing upon its morphogenetic importance in relation to earlier hegemonic forms of socio-legal regulation.

Why Morphogenesis and Normativity Part Company

Bureaucratic Regulation as Anormative Social Regulation

Historically, legal philosophy and social theory have cut the same very broad theoretical swathe from early societies to the social order at the beginning of this millennium when accounting for social regulation. Despite considerable variations and deviations not examined here, this is a trajectory where 'culture' is gradually displaced from the driving seat and steering the social order once (Durkheimian) 'organic solidarity' prevailed, diminishing further with 'the diversity of morals' (Ginsberg 1962)[7] and yet further as it confronted *fin de siècle* 'multiculturalism'.

Although fragmentation can be exaggerated if it makes no allowance for the growth in international law, human rights law, and the definition of new universal legal prohibitions (for example, 'Crimes against Humanity'), all the same these developments do not nullify the fragmenting bindingness of normativity in most parts of the life-world (locally, regionally, generationally, sexually, ethnically, linguistically etc.) and that the bonds of social solidarity have shrunk accordingly. This is what Doug Porpora has persuasively and pertinently diagnosed as the 'macro-moral disconnect', where the guidelines for behaviour show a growing detachment from systems of social normativity (religious and secular alike), which are increasingly confined to the private domain (Porpora 2001, 2013).

Within in our lifetimes, the phrase 'rules and regulations' was common in ordinary speech; one aspect of the bigger 'moral disconnect' is that they have come apart. Today, 'regulations' – which are one form of rules – are not accompanied by normative justification and a sense of obligation has been displaced among those conforming to them, along with feelings 'shame' for or 'guilt' about their infringement. Instead, these moral responses have been replaced by considerations of escaping detection, cost-benefit analysis of the price of the fine versus one's personal convenience (for those who can afford it) and a general disgruntlement about intrusion. This is what I mean by social regulation having become increasingly anormative. What remains to be done in the present section is to *justify attributing this social tendency to morphogenesis.*

[6]The terms 'bureaucratic' and 'administrative' regulation are used interchangeably in this chapter and 'bureaucratic' does not refer to Public Bureaucracies alone.

[7]An evolutionary exploration that is matched by many in legal philosophy texts on moral development (Joyce 2007; Krebs 2011; Tony Lawson's Chap. 11, in this Volume).

However, firstly it is necessary to detail in what ways 'regulations' differ from laws by their absence of grounding in any normative appeal – or sometimes the palest nominal one. In other words, their very *anormativity* has to be substantiated before moving on to discuss why bureaucratic regulation is the resort of so many agencies (not confined to governmental authorities), given the intensity of morphogenetic change in late Modernity.

A preliminary caveat and a caution are necessary; the distinctions between Government, Public Administration, Regulatory agencies and Independent ones plus the self-assumed powers of entirely Private agencies[8] vary in different countries for historico-structural reasons.[9] Thus, crude comparative metrics such as the number of laws passed or of civil servants employed, need to be taken in the context of the consistent growth of administrative bodies in the twentieth century's developed world (as governments assumed new responsibilities in welfare and taxation etc.). However in the 1980s, independent authorities mushroomed, fostered by neo-liberalism, which produced a great wave of privatisation, contracting-out and outsourcing, that many held required regulatory measures. Nevertheless, there is an important distinction between regulatory agencies that are usually a part of the executive branch of government and answerable to legal review, compared with 'Independent Regulatory Agencies'. For example, France differentiates *autorités administratives indépendantes* (*AAI*), which may not be instructed or ordered to take specific actions by government from others that can.[10]

The main reasons given for this proliferation and corresponding shift in the balance of power, often held to represent a fragmentation of the state, are similar for different countries. They are summarized in a Cabinet Office paper (2013), significantly entitled 'When Laws become too complex', showing that from 1979 laws have decreased in number, though increasing in volume, whilst Statutory Instruments have more than doubled from the late 1980s to 2006. Complexity reflects the increased expertise required, especially in sensitive or highly technical sectors. Casini's choice of words is revealing of the shift from '*legitimacy*', the historic pre-occupation of legal philosophy, to the fact that for these proliferating and differentiating bodies, 'their *legitimation* resides in the need for expertness and advanced technical competence' (Casini 2007: 21). It is here that the connection with the novel practices and techniques introduced through morphogenesis in the last three decades is situated.

---

[8]Such as the British hotel that unilaterally imposed fines on clients who posted negative reviews of it by deducting £100 from their credit cards (BBC Radio 4, 19.11.2014).

[9]For example, Woodrow Wilson's famous essay (1887) 'The Study of Administration', emphasized 'the separation of politics and administration', but this dichotomy remains contentious and delineated differently from state to state.

[10]The same principle of independence obtains in the U.S., e.g. the Federal Trade Commission, defined as a body of experts working 'independent of executive authority, except in its selection, and free to exercise its judgement without the leave or hindrance of any official or any department of government' (Casini 2011: 20).

However, it is salutary to note that within legal studies, where the growth of regulatory bodies has captured considerable attention, discussion has been restricted to an 'in house' debate about whether or not their increase subtracts from the powers of the state through 'decentering' control and results in its 'polycentricity', often referred to as the 'hollowing out of the state'. This is a debate largely without a social context because, at most, references are made to the changing political philosophies of those in Office. Moreover, the concern of 'regulatory studies' is with the workings of regulation in terms of 'good governance' or the opposite, rather than with the explanation of its growth, social form or relation to normativity.[11] Considerations of efficacy and efficiency displace the latter. Consequently, there is little meeting point between this corpus of work and my present concerns. Perhaps it is worth briefly outlining the three main positions adopted in 'regulation studies', which are broadly sequential, in order to account for why they are of little service to the sociological issues under discussion.

(a) Regulation by 'command and control' (CAC) is the preserve of the state, using legal rules backed by criminal sanctions. 'It is "centred" in that it assumes the state to have the capacity to command and control, to be the only commander and controller, and to be potentially effective in commanding and controlling. It is assumed to be unilateral in its approach (governments telling, others doing), based on simple cause-effect relations, and envisaging a linear progression from policy formation through to implementation.' (Black 2001: 106). These substantive assumptions are rejected here and also by those advocating position (b).
(b) Conversely, in the 'decentred understanding of regulation, regulation happens in the absence of formal legal sanction – it is the product of interactions not the exercise of the formal, constitutionally recognized authority of government' (Rhodes 1997). Partly based on the manifest failures of CAC, partly on the simple recognition that regulation has many locales (polycentrism), taking place 'in many rooms' (Nader and Nader 1985), and partly on Teubner's anti-centrist systems theory (Teubner 1993: 19–34), this popular approach also eschews any explanatory generative mechanism producing decentred regulation and settles for a list of contributory factors such as 'complexity', 'fragmentation of government', 'loss of steering power', 'new knowledge', 'novel networks' and so forth, whose permutations result in diverse sources of prescriptions.
(c) Finally, there is the millennial hybrid that combines the above positions, by accentuating the combination of institutional centralization with decentred regulation. Hence, in the quest for enhanced steering capacity, Moran argues that the state spearheads a 'drive towards synoptic legibility: installing systems

[11]Typical of this genre is Robert Baldwin (2005: 5) whose 'Is better regulation smarter regulation' dwells upon the Blairite move away from 'deregulation' (of business), and towards 'Better Regulation'. Contextual references are confined to the statement that 'UK governments have given high priority to reducing unnecessary legislative requirements ever since the modern movement to reform regulation commenced in 1985'.

of comprehensive reporting and surveillance over numerous social spheres; the consequential pressure to standardize and to codify, which is to make explicit what had hitherto been tacit; and the creation of new institutions (notably specialized regulatory agency) to help enforce all of this'; the best example being the Financial Services Authority in Britain (Moran 2004). As his title indicates, *The British Regulatory State: High Modernism and Hyper Innovation*, Moran's preoccupations come closest to my own, but not his conclusions. The development of what he terms 'meta-regulators' would represent a 'thickening of the centre' (Black 2007:4), meaning an enhanced role for the Treasury and Cabinet Office in Britain. However, are these not most effective against the weaker self-regulating groups (the professions), and ineffectual where advanced research with unknown applications is concerned (genetic engineering). Equally, isn't the professed aim of giving regulators a significant degree of operational autonomy a confession of governments' inability to regulate the regulators (state and non-state) in a co-ordinated manner? Finally, 'hyper innovation' (the result of the synergy I have already discussed) is neither going to go away nor to become predictable. It would leave any 'meta-regulator' in the same position as the law – running faster to catch up but necessarily remaining behind.[12]

The unhelpfulness of these positions (a) to (c) can ultimately be attributed to their empiricism. Such 'tendencies' are merely extrapolations from current data; there is no mention of generative mechanisms. All the same, it was hoped that this corpus of literature would have furnished a brief lexicon of fairly consensual and useable definitions. Yet as Black admits, 'definitional chaos is almost seen as an occupational hazard by those who write about regulation' and she provides a long and helpful guide to the variety of usages (Black 2001: 129–144).[13] Instead, I have resorted to self-help in the Ideal Type that follows, with the aim being to accentuate the most salient features that are distinctive of 'anormative regulation', without pretending to exhaustiveness or to having eliminated all overlap with other concepts. The bullet points below are intended to initiate a discussion of administrative regulation that is at least partially constitutive of the 'macro-moral disconnect', but they are hardly the last word.

---

[12]Those who advocate the advent of a tough new administrative law are falling into the same trap.

[13]Compare the following three definitions:

1. To the OECD regulation is 'the full range of legal instruments by which governing institutions, at all levels of government, impose obligations or constraints on private sector behaviour. Constitutions, parliamentary laws, subordinate legislation, decrees, orders, norms, licenses, plans, codes and even some forms of administrative guidance can all be considered as 'regulation'' (OECD 1995)
2. To the UK government's Better Regulation Taskforce, regulation is 'any government measure or intervention that seeks to change the behaviour of individuals or groups, so including taxes, subsidies and other financial measures'. (BRT undated)
3. Hall et al. (1999) provide the broadest and vaguest definition when they simply talk of people being regulated by culture.

- Regulations do not attempt to meet any form of 'normativity requirement', legal, conventional or personal (such as Korsgaard's 'reflective endorsement' 1996, 2009), but are the means of avoiding such appeals, yet they still remain regulatory.
- Regulations exert a *causal force* not a *moral one*. They are unrelated to the approbation, approval or assent of those to whom they apply (in some of their actions), but whose agreement to any given regulation is rarely directly sought. Derision from the population in question is a more likely response (to, for example, the intricacies of refuse collection) but not one associated with a high rate of non-compliance.
- Regulations do contain 'normative operators', words such as 'ought' or 'must' and is 'required'/'prohibited' or 'permitted' under certain conditions. However, they work – insofar as they do – through the instrumental rationality of the subjects in question, who feel no obligation but, rather, are calculative or prudential in their responses according to their means.
- Regulations have a heteronomous character, depending upon fines, penalizations and prohibitions, which are punitive without the subject concerned incurring either a criminal record or involving social sanction.
- Regulations have to be actual (it would sound odd to talk of the 'dead letter of the regulation'), but they can be displaced and replaced overnight without any appeal to the 'democratic defence of validity' (see my Chap. 1).
- Regulations do not necessarily stem from authorities within the legal order or that of their officers. Many do (as in planning regulations), but many others originate from retailers (concerning conditions for return, reimbursement or recompense for products), train and bus services, private utilities, landlords (no pets), hotels, companies, banks, financial services, libraries and taxi drivers. The law may or may not uphold any of the above.
- Regulations do not depend upon such social conventions as do maintain; indeed, often their avowed aim is the opposite, as in combatting discriminatory practices or policing acceptable vocabulary and behaviour. (It is not illegal to swear, conventionally many do, but we are sternly warned not to affront railway personnel or cabin crew in this way). *In fact, convention is now more frequently re-made by regulation than* vice versa.
- Regulations are basically concerned with the social co-ordination of action and practices rather than with issues of social co-operation or re-distribution. As such, they are at most binding (without entailing a sense of obligation) but never socially bonding. Hence the connection with a decline in social integration.
- Regulations differ from laws or other forms of rules in terms of what makes them social. In the latter cases, this depends upon their internal relations within complexes of roles and rules. For example, postmen/women do not read the mail of recipients (Al-Amoudi 2010). Conversely, bureaucratic regulations have an external not an internal social impact. What makes them social is simply that people (largely) behave in conformity to them, thus producing a manifest social regularity.

- Regulations are ultimately intrusive of previously unregulated (or more loosely regulated) domains, such as EU regulation No. 730/1999 on the retail of carrots, banning the public sale of forked specimens or those with secondary roots.

Anormative Social Regulation Takes Over

In forging the link between anormative bureaucratic regulation and the intensification of morphogenesis one socio-political characteristic of regulations is crucial. Regulations themselves can be innovatory, independent of any previous precedent and faster to introduce than legislation. Since they do not rely upon consensus among or consultation with the public affected, neither are they dependent upon the relatively slow development, typical of social conventions and of norms. *This feature recommends their suitability for ready response to the novel changes introduced through morphogenesis and its generic tendency for new variety to generate more variety*. Nevertheless, more than ready regulative capability is required to explain why they became the weapon of preference for governance over the last three decades. In the points listed above, various negative aspects were associated with regulatory governance: its heteronomy, undemocratic imposition, intrusiveness and the arbitrary if not absurd nature of some of its stipulations – as well as their very proliferation. What precipitates governments increasingly to favour administrative regulation over normative legislation, whichever political party is in office? What induces governments broadly to countenance other agencies issuing their own regulations (in commerce, transportation or even animal rescue[14])?

The background answer to the first question was discussed in Volume III (Archer 2015, ch. 7). The post war 'golden age', prior to multinationalism and financialization of the economy was the product of mutual regulation between industrial employers and their workforce, the state of one mattering to that of the other and the two sides enjoying the sponsorship of political parties alternating in government and opposition. Thus, Western democracies could fairly be characterized as 'lib/lab' (Donati 2000).[15] Enduring class differences were mirrored by 'lib' parties favouring neo-liberal policies, in the interests of the middle classes, and 'lab' parties sponsoring redistributive measures, of which welfare provisions were the most important, appealing to ordinary working people. The regular alternation of such parties in government (or the equivalent alternation of centre-right and centre-left coalitions) gave half a loaf of bread in turn to those they represented. In the turn-taking between 'lib/lab' parties, not everything introduced by a predecessor

[14]Now requiring a satisfactory home inspection in Britain.

[15]Donati also uses the term to refer more broadly to the *lib-lab* configuration of society, one that is a compromise between the liberal (lib) side of capitalist markets (free economy) and the socialist (lab) side of the welfare entitlements and 'equal' opportunities funded by the state (political system). See also Chap. 10 in this Volume.

was overturned by the successor when assuming office. However, such mutual regulation between these distinctive political parties was a formula for restrained *morphostasis*.

It did not last because voter turn-out in general elections plummeted throughout Europe as electorates recognised the diminishing powers of national governments, given international finance capitalism, multi-national corporations and supranational institutions such as the EU. A decade later, with the onset of the economic crisis, any residue of 'lib/lab' oscillation had disappeared to be replaced by a politics of 'centrism'. Very few (an exception is Bobbio 1996) still maintained that 'right' and 'left' retained any meaning – unless prefixed by the term 'ultra'. Slogans of the 'We are the 99 %' variety indicated that the economic crisis and the response to it of 'austerity' had eroded the residual class basis of political support in Europe and with it the 'lib' versus 'lab' distinctions between parties. At that point, its successor, 'centrist' politics had no alternative to attempting to cope with the consequences of *morphogenesis* that were no respecters of national boundaries. It was this above all (though not alone) that enhanced the appeal of administrative social regulation.

Politics Without Conviction: From Strategic to Tactical Government

Politics without conviction means a drastic shrinkage (*crispation*) of normativity in political life. Political parties are preoccupied with tactics; with a Saint Simonian 'administration of things' – the day to day management of austerity and the reduction of public spending with minimum backlash – not the 'government of people' based on a normative conception of the good society. Tactical governance, with its 'about turns', absorption in today's latest 'scandal', and the announcement of a 'quick fix', behaves like the fire service attending only to emergency calls. It ejects commitment from the political domain, whether in the form of expansive political philosophies or explicitly normative organizations with a broad conspectus on the good life. Thus, religion in general is banished from the public domain (Trigg 2008, Gorski, Chap. 3, in this volume), henceforth supposed to be a depoliticized matter of private belief and practice. *If functionalists had once held that values articulated every system of social action, they have become the antithesis of today's political aversion towards social normativity.*

Tactical politics favours dealing with (and fostering the development of) increasingly specialized single-issue groups, promoting or defending 'X', who can be allowed voice if and when a scandal concerns the 'X-zone'. Then, the media airing of their views stands for democratic consultation, but otherwise they are left in the wilderness of political lobbying. Tactical governance works through bureaucratic regulation whose highest aims are manifest (meaning measurable) efficiency and effective control. Institutionally, the public domain is carved into decreasingly small pieces, each with its own Regulator, meaning that the problems occurring in any fragment can be addressed technocratically. As a result, the pieces are never put back together and assessed for their coherence, let alone for their contribution to or obstruction of any normative definition of the good society.

Ultimately, politics without conviction generates a huge shrinkage of normativity itself within public life. What matters is that espistemically we, the people, live together in overt 'political correctness'; real ontological differences are not acknowledged, addressed, assisted, or ameliorated, where possible and desirable. This is a semantic displacement manoeuvre. If those lower down the social hierarchy are not addressed as 'plebs', 'slags' or 'pakis', then a veneer of civility conceals the endurance of real inequalities of class, sex or ethnicity. By implication, any form of society could claim to be 'good' provided it had somehow eliminated improper speech. Thus, the role of political correctness is to mute the expression of normative differences and places a stranglehold on their potential to justify demands for greater justice. *Anormative regulation inserts a solid wedge between norms and values.* This is a major means through which the 'macro-moral disconnect' is brought about, but its effects are even more evident at the meso-level.

Social Institutions and Governance by Performance Indicators

From their emergence in Europe, the distinctive feature of the professions was the adherence of each to a specific and demanding code of ethics, departures from which were usually disciplined by a governing body of peers (generally the case for doctors, lawyers, and academics). This ethical regulation, symbolized by the Hippocratic Oath, approximated to a secular vow of service. It both bonded members of a profession together and provided assurance to those they served that the skills in question were being used in their interests and thus that their relationship differed from a market transaction – as illustrated in the stock characters of the family doctor and lawyer. Undoubtedly, personal status accrued to them but it was counter-balanced by obligations (such as doctors turning out in the middle of the night). It was this version of institutionalized professionalism to which those Etzioni (1969) termed the 'semi-professionals' had aspired (teachers, nurses, social workers etc.), as they sought certificated and later graduate status.

Over the last quarter of a century, all of the above groups have become subject to governance by performance indicators. Schools, hospitals, universities and so forth became managed by 'objective' performance indicators with results published in League Tables, which undermined the solidarity amongst 'free professionals' and the relationality between them and those they served. The use of performance indicators represents an extension of the *logic of competition* from the business world to one previously held to consist importantly in the quality of human relations. The indicators deployed could capture measurable quantitative differences in crude empiricist terms (hospital through-put, waiting times for operations and so on) but were incapable of assessing the quality of care, of teaching or of research.

Both internally within each organization (schools, medical centres, hospitals and universities) and externally between the potential public of users, the *logic of competition* constituted an assault upon solidarity. A new conflict of interests had been introduced between professionals and the growing ranks of administrators; one damaging to the professional ethic and, in turn, to those who were being served. In extreme cases, such as the Report issued on the Mid-Staffordshire Health Trust in G.B.,[16] meeting performance targets had taken precedence over patient care. Robert Francis QC, leading the investigation, commented in his report that patients were 'left "unwashed, unfed and without water" while staff treated them and their relatives with "callous indifference". "There was a lack of care, compassion, humanity and leadership," he said. "The most basic standards of care were not observed and fundamental rights to dignity were not respected." It seems that a measurably excessive death-rate was required before the relational evils developing between staff and patients were officially addressed.

Externally, the effects of governance by performance indicators may not be fatal but they do damage the social solidarity among users. In seeking school placement for their children in establishments highly ranked on the League Tables for their measurable results, English experience shows parents moving house in order to be eligible for entry and cases of legal prosecution for some who lied about their addresses so as to place themselves in the desired catchment area. Parent is thus placed in competition with parent and their children under an obligation of gratitude for these manoeuvers. It is unnecessary to mention the transformation of our students into 'consumers', reluctant to undertake any module or to do more than minimal reading unless this 'counts' towards their results. Lecturers now hesitate about awarding low marks, and thus the expectations of undergraduates become inflated and a new competition is unleashed amongst the student body over constructing a CV that will prove attractive on the employment market. Corporate employers raise the non-academic stakes by the expansion of seductive internships, the appointment of 'student Ambassadors' and other forms of colonizing the campuses.

Internal and external effects coalesce. The use of Journal 'impact factors' by Heads of Department to control where colleagues publish, the appearance of Google 'hit' rates in academic references (common in Switzerland), the expectation that research grant holders must demonstrate its 'impact' before the research is even completed, embroil all in the *situational logic of competition*. Collegiality gives way to mutual suspicion, collaboration to strategic considerations, and peer review segues into a procedure for enforcing academic correctitude. *Cui bono* from this competetive turn? The answer is hardly anyone, except those – usually not the most creative – who have re-invented themselves as academic administrators, but not the state of research and not academia as a solidary body.

[16]The headline of *The Independent* (09.02.2013) read 'NHS's darkest day: Five more hospitals under investigation for neglect as report blames 'failings at every level' for 1,200 deaths at Stafford hospital'.

Nevertheless, the spread of performance indicators and the standardization of institutional practices in conformity with them (a national curriculum, testing at designated ages, syllabus deviation constituting self-harming) do have a cumulative numbing effect upon the professionals involved. Listening to the discussions at the annual meeting of the National Union of Teachers, for example, reveals that all of the above is already taken-for-granted and most interventions consist in nothing beyond tweaking the performance indicators themselves. By working under this form of governance, professionals become inoculated against the robust normativity that was their patrimony.

Governance by Bureaucratic Regulation

Whether we are talking about Local Authorities, National Governments or the E.U. most people would agree that bureaucratic regulation has increased during their lifetimes, despite the nineteenth century fulminations of Thomas Carlyle, Charles Dickens and later Ford Maddox Ford against 'red tape'. It is also worth noting that Canada, the U.S. and the E.U. have commissions or committees whose aim is to reduce it. In other words, bureaucratic regulation is a strange animal in the sense that some of the agencies most responsible for its proliferation, such as the E.U., at least wish to be seen to be unenthusiastic about it. What accounts for this paradox?

Certainly, bureaucratic regulation is about control and no democratic institution wants to be seen as a 'controller'. Yet, there has to be more to it because so many organizations that increasingly operate through this form of regulation make no claims about their governance being democratic: public utilities, banks, supermarkets, manufacturers, public transport, leisure facilities and hotels amongst dozens of others. I want to maintain that one reason for this profusion and proliferation lies in low social solidarity amongst the relevant populations (of users, consumers, clients etc. See Al-Amoudi, Chap. 6, in this volume) and one consequence of its growth is to drive solidarity even lower. No claim is being made that this is the only cause or sole consequence of these regulatory measures.

However, the most salient feature of administrative regulation is that it must be respected but does not require respect from those who abide by it. Regulations are instruments of control, ones that are constraining and can be enabling (as in certain abuses sometimes being taken more seriously), but they do not rely upon commanding normative consent, endorsement or approval from those to whom they apply. If that is the case, then it might seem that the prevailing level of social solidarity amongst any group who will be affected by a new regulation is irrelevant, because everybody will be bound by it.

That conclusion appears premature because it is when normative consensus is lowest in a target population that bureaucratic regulation can be applied most easily. Were there higher solidarity, entailing shared concerns amongst group members, the basis exists for potential (organized) opposition to bureaucratic fiat. Although solidarity does not necessarily imply a state of affairs even approaching normative consensus, the holding of shared concerns cannot be devoid of normativity. Some of the same things matter to those with concerns held in common and the most important of them is that these *ought* to be fostered rather than damaged. Conversely, low solidarity signals heterogeneous concerns meaning that regulation will have a mixed reception, but one too fragmented for resistance. In that case, control is simply control.

Although it does not seem definitional to me that *social* regulations have to be internally linked to social relations, they do influence them, which is not inherently part of their objective. *A bureaucratic regulation is usually satisfied if each and every member of the target population behaves as specified* (e.g. not parking except in designated bays). What makes a regulation social is simply when a social outcome is its objective, such as avoiding a definition of overcrowding ('No more than 8 standing passengers permitted'). Nevertheless, regulations influence real social relations – specifically social solidarity – in excess of the behavioural conformity sought.

Let us quickly glance at an improbable instance, that of the (still current) E.U. regulation governing the sale of carrots. Commission Regulation (EC) No 730/1999 of 7 April 1999 states they must be "not forked, free from secondary roots". One consequence has been that horticulturalists have to dump or find some industrial outlet for their offending carrots, being paid by supermarkets for only perfectly straight specimens. Another is that the price of the latter rises. Farmers are disgruntled and so are customers. Yet, considering the price, customers may conclude that farmers growing carrots are doing very well. Meanwhile, the grower, returning home with a half a truck load of rejected forked carrots that have now lost freshness and value, curses customer perfectionism. Ironically, neither party may be fully aware of EC Regulation No 730/1999 and both, if consulted, might well be normatively opposed to it. The attitudes they do share are discounted bureaucratically and the practices imposed by regulation serve to diminish solidarity between them.

Can one generalize from this ludicrous issue? Perhaps, to the extent that when social solidarity is low the weaker are the networks along which information flows and the less the bonds that mitigate or offset a person or group behaving in a way that is the product of regulatory control. Conversely, bureaucratic regulation enables competetive individualism to infiltrate more readily with every new decline in solidarity, thus serving to promote it.

Social Life That Escapes Governance

Many novel social practices, promoted technologically, are distinctively morphogenic; they catch on fast through positive feedback and do not become readily stabilized through negative feedback. In other words, they escape *both* bureaucratic and normative regulation alike. Should these be regarded as 'new personal freedoms' or as 'new forms of social anarchy', thriving in the absence of social solidarity? Certainly, it takes time for norms to crystalize in relation to new inventions and the social practices stemming from their adoption and use (remember the man with a red flag walking in front of the first cars). In that case, it could be argued that common prudential rather than normative concerns prompted road widening and the convention of driving on the right or left.

Yet, some current practices appear resistant to governance and such norms as may eventually develop are not necessarily *universal*. Take the introduction of television into the home in the 1950s. At first, the TV remained on when visitors came *because* friends and family had been invited to experience the new domestic wonder. In the next half century, as 'everyone' acquired one, it stayed on regardless of the difficulties of competing with it conversationally. Eventually, a strange convention developed, particularly though far from exclusively among the poorer, namely that if asked to switch it off, say by a visiting nurse, the sound would be muted but the picture remained flickering. Should this be seen as the private domain making a stand against public intrusions or as a more sinister form of 'privacy' becoming re-defined to include a constant media presence?

However, some relatively novel practices appear resilient if not hostile to regulation. Mobile phone users do not adapt existing conventions (such as moving out of others' way to re-tie a shoelace) but body-block, interrupt conversations to take calls, leave the dinner table, or broadcast to the entire restaurant. At concerts, in lectures or in church regulatory reminders have to be issued; the creation of a single Quiet Coach on trains is not respected but often contested by the same passengers who act in conformity with the adjacent 'no-smoking' sign.

I venture that such responses represent neither resilience nor resistance but are grounded in the 'macro-moral disconnect', intrinsic to social regulation by anormative *bureaucratic governance that systematically divorces norms from values*. On the one hand privacy itself is no longer a value, if it stands in the way of competition or control. Unregulated 'cold calling' by phone on the part of commercial enterprises is disruptive, disingenuous and often dishonest, but acceptable because profitable.[17] In parallel, official access to our telephone records (and e-mails and websites visited) is no longer confined to specific police inquiries but has recently been governmentally advanced as a universal surveillance strategy in the 'war on terrorism'.

On the other hand, anormativity and its moral disconnect positively encourage an anti-reflexive 'expressivism' in the general population. Put the intensive ownership of mobile phones (93 % in Britain) and their use (an average of 65 text messages per day by the young in the USA),[18] daily use of social media, together with the

[17]In Britain, the original (monopolistic) telephone company BT (now suffering from competition) lodges no complain against this use by commercial users; it profits from it and then capitalizes on the unwanted disturbance by selling its own brand phones with a so-called 'Blocking feature' that works (apart from blocking a single stalking caller) by such useful features as 'Block all international calls'! Cold calling is also how the intrusive practice becomes globalized because it provides employment for those in developing countries who actually place the cold calls.

[18]http://www.pewinternet.org/~/media/Files/Reports/2012/PIP_Teens_Smartphones_and_Texting.pdf

European average of 28 hours of television viewing per week and rising,[19] and time for serious Internal Conversation diminishes accordingly. Especially given the subordination of values, younger subjects cumulate the conditions conducive to 'fractured expressive reflexivity' (Archer 2012: 277–290): preoccupation with today's ephemera, inability to design purposeful courses of action; undeveloped personal 'concerns', displaced by fleeting absorption in fashion, fads and fabricated celebrities; and consequent unreadiness to make commitments to social or political action. In short, they are induced to become passive subjects, people to whom things happen, not those who make things happen. Some may also come to see themselves as victims of what are effectively new unregulated opportunities for cyber-bullying, relational deception, flaming, trolling and blackmailing.

When anormative regulation increasingly prevails, anormativity is what is also increasingly reflected back; and the situation is not improved by the multiplication and proliferation of new bureaucratic regulations. I repeat what I speculated in 2012, that such conditions 'open up the prospect of an increase in expressive reflexivity during the transition to morphogenic society, especially amongst the victims of modernity who are worst placed to avail themselves reflexively of the situational logic of opportunity' (Ibid: 289–90).

So far this chapter has tracked how sources of normativity within the legal order – laws, rules, norms, conventions and etiquette (Abrutyn and Carter 2014) – responded to the intensification of morphogenesis over the last three decades. I have maintained that the task of normative control has passed to processes of *anormative* bureaucratic regulation. These can respond faster to novel social changes but have largely severed their links to traditional legal concerns about *legitimacy*, yet are not imbued with social concerns about *legitimation*. Consequently, the legal and social orders are linked *instrumentally* meaning that instead of supplying normative guidelines for action, that are both constraining and enabling, social regulation is increasingly sought through regulative prohibitions and sanctions that are *anormative*.

In terms of the three main tasks that legal instruments can perform for the social order – assisting co-ordination, co-operation and redistribution – bureaucratic regulation focusses exclusively upon *co-ordination*, working causally to promote conformity rather than supplying guidelines fostering how we live together in fairness. It represents a 'moral disconnect' between norms and values and a privatization of morality. Moral concerns cannot be obliterated but their social diffusion is discouraged as voluntary initiatives prompted by them are colonized, economic philosophy is curtailed into 'There is no alternative', political philosophy

[19]According to Ofcom, the independent Regulator for the UK communications industries, 'the average number of hours of television watched by individuals in the UK has risen over the past eight years from 3.7 hours a day in 2004 to 4.0 hours a day in 2011.' 'The average American over the age of 2 spends more than 34 hours a week watching live television, says a new Nielson report – plus another three to six hours watching taped programs', https://www.nydailynews.com/entertainment/tv-movies/americans-spend-34-hours-week-watching-tv-nielson-numbers-article-1.1162285#ixzz2KgAqQ1QM

truncated into 'getting by' without vision, and human philosophy reduced to political correctitude unrelated to humanistic ideals of flourishing. In consequence, all the resources most capable of fostering eudaimonia, are repressed by the top-down imposition of anormative social regulation. They are fragmented into the specific remits of each regulative organization, which at most stimulates single-issue pressure groups as the form of opposition. These are hampered from coalescing because they compete for governmental recognition at election time in relation to their numerical strength. This is reinforced because the majority of the population is left to the anti-normative mercies of the media and the triviality of its contents. However, normative sources of contestation are not eliminated.

In sum, the major top down effect is to augment the overall decline in social solidarity, since bureaucratic regulation operates through instrumental rationality and is therefore fundamentally individualistic. Thus, there is no encouragement for the majority to become reflexive relational subjects (Donati and Archer 2015) but, rather, anormative social regulation constitutes both structural and cultural barriers against effective relationality and creative reflexivity. It follows that we should not be surprised that 'those born here' can be recruited as jihadists, that migrant groups form residential enclaves, and that the affluent retired are retreating into gated communities. These, at least have some form of social integration surpassing the absence of solidarity encountered in the developed world and a source of values sustaining normativity, albeit not ones promoting the common good.

Such are the results when the generative mechanism fueling intensive morphogenesis becomes systematically skewed towards market competition, with its intrinsic tendency to produce winners and losers, but one that increases the disproportionality between the two ('We are the 99 %'). From this perspective, the potential for the same generative mechanism to diffuse 'win-win' contexts cumulating in an integrative Commons is overshadowed by the proponents of the *situational logic of competition* having made common cause with social regulation. Consequently, the prospects of a eudaimonic morphogenic social order appear to be paralyzed.

Resurgent Values: The Countervailing Influences of Digital Diffusionism

So far in this Chapter I have presented anormative social regulation as a 'push-over', working from the top down and promoting financialized interests – one that feeds upon low social integration and depresses it still further. It furthers divisive competition between a shrinking proportion of global mega-competitors (the 1 %) rather than fostering co-operation among the wider constituency (the 99 %). However, if we return to the generative mechanism that has been advanced as underpinning Late Modernity and its transformation – that of economic competition working in synergy with digital technology – I have repeatedly maintained that these pull society morphogenetically in two different directions (Archer 2014a). However, the bottom-up normative influence of digital diffusionism is neglected simply, I suspect, because it fails to conform to entrenched expectations that contestation will be expressed through the emergence of social movements (Carrigan, Chap. 9, in this volume). Social scientists have become accustomed to this trajectory, which was indeed pronounced over the last two centuries. But it was merely a tendency sustained by a structural and cultural context lacking in ready means for communication and thus for rapid mobilization. That today's form of contestation is novel and does not resemble the social movements of the past in form, content, workings or consequences has nothing to do with whether or not it is normative and effectively confronts our one global society with the reanimation of values.

In fact, it is precisely in the conditions that are now increasingly hostile to the social movement as we knew it, that the new, current forms of normative contestation can be understood. To do so entails taking the Realists' conception of the stratified ontology of the social order very seriously indeed because the novel re-presentation of values challenging anormative social regulation cannot be restricted to the confines of the 'meso-level' that was the terrain of the customary social movement: it entails the micro, meso and macro-levels.[20]

Leaving Old-Style Social Movements Behind

It is not disputed here that current conditions are inimical to the development of old-style social movements. Highly regulated social orders, characterized by low social integration, where values are repressed in public life, are three social features that constitute barriers to their development. Empirically, the most familiar and relatively enduring ones are experiencing numerical diminution and either incorporation or marginalization: the membership of political parties, of trades unions and of churches and denominations. Newer voluntary movements in civil society are frequently 'colonized' from above and have their normativity stifled in public-private partnerships or by tightly regulated outsourcing (as with care in the community). Alternatively, they are used from below by those for whom they were designed, but are misused from above to supplement the deficiencies of political policies of austerity (as is the case for Food Banks[21]).

This does not deter new pro-social initiatives, indeed it is an incentive to them, but they confront the 'paradox of diffusion', namely the more successful they are

[20]This has been one of the main contributions of Emmanuel Lazega to our collective enterprise, namely his quiet insistence that networks require inter-level investigation if we are to grasp their dynamics and outcomes. In a sense, this renders 'intersectionality' not unimportant but allied to the familiar preoccupation with the formation of meso-level social movements alone.

[21]British Prime Minister David Cameron denigrates the normativity of food donors and volunteers by stating that they are simply enlarging the ranks of 'benefit scroungers'.

the more vulnerable to colonization they become. Thus, it is not old-style social movements that prosper but, on the one hand, those voluntary initiatives that start small by confining themselves to circumscribed geo-local areas. The (admirable) Italian venture of developing 'Social Streets' will provide a good test case; they are likely to proliferate globally because of the relational goods they generate at low cost but are vulnerable to the withdrawal of public resources if such self-help provides facilities 'for free'. Such initiatives diffuse digitally and fast: in Volume II the number of Food Banks that had spread to Britain could be enumerated (over 300); now they are everywhere.

If this is the case for social movements as we have known them, then for digital diffusion to make a normative impact, its re-assertion of social values must take a different form. It seems that it already has done so, although sociologists have been far more intrigued by its phenomenal characteristics than by explaining its underlying generative mechanism and dynamics.

Digital diffusionists, (whose genealogy goes back to the original 'hackers'), have to follow the imperative of diffusion itself; otherwise their normative message goes unheard. They need to broadcast the universal value of the Commons; that intellectual property rights are matters of artificially contrived cultural scarcity; and to show that 'win-win' cooperation is in the interests of all, as with Open Access. The problem is how to follow this imperative, given that their opponents gain a much higher public profile (through the films, books and media coverage given to internet billionaires) by collaborating with global capitalism. Given Porpora's 'macro-moral disconnect', the answer is certainly not to preach. The Bible-belt fundamentalists have been running their radio and television stations for several decades in the USA but these do not get beyond preaching to the converted. In part, the answer is to let the quality of relational goods 'speak for themselves', as does Wikipedia to its regular users.

On the other hand, it appears that their values have to be vaunted in acts of outrage or expressed in *outré* forms that ensure their diffusion by the media as a whole. This is not novel, though its scope is vastly augmented. The visual arts, ironic poetry and novels and especially the performing arts have 'traditionally' employed such shock tactics, but to a fairly circumscribed audience and these, too, have become increasingly outrageous in order to make an impact. Castells' 2012 title, *Networks of Outrage and Hope*, seemed promising in this respect, but his exclusive and optimistic concentration upon the 'Occupy' protests veered off towards considering them in the light of nascent old-style social movements. Instead, the 1968 *événements* in Paris come closest as a prototype of today's 'outrageous' manifestations. Nevertheless, the link needs forging with Pussy Riot, the Slut Walk marches, the Copenhagen cartoons and those of *Charlie Hebdo* before and after the assassinations. Yet, if no social movement issues from the million plus demonstrators in Place de la République in 2015, do these protests equal more than the instant but transient responses to natural humanitarian disasters such as in Haiti, the Philippines and now Nepal? Certainly, they gain diffusion, as slogans and cartoons go global in close to real time, but is their impact ephemeral? After all, the Paris *événements* were a failure in terms of their immediate impact and subsequent lack of institutionalization: the Fifth Republic did not collapse, De Gaulle returned to office and the higher education reforms reneged on delivering the autonomy and participation promised but managed to get the protesters off the streets.[22]

If the answer is determined by the criteria applied to old-style social movements, then it will affirm their evanescence. If the arguments behind that conclusion note that the coordination costs of protest are nearing zero and that demonstrations are now 'ten a penny', that hash tag reactions may spell reciprocal communication but lack the reflexive deliberation needed for the clear articulation of goals, and that their impact is as transient as media attention, then I suspect that new wine is being put into old bottles.

Personal Morphogenesis; the Micro-level

Consider the Campaign for Nuclear Disarmament in the pre-diffusionist era of the late 1950s and 1960s. We marched to bring about unilateral disarmament and we failed. We also had little success in melding European CND into a movement or in convincing any serious contender for Governmental Office to endorse unilateralism. If analysis is riveted on the meso-level of organizational formation and change alone, this is a story of complete failure – as an old style social movement.

However, it is not the whole story if we go 'down' to the micro level and examine the experiential effects on marchers, their values, and subsequent life-courses. We did not march as lone subjects, but exchanged with our fellows protesters and from them learned a great deal that had no direct connection with nuclear warfare: about literature, music and painting; about philosophy, meditation and vegetarianism; about accepting breast-feeding in public, taking communal showers and sharing brown rice. Does this matter societally? Undoubtedly it did personally for we baby-boomers, reared in straightened circumstances and growing-up surrounded by the petty bourgeois values dominant during post-war reconstruction.[23] Without these exchanges *en route* I would not have become a sociologist but the conventional 'Girton girl', successfully deconstructing *Beowulf* at Cambridge, as home and school expected. Not only did it play a profound role in personal morphogenesis, but we also became alerted to the fact that this was not simply a single issue demonstration. The values of co-marchers linked up both morally and organizationally to anti-apartheid, civil rights and nascent ecological concerns – some of which did become social movements although I am arguing that this is not the litmus test for protests having a morphogenetic impact on the social order.

---

[22]La loi d'orientation de l'enseignement supérieur; for its promises and how these were clawed back see Archer (1972:127–153).

[23]Food rationing in Britain ended as late as 1954.

Personal morphogenesis is not individualism nor amenable to explanation in terms of Methodological Individualism. Those who participate in demonstrations come *from* a social context (natal background, current employment, associations to which they electively belong) and they do not *return* there completely unchanged as they probably do after a weekend at Disneyland. Every protest invites a reconsideration of personal values. As reflexive subjects, all participants respond to some degree and according to their dominant mode of reflexivity. The effect may simply be to reinforce those values that prompted them to be present but, as Emmanuel Lazega pointed out, they re-enter their current organizations not quite the same attitudinally as they were. Moreover, we all build up a biography of social action and, given the normative connections between issues signaled above, different trajectories of social involvement are constituted over everyone's life-course that play a part in shaping and reshaping personal normativity (Archer 2000: 301–303).

In my chapter in Volume III, 2015, the growth of passive Pimary Agents at the expense of active Corporate Agents was accentuated [24] and it is not retracted here because *inter alia* social integration continues to plummet, which in turn reduces those willing to join organized pressure groups with well-articulated agendas for change. It follows from this that *the main, initial effect of participation in protest will be an aggregate one*. This is the case even though many if not most Primary Agents are not lone individuals but 'Relational Subjects' (Donati and Archer 2015); it is simply that their relationality does not extend as far as becoming members of groups organized for the pursuit of a particular kind of morphogenesis.

Thus, at the micro-level, '*digital diffusion*' *works predominantly through aggregation in effecting normative change*. In this it is identical to Wikipedia, which introduces the value of the Commons to its free users, who are not asked to sign up to any form of membership. Significantly, this also parallels the social media, despite their deceptive harping on communication between 'friends'; typical users are people home alone. Of course, Realists have never denied aggregate effects, merely the reduction of all social causality to them. Here, the structural/cultural emergent properties constituting the generative mechanism are being combined with the aggregate form that their causal influence assumes at the micro-level in the current structural and cultural context.

How does it work? This is mainly through the effect of collective protest upon personal reflexivity. First, the dominant modes of reflexivity practiced by subjects act as a filter on those attending demonstrations or being attentive to them. Thus, Communicative Reflexives will tend to be a small percentage of participants as people restrained by their dense network of 'similars and familiars', unless these

[24] 'Primary Agents' are collectivities of people who share the same life-chances. They are aggregates, but these can have important social consequences. However, they are different from 'Corporate Agents' who are never aggregates because they have organized themselves in pursuit of certain goals and have articulated the changes they seek.

interlocutors happen to come from 'activist' backgrounds.[25] Autonomous Reflexives tend to shun collective action and fractured Expressive reflexives may turn out 'for fun', but since their fracturing extends to their normativity and disables them from prioritizing their 'concerns', they are unlikely to remain affected beyond the duration of the event. Second, it will thus be the Meta-reflexives among whom the normative issues highlighted and messages received will resonate most, by posing questions for further deliberation rather than by some blunt force, usually labelled 'group pressure'. Their mediatory internal conversations will not arrive at the same conclusions for all, partly because their concerns are at least differently nuanced and partly because they have differing biographies of involvement. However, the fact that they are temporarily focusing upon the same issue will serve to concentrate any normative impact upon that and related areas.[26]

Thus *the 'digital diffusion' that enables demonstrations to be organized much more easily than in the past exerts its first effect through changing the normativity of participants themselves*, even if this means only the intensification of previous values (including reinforcing contra values). However, although some collective endeavors will usually follow (new Websites, Magazines and bands) these, at best, represent what Mark Carrigan calls 'fragile' Corporate Agents (Chap. 9). The impact of normative change, by those who have been changed, does not follow the 'old' route into the development of social movements. Instead, we need to take institutional 're-entry' much more seriously and to examine the networked link-ups and link-downs that are the channels through which normative change flows and can amplify, although it will meet with constraint and contestation.

Networking: At the Meso-level

Certainly, *qua* individual persons, most will return to their pre-existing roles (in work, the family and civil society), but they will *personify* their role occupancy rather differently because of their enhanced normativity. For example, teachers are likely to introduce new topics for discussion in class and in essays, whilst academics will display posters that symbolically affirm their enhanced commitment to given causes. Yet, beyond these micro-level manifestations of their values, the relationality of those most affected will change, not simply in their face-to-face collegial relations (for example, who now gravitates towards whom and avoids others in an office or common room). In the last Volume (2015) Donati discussed the trajectory of relations in a couple, where relational morphogenesis in this dyad depended upon Ego making a proposal to Alter that could only be morphogenetic, rather than

[25]This was not unknown in old-style social movements such as CND, where the Quakers, as pacifists, who had been Conscientious Objectors, during war time, played a significant role.

[26]This 'focusing effect' is quite well illustrated by the fact that the issue of *Charlie Hebdo* after the assassinations had a print run of five million compared with previous sales of 30,000.

conflictual, if both endorsed the modification suggested (big or small). Since we never reflect in a vacuum, but always in a context, then the heightened normative commitment produced by participation in a protest – especially if the couple has done so together – may well be the source of Ego's proposal and Alter's assent.[27] Henceforth, they might become a couple (partly) defined by their 'concern' about, say, climate change.[28] (Alternatively, serious disagreement over a normative issue could lead to their break-up as partners or close friends).

However, these micro-level dynamics are also intertwined with meso-level changes that are the direct effect of digital diffusionism. The old-style social movement could foster constancy of commitment only amongst those who volunteered for continuous involvement through some version of 'membership'. Even then, normative commitments could grow cold between one protest event and the next, always supposing the movement had become enough of a Corporate Agent to organize another. Digital diffusion has succeeded in transforming this major normative constraint by replacing 'membership' and its sporadic services (through postal leaflets) by the continuous if convoluted networks that operate 24/7. For any given cause, a plurality of websites exist supplying constant contact, supplemented by independent blogs, and serve to reinforce as well as to refine the normativity of those drawn to thousands of causes. Inter-network communication promotes both collaboration and conflict, but there is room for all, at no expense and at their users' convenience, whilst conjointly maintaining the salience of the normative issue.

At the meso-level, it is crucial to stress that digital diffusion is continually innovative; *the new variety it constantly introduces is the main normative weapon in its arsenal* because this extends the range and reach of networks of users. This role is underplayed by those riveted by the numerical growth of Google, Amazon, Facebook and Twitter and the accompanying increase in hours devoted to television are seen as the normative allies of financialized capitalism and guarantors of neoliberal values. What is systematically under-emphasized is that simultaneously, digital diffusion is quietly dismantling the whole mainstream media structure – its Orwellian hegemony, the contribution that distraction makes to quietism and to fostering consumerism. Certainly, many have noted the decline in both newspapers and their readership, especially among the younger age groups. Yet, few have linked up this decline to the frenzied descent into illegal activities (particularly phone-hacking) promoted by news moguls who do recognize that they are now on the run.

The biggest success of digital innovation is the doomed nature of television, monopolized by the state and market, despite new ventures into streaming, podcasts and the sale of 'boxed series' on Amazon. Big plasma screens are for pubs and football, for beer and conviviality. Home viewing of scheduled programs is the resort of the elderly and the poor. It is rapidly being replaced by an elective combination

[27]This proposition could be checked empirically.

[28]I define our identity as determined by our 'constellation of concerns' and the prioritization of these concerns. For no relational subject are these 'things that matter' to them fixed but ever open to experience, learning and (re)evaluation, which are all reflexive exercises (Archer 2000, 2007).

that is self-mixed from an increasing array: gaming and gambling, films and music, blogs and news sources, retail and sport– any walk through a train or plane reveals the electronic resources people own and use that enable bespoke reception. In short, most of us now have the means to put together what matches our concerns and to deepen them by searching for further information and commentaries. As strong evaluators, we can now exercise our values by self-selection from options that grow almost daily. This is one of the most important practices through which people increasingly avoid normative regulation and means that more of us become normatively un-herdable cats rather than regulated beings.

Macro-level Normativity

One further nail in the coffin of 'methodological nationalism', which was touched upon earlier when discussing political 'centrism', is that nation states are no longer the seat of anything that could be called national normativity. While governance has become the preserve of bureaucratic social regulation and co-ordination, Government without conviction is more concerned with muddling through, balancing the books, business as usual and the management of austerity than with the pursuit or defense of values. Western attempts to define national 'identity' are dropped with embarrassment. Moreover, the US, Britain and the EU do not want to fight anymore – the political value of returning body bags being negative. Earnings from prostitution and drug dealing are now included in many countries' calculations of GDP. Europe very belatedly (2015) acceded to assisting Italy with the 'graveyard of Lampedusa'; though some EU members, such as Britain refused to play their part in accepting a modest portion of the refugees. The list could go on and it would seem to highlight the novel absence of normativity at the macro-level – except that nation states are no longer the only serious macroscopic players.

Increasingly, the digital protagonists of values are converging upon the INGOs, seeking their endorsement for resisting Climate Change, Human Trafficking, exploitation of children, female genital mutilation, organ harvesting among many other issues. To have a particular cause listed among the UN's Sustainable Development Goals – especially as a self-standing SDG – is the acme of success for 'normative organizations'.[29] Why? Neither SDG's nor Protocols are enforceable, but require national ratification and then legislation that can fall far short of the normative intent; and some nations simply refuse to sign (such as the lasting refusal of the US to endorse the Kyoto targets for reduction of carbon emissions). Why has the buck of humanitarian concern been passed to the INGOs?

[29]This (early 2015) was a good time to observe the phenomenon as the list of SDG's for 2030 was the subject of heavy negotiation. On August 31st 2015, the abolition of Human Trafficking and Forced Labour were incorporated in Clause 8.7 of the final list of SDGs.

Here, I will venture the bare bones of an explanation in terms of the two directions in which the generative mechanism is pulling morphogenesis and illustrate it with reference to pressures for the elimination of Human Trafficking. Since this growing and lucrative practice is referred to as 'modern slavery' in many current declarations, how is it that in countries such as Britain and the United States, which abolished and abominated human slavery more than 150 years ago, human trafficking continues to flourish in the twenty-first century?

In the Western world, governments and political parties have a divided stance towards Trafficking. On the one hand, electoral considerations encourage attending to the strength of resistance to migration, as evidenced by the growing popularity of ultra-right parties. On the other hand, most of these countries are economically compromised by the use of cheap, exploited and often trafficked labour in *their* multinational enterprises in the developing world. At home, they are not immune either, given disclosures of 'sweatshops' producing clothing, for example, for well-known multi-national brands. Although these are usually dismissed as bad tales from the last century, new disclosures continue to be made in Europe and the US. In other words, the black economy is still needed for the white economy to be competitive and, in Western countries, trafficked forced labour plays its part, now including boosting the statistics of GDP. This is why they dragged their feet and how the INGOs became the largest Corporate Agents to oppose Trafficking (Archer 2014b).

The criminalization of human trafficking is a phenomenon of the new millennium. All of the protocols and conventions branding it a criminal offence date from 2000. Why was this so late? Why was it spearheaded by the United Nations (UNODC) and other INGOs, especially the ILO? Why did 166 nation states 'hurry' to sign up to the Palermo Protocol within a decade? If the response is that trafficking had intensified, then its profitability served only to indicate the growing demand for it in developed and developing countries alike.

The answer seems to be that the INGOs as supra national bodies were an organizational focal point; the ILO had already registered its opposition to trafficking as part of forced labour in 1930[30]; the UNODC (founded in 1997) moved fast when the connection between drug smuggling and human Trafficking became undeniable, with the UN General Assembly passing its Protocol that came into effect in 2003 as a legal instrument to combat organized transnational crime. These and subsequent instruments were far from ideal and meet with dilution and resistance at national level, but they do exert leverage against Trafficking whilst the vast majority of countries have been minimalistic in their responses.

[30]The International Labour Organization's (ILO) 'Forced Labour Convention' (1930, no. 29) had defined 'forced labour' as covering 'all work or service that is exacted from any person under the menace of any penalty for which the said person has not offered himself voluntarily'. This definition has its defects because 'forced labour' subsumes 'trafficking' and *also* illegal migration, if and when 'fraud and deception' effectively defy voluntary action.

Consequently, voluntary associations from small groups of humanitarians to large digital groupings and the Catholic Church have begun to collaborate and converge upon the INGOs and especially to target the UN after the novel formulation of Millennium Development Goals in 2000. Now, since these are to be reformulated in 2015, this represents a magnet inducing co-operation between diverse groups sharing this normative concern. There is collaboration between different clusters seeking agreement on the formulation of a Sustainable Development Goal for eliminating Trafficking, which was successful on August 31st 2015.

What this illustrates is an opportunity being taken to reverse the 'Macro-moral disconnect'. Although the attempt to confine religion to the private domain is fierce, it does not deprive the Churches of their organizations and these are a crucial part in the development of Corporate Agency. Since Trafficking is a humanitarian concern, it accommodates global ecumenism and joint declarations by leaders of different faiths.[31] Equally, as such, there is no barrier to collaboration with secular humanists and their digital platforms. As synergy grows between them so digital diffusion increases, swelling support and encouraging the precise articulation of shared goals. This Corporate Agent is growing more robust, there are some points of divergence but they have not induced 'fragility' but represent items for the future agenda.

Conclusion

Why is this illustration of the bottom-up impact of digital diffusion important? Because it demonstrates that the crucial element that escapes anormative bureaucratic regulation is our 'concerns'. As Charles Taylor once put it, we are 'strong evaluators' (1985: 65–68) and whilst we may live as instrumental rationalists with the barrage of socially regulatory measures confronting us in everyday and professional life, our humanistic concerns cannot be eliminated and they can even override what were once divisive normative differences, such as divisions amongst the world's faiths. If the example I have used of Trafficking seems to be an 'easy illustration', exactly the same account – though with its own scientific complexities – could be offered for Climate Change, which also seeks designation on the list of UN priorities. In other words, digital diffusion can be an effective contestant, and one capable of generating Corporate Agency at the Macro-level as well as its effects at the Meso- and Micro-levels. In sum, anormative bureaucratic regulation is an attempt to drive a wedge between norms and values, but cannot eliminate normative concerns; digital diffusion provides them with a novel variety of means for their social expression and influence.

[31] See www.endslavery.va for the text of the 2014 ecumenical 'Joint Declaration Against Modern Slavery'

References

Abrutyn, S., & Carter, M. J. (2014). The decline in shared collective conscience as found in the shifting norms and values of Etiquette manuals. *Journal for the Theory of Social Behaviour, 43*, 2.

Al-Amoudi, I. (2010). Immanent non-algorithmic rules: An ontological study of social rules. *Journal for the Theory of Social Behaviour, 40*(3), 289–313.

Archer, M. S. (Ed.). (1972). *Students, university and society*. London: Heinemann.

Archer, M. S. (1985). The myth of cultural integration. *British Journal of Sociology, 36*(3), 333–353.

Archer, M. S. (1988). *Culture and agency: The place of culture in social theory*. Cambridge: Cambridge University Press.

Archer, M. S. (2000). *Being human: The problem of agency*. Cambridge: Cambridge University Press.

Archer, M. S. (2007). *Making our way through the world: Human reflexivity and social mobility*. Cambridge: Cambridge University Press.

Archer, M. S. (2012). *The reflexive imperative in late modernity*. Cambridge: Cambridge University Press.

Archer, M. S. (2014a). The generative mechanism re-configuring late modernity. In M. S. Archer (Ed.), *Late modernity: Trajectories towards morphogenic society* (Vol. II). Dordrecht: Springer.

Archer, M.S. (2014b). *Being trafficked to work*. http://www.casinapioiv.va/content/accademia/en/publications/extraseries/sustainable.htm

Archer, M. S. (2015). How agency is transformed in the course of social transformation. In M. S. Archer (Ed.), *The generative mechanisms transforming late modernity*. Dordrecht: Springer.

Baldwin, R. (2005). Is better regulation smarter regulation?. *Public Law*, 1–19.

Better Regulation Taskforce. (undated). *Principles of better regulation* (p. 1).

Black, J. (2001). Decentering regulation; understanding the role of regulation and self-regulation in a post-regulatory world. *Current Legal Problems, 54*(1), 103–146.

Black, J. (2007). Tensions in the regulatory state. *Public Law*, 58–73.

Bobbio, N. (1996). *Right and left*. Cambridge: Polity Press.

Cabinet Office Paper (2013). www.gov.uk/government/publications/when laws become too complex (downloaded 21.11.2014).

Casini, L. (2007). Models of public administration. Comparative analysis of administrative organisation. In *Formez, Innovazione amministrativa e crescita. Rapporto con raccomandazioni* (Ricerca Giannini-Formez II Fase, Volume VIII). Rome, Formez: International Comparisons.

Donati, P. (2000). *La cittadinanza societaria*. Laterza: Roma-Bari.

Donati, P. (2014). Morphogenic society and the structure of social relations. In M. S. Archer (Ed.), *Late modernity: Trajectories towards morphgenic society*. Dordrecht: Springer.

Donati, P., & Archer, M. S. (2015). *The relational subject*. Cambridge: Cambridge University Press.

Elder-Vass, D. (2007). Reconciling Archer and Bourdieu. *Sociological Theory, 25*, 4.325–346.

Etzioni, A. (1969). *The semi-professionals and their organization: Teachers, nurses and social workers*. New York: The Free Press.

Ginsberg, M. (1962). *The diversity of morals*. London: Mercury Books.

Gouldner, A. (1971). *The coming crisis of western sociology*. London: Heinemann.

GOV-UK. (2013). *When laws become too complex*. Cabinet Office and Office of the Parliamentary Counsel, https://www.gov.uk/government/organisations/publications/when-laws-become-too-complex (downloaded 21.11.2014).

Hall, C., Scott, C., & Hood, C. (1999). *Telecommunications regulation: Culture, chaos and interdependency inside the regulatory process*. London: Routledge.

House of Lords. (2011). House of Lords, Library note, LLN 2011/028.

Joyce, R. (2007). *The evolution of morality*. Cambridge, MA: MIT Press.

Kelsen, H. (1945). *General theory of law and state*. New York: Russell and Russell.

Korsgaard, C. M. (1996). *The sources of normativity*. Cambridge: Cambridge University Press.
Korsgaard, C. M. (2009). *Self-constitution: Agency, identity, and integrity*. Oxford: Oxford University Press.
Krebs, D. (2011). *The origins of morality*. Oxford: Oxford University Press.
Moran, M. (2004). *The British regulatory state: High modernism and hyper-innovation*. Oxford: Oxford University Press.
Nader, L., & Nader, C. (1985). A wide angle on regulation: An anthropological perspective'. In R. Noll (Ed.), *Regulatory policy and the social sciences*. Berkeley: University of California Press.
OECD. (1995). Recommendation of the Council of the OECD on *Improving the Quality of Government Regulation*, OECD/GD(95)95, Note 1.
Parsons, T. (1951). *The social system*. London: Routledge and Kegan Paul.
Porpora, D. V. (2001). *Landscapes of the soul: The loss of moral meaning in American life*. Oxford: Oxford University Press.
Porpora, D. V., et al. (2013). *Post-ethical society*. Chicago: Chicago University Press.
Rhodes, R. (1997). *Understanding governance*. Buckingham: Open University Press.
Social Streets – Italy see www.socialstreet.it.
Taylor, C. (1985). Self-interpreting animals. In C. Taylor (Ed.), *Human agency and language*. Cambridge: Cambridge University Press.
Teubner, G. (1993). *Law as an autopoietic system*. Oxford: Blackwell.
Trigg, R. (2008). *Religion in public life: Must faith be privatized*. Oxford: Oxford University Press.
Turner, S. P. (2010). *Explaining the normative*. Cambridge: Polity.
von Pufendorf, S. (1964) [1688]. *On the law of nature and nations*. London: Wiley.
Wilson, W. (1887). The study of administration. *Political Science Quarterly, 2*, 197–222.

Chapter 8
Joint 'Anormative' Regulation from Status Inconsistency: A Multilevel Spinning Top Model of Specialized Institutionalization

Emmanuel Lazega

Weak Culture: Proliferation of Anormative Rules and the 'Democratic Deficit'

Margaret Archer (this volume) argues that social regulation becomes anormative with social morphogenesis: "[...] 'Anormative Regulation' of the contemporary social order or, if preferred, its 'Bureaucratic Regulation' – replete with Weber's 'iron bars'. In other words, normativity plays a much reduced role in furnishing guidelines for social action because the law and social custom diminish proportionately in relation to non-normative forms of regulative social control". From a neo-structural perspective, this link between anormative regulation and morphogenesis has far-reaching implications. This chapter argues that this link sheds a strong critical light on joint regulatory processes driven by the two most powerful actors in contemporary societies: states and business (i.e. mostly large multinational corporations and their industrial representatives). Indeed business usually tries as much as it can to participate in the governance of its markets, as well as in the governance of society at large. As a consequence, the staggering number of specialized, unelected, and taken for granted rules (bundled in complex systems of rules) that organize society based on both public administrative law and private standards has created a situation in which institutions of electoral democracy are strongly challenged by a new political economy.

I examine the construction of such "joint regulatory institutions" (as differentiated from what the sociological tradition considers to be public institutions) by looking at how specific institutional entrepreneurs, who are part of collegial oligarchies mixing public and private elites, use 'weak culture' (Breiger 2010) to

E. Lazega (✉)
Institut d'Etudes Politiques de Paris, CSO-CNRS, SPC, 19 rue Amélie, Paris, 75007 France
e-mail: emmanuel.lazega@sciencespo.fr

M.S. Archer (eds.), *Morphogenesis and the Crisis of Normativity*,
Social Morphogenesis, DOI 10.1007/978-3-319-28439-2_8

produce and rank specialized norms in the organizational society. Both the state and large business corporations and industries create their own normative spaces and work on extending them to the whole of society, most frequently via entire populations and occupations of 'dual alters' or brokers in multilevel networks (Lazega et al. 2013). Among institutional entrepreneurs, the most central in this creation are "multistatus oligarchs" (MSO), i.e. central players in the accumulation of different, socially incompatible powers and resources, and skilled at creating closed normative spaces that they can misleadingly present as public spaces operating in the public interest. This institution represents a form of joint governance or a combined regime of endogenous and exogenous conflict resolution in markets. The label 'joint' refers to the fact that governance is mainly a combination of self-regulation and exogenous regulation, a combination in which costs of control are shared. The joint element in 'joint regulation' can be defined as the coexistence of several sources of rules and constraints, both external and internal, that weigh on the actors in charge of solving conflicts by making, interpreting and enforcing the rules. Thinking about joint regulation in those terms follows both an organizational and a broadly conceived neo-structural approach to economic institutions (Lazega and Mounier 2002; Lazega 2009).

As outlined by neo-structural sociology, the joint regulatory process stresses the ways and means used by this oligarchy, often in situations of conflicts of interests and making use of status inconsistencies, to build/buy a form of legitimacy that does not require election and constitutencies, and that cuts across the boundaries of Montesquieu's division of powers. This political activity is based on multilevel institutional entrepreneurship, in which the collegial oligarchy includes heterogeneous professionals and experts of various sorts, high level bureaucrats, technocrats and civil servants. All represent both the organizations to which they are affiliated and themselves as committed persons taking political initiatives.

In this chapter, I look at an extreme case of how business gets organized collectively to do so by creating a judicial institution that is both public and "captured" as the result of a complex historical and institutional process. The focus is on the dimension of this process that is brought to light by social and organizational network analysis and a neo-structural approach. This multilevel regulatory process is represented by the image of a multilevel spinning top. Without any 'conspiracy', organized and superimposed levels of collective action neutralize public debate in democratic institutionalization mechanisms based on electoral politics. They do so by enrolling and promoting small networks of institutional entrepreneurs using boundary work, personalized social relationships and social alignments in lobbying to impose selective and narrow choices of weak culture, thus framing normative judgments epistemically.

In turn, this weak culture is taken for granted and gives individuals the opportunity to develop pragmatic decision making that, under specific conditions, is equivalent to procedural norms bringing joint regulation closer to institutional capture. This capture has often been defined as "the efforts of firms to shape the laws, policies, and regulation of the State to their own advantage by providing illicit private gains to public officials" (Hellman et al. 2000). I suggest that this definition is too quickly focused on individuals. The definition of the process of institutional capture should be broadened to involve corporatist efforts to design or redesign institutions themselves, to frame issues and set premises for decision making in rule enforcement and to obtain systematic collective gains for interest groups in these institutions. These elements add to the capacity of collective actors to gather invisible advantages. A court can thus be captured in as much as interest groups are successful in using their influence to benefit systematically from its decisions based on 'anormative rules' (Archer 2016).

Production and Ranking of Specialized Norms in the Organizational Society

The "regulatory" mechanism in society is a political process by which interdependent but conflicting and competing actors try to control their own normative space. This process of promoting new rules involves both bottom-up and top-down dynamics. Participation in institutionalization and the regulatory process are unequal at best. Competing parties have different definitions of what the public interest is at each level. In order to participate, they count on their networks of relationships, on their own power and influence in their system of interdependencies. The formation of norms is meant to stabilize participants' commitments and exchanges to deal with the risks and dilemmas associated with individual and collective action. This regulatory process is in fact a process of institutionalisation, of institutional adaptation, most often entailing institutional redesign. The internationalization of law, for example, is an highly complex set of regulatory processes characterizing organized forms of collective action at a level unprecedented in terms of sheer size and complexity. A sociological theory of the regulatory process may be of help to think about this complex set of processes.

A broadly conceived neo-structural theory accounts for collective actors' built-in dependence on cultural processes, which are normative in kind. Saying that status provides a position of strength to define terms of exchanges is equivalent to saying that it helps define or select the values, norms, and rules from which such terms are consciously or unconsciously derived. In early structural sociology, the conceptual relationship between relational structures, on the one hand, and rules, norms and values, on the other hand, was elusive. In narrow structural approaches, resource interdependencies, more than norms, were considered the only principle of social order. A neo-structural approach, however, aligns itself with a more institutional perspective when it emphasizes the interpenetration of the interactional and normative realms in order to explain social change or stability (Lazega and Favereau 2002). Institutional theories of action have long stressed organizational values, norms, and rules as restraints on opportunistic behaviour and brutal exercise of power. Such values are debated, contested, and permanently redefined by members. In transnational as in intranational institutionalization, stakeholders try to shape each other's reasoning and framing in order to define juridical roles. They do so by combining rules and networks, conventions and relational infrastructures (Lazega and Favereau 2002).

Collectives change in part because they can redefine their formal and informal rules. Any regulatory process – or process of redefinition of rules governing the collective – is a form of change that involves broken promises in the redistribution of resources (Reynaud and Reynaud 1996). When the rules of the game are changed; some parties lose resources and others win resources compared to the *ex ante* distribution and commitments. This is why, in organizations as in any political community, regulatory changes need the support of members with both power and legitimacy to push for these changes. Specific members, those with multiple and loosely connected forms of status, are the key in such changes, because they can use such dependencies and legitimacy in the regulatory process. This institutional level of organization was explicitly formulated by many sociologists (for example Merton 1959) and by studies of political or micro-political efforts, by competing interests, to change the rules. Such efforts may or may not be successful, and social arrangements are often stable enough to hide underlying contests. But neo-structural analysis can help in identifying them.

Specifically, two notions combine a neo-structural and an institutional perspective: Selznick's idea (1957) of 'precarious values' and the notion of 'multi-status oligarchs' (Lazega 2001). A value is precarious because it is always in danger of losing its representatives, that is, the active support by organized interest groups and elites that help preserve it as a candidate for top priority on the list of all competing values. 'Multi-status oligarchs' are precisely the members of a collective with enough status to redefine priorities between precarious values and derived policy options. Indeed, regulatory changes need the support of members with several forms of status. These oligarchs must have the capacity to promote regulatory changes and deal with the negative effects of broken promises and betrayed commitments induced by social change. Particularly when differences in power are not huge among members, this capacity often rests on the 'sacrifice' of resources by such multi-status oligarchs, and on the legitimacy obtained from such 'sacrifices'. Those who can afford to give up resources, presumably for the common good, while not losing power are people with several inconsistent forms of status. Thanks to this inconsistency, or loose coupling, losing one form of status does not entail losing another. Multistatus oligarchs can thus drive change (the redefinition of rules) while staying in power.

In sum, competitors very often cooperate in order to establish a common language of reference and common rules. In this area, status competition is an essential element of the regulatory process, whether leading to real changes or to resistance to change. From a neo-structural perspective, special dynamics characterize regulation: that of oligarchic negotiation of precarious values and the construction of legitimacy through relative (often false) sacrifices (Lazega 2001). The regulatory process for markets, for example, shows that entrepreneurs can become "institutional entrepreneurs" active in the social construction of their markets. Even in an egalitarian system, everyone does not defend their regulatory interests with the same efficiency. It is not simply a question of stating that the strongest impose their rules: rather, neo-structural sociology shows that actors with multiple and inconsistent forms of social status can be the most influential in this definition of the hierarchy of rules because they combine a form of legitimacy (an ability to speak on behalf of the collective in a credible manner) with their power (the control of resources that others need) precisely by using the rhetorics of this very relative 'sacrifice' to build/buy legitimacy.

Joint Regulation of the Economy by Collegial Oligarchies

Regulation of business is of particular interest in market societies. It is today openly characterized by a great polynormativity. Faced with quantities, coordination in a market involves prices and calculations, but also qualities and interpretation. It is notably through competition by quantities that a plurality of partially autonomous normative orders provides the business world with numerous sources of regulation. The relative weight of the law versus other types of norms depends on the force that the State and public institutions muster to influence this joint regulation in concrete situations of economic action. In the business world, the law occupies a position of primacy with respect to other norms not only because of the primacy of the State, but because the corporate actors in the economy, especially business, have the ability to participate in the definition of the law via processes of lobbying and joint regulation.

Business intervention in the regulatory process has always existed. But it is becoming increasingly more systematic today, as the so-called "regulatory" State tends to establish – in all the domains of public policy – general and vague legal frameworks, leaving the task of defining the substance of the rules to the discretionary interpretation of stakeholders who contribute to governance. Professions such as business lawyers, investment bankers, or consultants play a role of mediation that is significant from a regulatory point of view, especially at the international level. This mediation role is all the more important in international commercial contracts in the absence of stabilized market rules (Flood 2007). Through various forms of lobbying, enterprises greatly contribute to the campaigns of political parties in nation-states, and in exchange they obtain the right to discreetly fill in the void.

The fact that the regulatory deliberation is dominated by such "important" members is not sufficient in itself to account for the social mechanism of negotiation of precarious values. In effect, issues of status consistency must be brought in. As suggested by Frank (1985), the price of status is high when members interact intensively. Cumulating several forms of status, multi-status members muster added legitimacy by showing that they 'sacrificed' resources when siding with specific – and costly to some – policy options) to drive the negotiation of precarious values. Several dimensions of status can be described in social life, both exogenous and endogenous. The role played by members cumulating such heterogeneous and inconsistent forms of status has been shown to be a key one in the regulatory process as a social mechanism (Lazega 2001). Inconsistency, or at least loose-connectedness, of the multiple forms of status is functional. In effect, it allows "oligarchs" to lose resources along one dimension, while still maintaining prominence and concentration of resources along other dimensions. Correlations between forms of centrality in different elite networks, for example, show that persons with such loosely-coupled forms of status are present in any community or society.

Negotiating precarious values is thus the ultimate way for actors to politicize their exchanges. Actors who are strategic and polemical in their appropriateness judgments can argue endlessly about changes in the rules of the game. Multi-status actors, with such relatively loosely coupled – or 'inconsistent' – forms of status control and stabilize the regulatory process. The source of their influence is both control of resources and bureau-professional legitimacy. Since any such change means broken promises, they are in a better position than others to handle the effects of these transformations among members. They can legitimize them by (pretending that they are) sacrificing resources of their own for the collective good, thus reaching a position where they can ask for similar sacrifices from others as well. Taking this high road, however, may not be efficient in itself (the losing party may object that 'similar losses' are relative, and may not be equally bearable by all), which is why multi-status actors are also in a position to force these changes by using their control of resource dependencies. Both legitimacy and power go hand in hand in the management of social change.

Participation in institutionalization and the regulatory process is unequal at best. However, conflicts of interests provide a specific competitive advantage in this process. Conflicts of interests are situations – often incompatible from an ethical perspective – that help specific actors to cumulate inconsistent forms of status and concentrate resources and legitimacy that provide a competitive advantage in the regulatory process. This is particularly visible in certain professions that have played a central role in the political history of Western societies, such as lawyers. Conflicts of interest are a classical ethical preoccupation for many professions: for lawyers who represent successively or concurrently potentially competing clients; for medical doctors who, for instance, own a laboratory to which they send their clients for medical tests; for industrial engineers who move from one employer to another and have to sign agreements preventing them from working competitively on the same matters for at least 2–5 years; for U.S. bankers who are allowed to underwrite securities. And so on: the problem looms large when conflicts of allegiance divide actors invested with some discretion and trust. These professions have traditionally tried to deal with this problem by formulating codes of deontology that are meant to protect confidentiality and secrecy in the relationship between the professional and the client. However, recent growth of organizations (both private and public) employing professionals and semi-professionals (law firms, hospitals, advertising agencies, financial institutions), their increasing specialization, increased mobility of their members and flexibility of their labour markets, all contribute to the need to redefine this problem and to design new measures to deal with it.

It is thus possible to argue (Lazega 1994, 2012) that such organizations actively *seek* conflicts of interests, then put their members in what could be called a 'situation'. Situations of conflicts of interests are opportunities for organizations to increase brokerage capacity, access to resources and to power. As long as they can hide the fact that they are exposed to conflicts (Katz 1977) or as long as they can blame their individual members for unethical behaviour when they get caught, organizations look for network positions that help them span multiple boundaries, mediate between conflicting interests, create procedures that become a form of 'weak culture', in Breiger's sense (Breiger 2010). These positions help them reframe so as to control the interpretation of the substantive issues. Individual members are then expected both to put the interests of the organization first and not to behave like ethical heroes.

Large corporate law firms' role as brokers, mediators and boundary spanners in international business is particularly important in the absence of true business law and stabilised market rules.[1] Large corporate law firms can be regarded as powerful players in modern globalisation. Sellers (1991) calls them the 'shock troops of capitalism' imposing standards in international business and providing 'trust' for deal-making in very uncertain situations. Because they are permanently in situations of conflicts of interests, they have an important power of arbitration in commercial contracts between multinational firms (they hold information about the two sides) and play a part in their enforcement or possible renegotiation. In the absence of clear and applicable law, they provide formats for documents, contracts and written agreements or procedures. At the same time they contribute to building the international financial market and the market for legal services. In becoming experts and go-betweens in the field, they also take part in national or international regulation of business. This gives them a position of strength vis-à-vis their corporate clients and international regulation authorities. They are in a position of developers of law, promoting what Edelman calls an endogenous notion of law (Edelman and Suchman 2007). This set of roles heavily depends on being as often as possible on both sides, i.e. on using conflicts of interests strategically.

Joint Regulation in Judicial Institutions

In the organizational society, it is this elitist regulatory process that produces "anormative rules" (Archer, Chap. "7", this volume) when the tragi-comedy of relative sacrifice by players with status inconsistency provided by situations of conflict of interest is successful enough to build a form of legitimacy for specialized rules that no longer make sense for non-expert citizens. In order to illustrate this argument, an interesting example is provided by the new rules being hammered out in similar circumstances to define property, in particular intellectual property,

[1]Flood (2002): "The rise of the international law firm is unconquerable. Why? State and supranational lawmaking have not been able to keep up with the rapid developments in the globalization of law. The only institution that has marched in step has been the large international law firm. No global transaction – contract, distribution agreement, securitization, franchise – can be done without them. They have colonized the world of global law".

a central institution in a society that needs to innovate in order to survive. This is the case of the construction of the European Unified Patent Court, a transnational institution, whose underlying regulatory process aims at defining "good patents".

Intellectual property (IP) is a key institution of contemporary capitalism. Current debates about such property rights are an example of such processes. These IP rights do not constitute a perfectly coherent and stable system. For example they bring together complex, heterogeneous rules and regulations protecting patents. Negotiating how IP rights can be established is a political compromise. Establishing property rights has always been one of the most decisive actions of governments and one of the main reasons to fight and use powers in society at all levels. Intellectual property is especially crucial in societies that have cornered themselves into a situation where they need technological innovation to survive. Negotiating a solution to the economic dilemma of knowledge (its non-rival nature in use and freedom for better diffusion on the one hand; and the high price of the production of knowledge goods and the establishment of price mechanisms inciting actors to produce them, on the other hand) is the goal of the definition of IP, especially of pragmatic definitions of patents. These definitions are historical and institutional constructions that change with technological evolution, but also with the capacity of players to steer the definition of a "good patent" in one direction or another. They thus respond to political and economic interests with legal, cultural and administrative rules and practices.

This example of the development of the knowledge economy and intellectual property law at the international level is based on a recent study (Lazega 2011) of an interesting process of ongoing internationalization of patent law in the European context. European States cannot agree on what is the right interpretation of the "good patent" and whether or not there should be a European Patent Court. Should Europe define patents as an 'exception' [very special protection against competition] or as a 'reward' [an ordinary return on investments for incremental innovators]? Industries and large corporations whose business models have patents at their core (food, medicine, semi-conductors, etc.) pushed for the creation of a new kind of court. The Unified Patent Court is a hybrid, semi-public institution that will operate as a public one. Here also, cross-level regulatory competition and regulatory cooperation among competitors involves many heterogeneous actors, some of who are able, thanks to their inconsistent forms of status, to build legitimacy through false/relative sacrifice and thus push through their priorities and rules. Building legitimacy helps them deal with the losers created by such changes in the rules of the game.

Courts are indeed a locus of joint governance. They are not static institutions making a-temporal and purely rational decisions. They are contested terrain, the prizes or objects of broader economic competition and conflicts that occur outside courthouses (Flemming 1998). This is especially the case in courts in which judges are themselves business people elected by their own business community – as will be the case of many technical judges at the UPC. Attempts at influencing what goes on in the court from outside the court come from various angles. Flemming lists five such angles: external stakeholders can try to influence jurisdiction (the range of disputes over which the court has authority), positions (actors formally authorized to participate in the disposition of cases), resources (the capacity to influence the decisions of other actors), discretion (the range of choices available to actors), and procedures (rules governing courtroom processes). Parties involved in that contest may not be directly concerned by all the conflicts that are dealt with by the court, but they may have indirect concerns, material or symbolic, in the decisions of the court, and thus attempt to influence what goes on.

Flemming's categories help focus on specific processes of influence. Indeed, collective actors involved in conflicts on markets, such as companies, whole industries (in class actions, for example) and even State administrations, may have strong incentives to influence who becomes a judge and what resources are available to these judges. For example, the more litigious these sectors are, the stronger their incentives to share the costs of conflict resolution. These collective actors are usually conceived of as external actors. Their incentives to influence the jurisdiction of the court are to protect their interests in the long run. They may do this by helping some of their own selected members in becoming judges. The stronger their incentives, the more they can be expected to take care of their representation among the judges. Such judges, once in a position to resolve conflicts between parties, may have combined incentives to influence the jurisdiction of the court: on the one hand, they represent the law and are meant to proceed in all independence; on the other hand, they may represent, and therefore protect the interests of the organizations that supported their becoming a judge in the first place.

Influencing who becomes a judge and what resources are available to these judges can be a very strong, although indirect, way of influencing the outcome of judicial decision making. In effect, collegial deliberation among judges is built into legal institutions. This deliberation – whether formal or informal – relies heavily on knowledge management by the court. This brings us to the second process (in Flemming's list above) by which influence characterizing joint governance is exercised in such organizations. One way to influence the behaviour of judges is to try to set the premises of their decisions by attempting to control the information and advice available to them while sitting in judgment. Judges coming from one sector of the economy may thus, as "judicial entrepreneurs" (McIntosh and Cates 1997), attempt to keep particular definitions of problems alive, or promote the ideas, customs, rules, and interests that are commonplace in their sector, although not in others. Control over the premises of decisions can be assumed to influence the probability of who wins even if this "framing control" by players is almost invisible to outside observers.

The law and the courts are aware of the fact that different types of actors in the environment of the court are involved in such attempted influence. Anticipating that the court will be the target of such external attempts at influence, the legal system provides rules concerning conflicts of interests for judges: when they are too close to one of the parties, for example, when they sit in judgment on a competitor, sometimes even of a business in the same industry as their industry of origin, they must self-disqualify or, if discovered, be removed from the case by their hierarchy. However, a neo-structural approach to joint regulation can question the success of such procedural attempts in neutralizing external influences, especially when the judges are elected or self-selected by ideological commitment to political ideas.

This approach is useful in part because it helps identify the small collegial oligarchies with particular influence in transnational institution building. They are enrolled to work on the professional hurdles linked to the diversity of approaches to the same issue in different countries. To describe social and communication networks during these 'field configuring events' helps explore the micropolitics of institution building among multi-status oligarchs. In particular, I look at the production of alignments in networking among collegial oligarchies. I argue that such normative alignments take place in combining norms and status, i.e. in alignments between epistemic leaders who are *primi inter pares*.

The Case of a Transnational Institution Specialized in Intellectual Property

The European Unified Patent Court (UPC) is an informative case for further exploration of these micropolitics of institutionalization. The main actors in this work of joint regulation are corporate lawyers and judges as institutional entrepreneurs. In this case, corporate lawyers create, on behalf of their clients, a social network of heterogeneous judges so as to pre-organize future normative alignments on the anormative rules selected as the procedural basis for the future institution.

During the last two decades, judges who specialized in patents in their own countries were brought together in a 'field configuring event' to network and get to know each other, learn about each other's logics and discuss substantive interpretation and procedural choices that will create the framing of this future European judicial institution. The event in which this process is examined is the so-called Venice Forum (VF), a microcosm that was orchestrated by the corporate lawyers representing large European companies (in sectors with patents at the core of their business model, such as pharmaceutical, biotech, semi-conductors, etc.) and organized in an association called European Patent Lawyers Association (EPLAW), the European Patent Office (EPO), the European office awarding European patents to companies),[2] and an association of judges (called IPJA, for Intellectual Property Judges Association) coming from all over Europe. The main institutional and long-sighted entrepreneurs driving the institutionalization process have been the corporate lawyers, whether large law firms or powerful in-house lawyers of large corporations. But the main actors at this event, the judges, are a heterogeneous set of judges in the sense that they can be top level judges as well as low level in the judicial hierarchy, specialized or generalist judges, and at different stages of their career, the structure of this career being different in various European countries

[2]EPO is the executive arm of the European Patent Organisation, an intergovernmental organisation that was set up on 7 October 1977 on the basis of the European Patent Convention (EPC) signed in Munich in 1973. It has two bodies, the European Patent Office and the Administrative Council, which supervises the Office's activities.

and legal cultures. At the time, and still today in practice (2015), Europe had 27 jurisdictions and 27 kinds of patent decisions. During this event, lawyers and judges got to know each other, gave conferences, organized mock trials and dreamed up the future institution and its procedure.

The Venice Forum had three general goals. The first was to facilitate communication and recognition among European patent judges who were likely to work together in the future Unified Patent Court (UPC). The judges who accepted the invitation to participate came from the lowest specialized jurisdictions as well as from the highest national courts in the European countries. The second was to help lawyers know the judges. Corporate lawyers participate in this effort to build a new market institution because it helps them get to know their judges and to observe mock trials in a way that allows them to prepare a toolkit of strategies, including a multilevel and sophisticated way of carrying out 'forum shopping' for their clients. The third was actually to promote a specific perspective on the European patent as well as the construction of the UPC as an expression of European legal patriotism that is meant to protect the economic interests of European innovation in the competition with other continents. The judges coming to the Venice Forum knew that their gathering was part of a broader political process.

The ambition of EPLAW and EPO is to create convergence towards a unified substantive interpretation of good patents. They however do not succeed in getting rid of interpretive differences in political economies and forms of capitalism as diverse as, for example, the UK and Germany. Redesigning the institutional framework of intellectual property is in fact an enormous political ambition. In addition, the regulatory activity of the judges is not simply aligned on the institutional model and constraints of their respective countries. The multilevel character of the structure allows for discretion and flexibility at the individual level. Judges from the same country can understand what a 'good patent' is in different ways. Their conception of the good patent in terms of goals and scope varies. These variations still exist today and our purpose is to examine the extent to which alignments on possible dominant views takes place through a set of processes bringing together conventions and structures, culture and networks, norms and status (Favereau and Lazega 2002).

Jettinghoff (2011) has provided a reconstruction of the history of the attempts to build a European patent and a European Patent Court in two parallel and competing political arenas (Venice vs. Brussels, to simplify), with a presentation of the underlying political dynamics, including a presentation of the stakeholders and an exploration of the influence of groups of "patent law experts" in the process, i.e. the corporate lawyers and judges who were, for the latter, our respondents. Jettinghoff argues that the Venice Forum mattered in the regulatory process. In 1973, a treaty called the European Patent Convention was signed and the European Patent Office in Munich created as an agency outside of the EU. The Patent was not a Community Patent, only a "Unitary Patent" for Contracting States, but EPO was allowed to bypass national patent offices in Europe. "The intention was that the integration of the patent system would be completed with a unitary patent and a common court of appeal." It took 40 years until a European judicial institution was created (in 2012) due to become operational in 2015. Rules produced in Venice as opposed to Brussels thus qualify as anormative rules.

In the core of the network and personalized collegial elite around which the Venice Forum is constructed, actors know that it is not likely that a single substantive interpretation and political consensus will emerge among them on the definition of what a good patent is. Their purpose is to start with the goal of creating procedural norms and the adhesion of European judges to these norms. For the members of the elite of judges, the job is to circulate the procedural norms that they are used to rely upon and that they want to champion. Mock trials are meant to stage the use of such norms, discuss them, compare them to other norms, and try to reach consensus on how to use them. In fact the core judges are mediators between their national interests and the other judges and their job is to circulate the norms. The more central they are in the VF network, the more successful they are in that respect. Open and direct political discourse is not allowed because European judges, as a principle, are used to defend their independence in that area; but the same ideas are framed in discourse on convergence between legal cultures and bodies of law.

The VF succeeded in enrolling and mobilizing a whole population of judges around a core of already committed judges, to recognize them individually as representatives of their countries, to create ties between them (i.e. build a personalized network of European judges who know each other well), to provide them with both epistemic leadership and the opportunity to meet, talk and rub shoulders with these leaders, and thus to construct the support of the less committed judges. This social exchange provides the semi-peripheral and peripheral judges with a chance to be listened to and with a chance to feel that they co-constructed the procedural norms coming out of these events as guidelines for the future Patent Court. It is well known that actors who contribute to construction of norms are much more likely to enforce these norms than actors who are simply subjected to them.

European countries have different judicial cultures, which allows for forum shopping by multinational corporations that select the courts of the country that interprets substantive patent law in a way favourable to their interests.[3] But IP related normative choices framing the future institution can be either substantive or procedural. Based on interviews (Lazega 2011), with respect to a personal substantive interpretation of the rule in the application of patent law, the judges were asked about their personal and substantive views on patents, in particular whether they think that they are exceptions to the freedom of copying which means that the validity of patents and the scope of protection are to be critically assessed; or whether they are rewards for the contribution of the inventor and therefore their validity is to be subject to a mild assessment and the scope of protection is to be broad. The results were that, on the one hand, 45.5 % of the polled judges believed patents to be exceptions to the freedom of copying. The reasons provided are not necessarily homogenous. For example a UK judge generalizes the definition: "patents are exceptions to the freedom of independent action". A French judge

[3]See for example the case of the "Italian Torpedo" (Franzosi 1997).

thinks that too many patents are delivered, and therefore judges should be more critical: "The problem is that there are all sorts of patents. In France, we have between a 50 % and 70 % cancellation rate for European patents awarded by EPO with an 80 % confirmation rate on appeal. In the awarding of patents there will be a need to show more rigor and requirements – of raising the bar (. . .) EPO's problem and solution approach is not always reliable in France, we are more demanding about an inventive step than EPO. EPO's budget depends on the number of patents awarded and we spend our time cancelling their patents". Another argument used in favour of critical assessment is that "allowing small changes or small innovations [to be patented] too often would increase the workload of courts and patent offices".

On the other hand, 27.3 % of the judges thought that patents are rewards for the contribution of the inventor. A Portuguese judge thinks that "progress and innovation should be promoted – it takes a lot of work to create something and this work should be rewarded by creating a calm environment". However a few judges express the opinion that the second part of the statement, "mild assessment of the validity of the patent and broad scope of protection" is not necessarily a consequence of the first part of the statement, and thus has to be balanced. This divide led 21.2 % of the judges to take a position "in between", a position often labelled "The European Compromise", i.e. to assert that they apply one rule or the other depending on cases: "Decisions are made on the merits of the case and whether they demand a strict or wider interpretation of the innovation".

Venice Forum judges thus disagree on the substantive interpretation of the definition of a good patent. This shows in the variations in responses to the question on the rule that they apply in patent-related litigation. There is however a considerable agreement between them, regardless of interpretive disagreements, on several procedural rules that should be used and that stem from the rules already used by EPO: first, the assessment of an inventive step; second, the determination of scope of protection; third, the involvement of technical experts. Procedural rules can be considered to be examples of 'weak culture', as defined by Breiger (2010), as well as anormative rules as defined by Archer (Chap. "7", this volume). Building procedural agreements is much easier than building substantive consensus in interpretation. Since national courts would often disagree about the solutions to provide for similar cases the process of transnational institutionalization depends, at least for a generation, on the consensus and jurisprudence that elite transnational individual judges, the first sitting judges of this court, will be able to build based on these procedural rules.

Measuring Alignment on Anormative Rules

Given the lack of agreement on substantive interpretations of patents and derived rules, the individual composition of the oligarchy of judges becomes extremely important in the institutionalization process of this transnational court. Indeed, the future judges of this institution will have to make individual decisions that will create a jurisprudence that is likely, derived from previous experience, to create the basis for future law. Therefore, personalized networks of mobilizing, learning, building personal adhesion to norms and alignments of the champions promoting these norms becomes a crucial process in the management of dissensus in substantive interpretation. During the interviews all the judges accepted to share their perception of who among them was personifying the future Uniform European position with respect to procedural rules, if they believed that any Uniform position would emerge over time. Nominating the judges who were closest to reflecting the future European norm in their discourse with respect to the controversial issues listed above was equivalent, in these judges' minds, to electing these opinion leaders to become the first sitting judges at the future European Court, if not the members of the future Court of Appeal under the control of which judges at the European Court would operate.

Figure 8.1 maps this Uniform network, providing information about how the judges position themselves and others with respect to a future possible uniform European doctrine on patent issues. As shown in this figure, the Uniform network is a highly centralized one.

Identifying the most central judges in this network shows that the Venice Forum judges perceived at least six judges among themselves, from five different countries, as colleagues whose positions on controversial issues are likely to reflect the future EU Uniform position. In this network, these judges are Dutch, German, British,

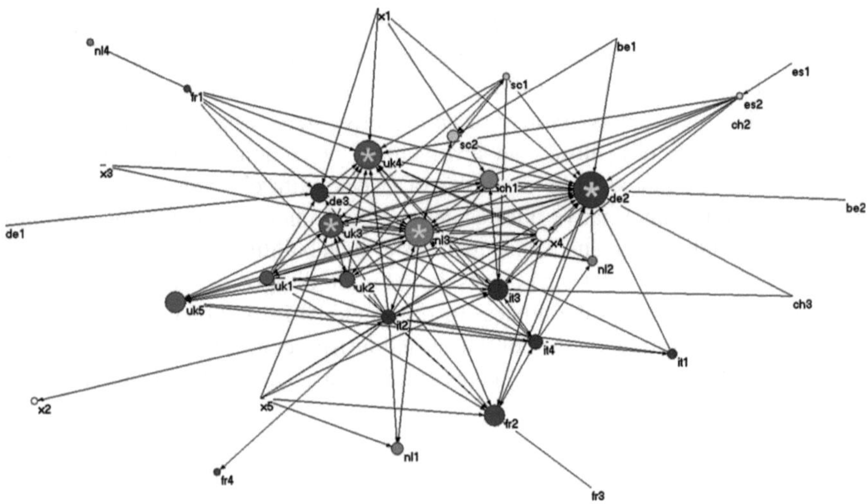

Fig. 8.1 Identifying super-central leaders (multi-status oligarchs) with inconsistent forms of status in a collegial oligarchy assembled by a transnational, public-private bureaucracy: the case of judges perceived by their peers as closest to the future Uniform European position (if any) on the interpretation of patents. The core of this network is defined as the most cited judges (indegree centralities) based on the number of citations above the 90th percentile. The core/periphery dimension of the structure of this system is confirmed by statistical analyses

Italian and Swiss. Many have different ideas with respect to 'harmonization' of positions in Europe, some even disapproving the idea of convergence, stressing 'circulation' instead of convergence, even if this must lead to diverging decisions and lack of judicial security. Thus, in 2009, convergence towards consensus on the EU uniform position in this network still remained uncertain. One can infer from this structure that field configuring events such as the VF do not necessarily, by themselves, lead to convergence of perspectives and uniform positions among IP judges in Europe. When countries are clustered into blocks that each represents a different type of capitalism (i.e. German, Anglo-Saxon, and all the others) based on the classification of types of capitalism identified by Bruno Amable (2003) in three categories,[4] this picture indicates very clearly that the UK and German forms of capitalism are at the core and that future alignments will go from the North and from the South of Europe towards these two dominant kinds of IP capitalism.

At the stage of development of this transnational institution, normative divergences among institutional leaders matter much less than the individual understanding that each of the judges gains from clarifying the differences between their own approach on these issues and that of their perceived institutional leaders. Combined analyses of conventions and relational structures in a complex institutionalization process show that this process consists in exploring with institutional entrepreneurs the price that they will have to pay, the concessions that they will have to make, in order to participate further. Experiments of role playing in mock trials with judges coming from different European countries were fleshing out these future alignments. In many ways the VF was preparing for the socialization of future European judges who will be the main powers in this institution, and signaling expected normative alignments on institutional leaders' procedural choices. The forging of new appropriateness judgments as a specific step in the institutionalization process depends on the choice of priority norms in a controversial context, and this step is successful when this choice is collectively personalized by a collegial oligarchy, a step that is easier to achieve in such elitist assemblies brought together in selective field configuring events. Progress in the negotiation of priority norms is achieved through these identifications, these creations of pecking orders and these alignments on the normative choices made by the members at the top of these pecking orders. Network analyses thus have a revealing effect on specific dimensions of institutionalization processes, such as the negotiation of priority anormative regulation combined with the identification of a leadership that will personify the reference group and the norms that are deemed common to its members.

For business, forging these common and personalized judgments is a largely invisible way of framing, building, ultimately 'capturing' a public institution. This

[4]Mainly the European continental capitalism (characterizing CH, NL, IR, BE, NO, DE, F, AT) with Germany, and in part the NL, as its leaders on this terrain of patent law – although the NL could also be considered in part as a representative of social democratic capitalism (characterizing DK, FI, SE); and the liberal market capitalism represented by the UK. Mediterranean or Southern capitalism includes GR, IT, Port, ES who also happen to be countries without strong IP specialization in their judiciary.

process facilitates the creation of a self-contained normative space where challenges are reduced to 'safe criticism' and exogenous control becomes very costly, next to impossible. The elitist nature of institution building has long been an issue for observers of a European 'democratic deficit'. Elitism can also be a way to protect the institution: very generally, when an institution dysfunctions, individuals are blamed, which is only accepted by elite individuals. Neo-structural sociology shows that if institutionalization processes are facilitated by this personalization, then the issue raised by this deficit may be how to design institutions that depend less on this personification.

There were no clear winners and losers yet in 2009 in this institutionalization process as measured through normative alignments, although it was already obvious that some would have to make more concessions than others to be retained in the future as judges in the upcoming court. In the case in point examined here, the conditions under which this process is successful still remain uncertain. The substantive 'European compromise' in interpretation of patent laws is still elusive: this lack of consensus is dangerous for this institution. For example, industrialists in the UK and Germany might fear being dispossessed of their own conception of IP to the benefit of their competitors' conception, a dangerous situation for their markets and profits that will lead to forum shopping. The future Uniform position is still unclear and replaced by procedural anormative rules. Without consensus on personal interpretation, only personified consensus on procedural norms is anticipated. These public/private institutions accept that the procedural rules will be formulated by highly selected judges who are considered epistemic and normative authorities by their peers before these rules are injected into and tested by the political process. The institution as a 'tool with a life of its own' (Selznick 1957) has this unpredictable element. But its specialized nature makes the process more capturable and safer for them than if the institution had been framed and built in the public arena, under the surveillance of the wider political spectrum.

Shedding this neo-structural light on regulation is thus equivalent to analyzing the production of anormative rules. These regulatory processes take new forms in contemporary society (Archer 2013, 2014) and involve hidden costs. Increasingly, organizational societies see secondary socialization to such anormative rules as the main source of social order.

Toward a Multilevel Spinning to Model of Institutional Emergence

To reflect more generally on the link between relational structures and the process of institutionalization, especially of anormative rules, it is useful to remember that social networks are systems of interdependencies between actors (individuals or organizational) capable of collective action. A complex social phenomenon such as the emergence of a new institution takes place at several levels simultaneously that must not be conflated but that co-constitute each other (Archer 1982; Breiger 1974;

Brailly and Lazega 2012; Lazega et al. 2008). Dynamics of such multilevel systems of collective agency assume, as also suggested by Berends et al. (2011) or Grossetti (2011), that the evolution of networks at one level of collective action is influenced by that of another level of collective action, and the other way around in recursive ways.

Such dynamics can be considered to be the outcome of a meta-process bringing together both individuals and organizations, in which the evolution of one level explains in part (in causal terms) the evolution of the other. Level 1 relationships can emerge as a result of the emergence of level 2 relationships. Actors of level 1 may be able under certain circumstances to change the structure of level 2, especially by bringing an intermediary level into the picture, a substructure such as workgroups between which individuals move and that includes individuals and is capable of collective action and is included in the organization, and therefore in the inter-organizational level of collective action. This kind of intermediary level substructure – including relational infrastructures such as status and niches– represents both a tool and a "decompression chamber" between levels.

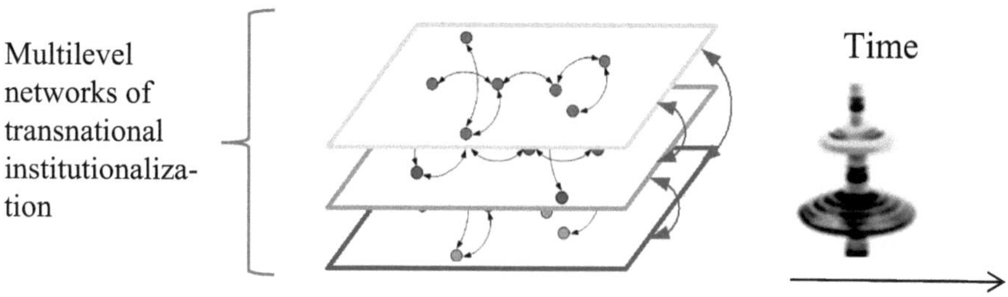

This image of a multilevel spinning top combines dynamic and multilevel perspectives on the institutionalization of norms and especially of anormative rules. In this metaphor, we find the ingredients of institutional emergence: decisions and normative choices made by individual actors and organizations, affiliations of individuals to organizations, networks of collective agency at each level, trajectories and more or less supervised circulations between places at the intermediary level (as in many labour markets in which competition is made increasingly open as one goes down the social stratification hierarchy), but also changing relationships between these intermediary level airlocks themselves as driven by relational turnover created by mobility (Lazega et al. 2006). This set of processes can perhaps become increasingly morphogenic when bringing together networks of different levels in which individuals' affiliations are thus dependent on their mobility in loops, as in carrousels. Evolution of a multilevel social space means, from this perspective, dynamics related to this third, intermediary level. To understand the dynamics of coevolution between collective actions at two levels, it is necessary to bring in an intermediary – but nevertheless, in our view, generic third level.

In many ways, the case in point of the emergence of the Unified Patent Court presented above is an application of this multilevel spinning top. It helps explain how a small network of institutional entrepreneurs with multiple and inconsistent forms of status uses, in its lobbying activity, multilevel networks and their dynamics to acquire the staying capacity and subsequent influence that is needed to frame, build and entrench a transnational institution. The image of a spinning top represents this process heuristically.

These circular movements and trajectories of actors (for example mobilities in loops (White 1970) and revolving doors from public responsibilities to private jobs, and back to public positions) create an informal pecking order (metaphorically: the shaft of the spinning top) that enables the most central among these institutional entrepreneurs to obtain central formal positions in the institutionalization process and to act as brokers between conflicting sides with different political definitions of the institution. The main idea of this mechanism is that when such individual, oligarchic and dynamic positions of institutional entrepreneurs are stabilized by a supportive inter-organizational network (hence the crucial dynamics of the multilevel dimension of the process), these entrepreneurs are able to maintain their centrality and interactions long enough to surf on – if not to avoid altogether – the unpredictable and conflictual politics of the electoral process. This mechanism thus helps them succeed in their institutionalization efforts in spite of being a small collegial oligarchy: the multilevel structure of the systems of interdependencies between the actors helps them keep their initial advantage as institutional entrepreneurs in selecting rules that will become priority rules for this institution. Here, the dynamics of multilevel networks are indicators of this mechanism that mobilizes superimposed levels of collective agency, interpersonal and inter-organizational at least, i.e. two meso levels that are added to the traditional national and international levels of agency and complexity.

Taking into account the vertical complexity of the social world requires differentiating and articulating these levels and their respective dynamics, adding a problem that can be called a problem of "synchronization" between levels. Synchronization is a task of scheduling and coordinating superimposed interpersonal and inter-organizational forms of collective agency over time at the cost of one level or the other. Synchronization between levels by building and maintaining social forms is much more costly for some than for others, especially for actors who are forced to be mobile – unless they can use this mobility to create new advantageous social forms. Stabilizing synchronization costs is rewarding for actors with a strong relational infrastructure because these costs are either shared or dumped on others. From that temporal perspective, the whole process of institutionalization examined above may in itself be part of synchronization dynamics characterizing a morphogenic society (Archer 1995).

Conclusion

In tracing complex institutionalization that often presents itself as specialized, it is worth using a neo-structural approach to joint regulation processes in which business and the state structure the context of interactions and thus create favorable circumstances for the emergence and enforcement of new collective rules, at the international level in the example used here. Tracing this process leads to a series of steps that provide a neo-structural approach to the determinants and proliferation of 'anormative regulation' (Archer, Chap. "7", this volume). The result of the regulatory process depends on the pattern of interactions between players with a specific structural identity, called multi-status oligarchs, especially on their capacity to use – thus undermining electoral democracy – their multiple, heterogeneous and inconsistent forms of status, as well as weak culture, to build/buy bureau-professional legitimacy. This register of legitimacy presents itself as both minimal and taken for granted when looking at each new and specialized rule promoted separately, but as impossible to change when looking at the system of rules bundled together. The role of this regulatory process in the recomposition of the political regime of Europe is sketched through the example of the creation and installation of the European Unified Patent Court and the question of the possible institutional crisis that could emerge from a constitutional conflict with the European Court of Justice.

In this case, failed internationalization of substantive interpretation of patent law in the European context ('patent as exception' [very special protection against competition] *vs.* 'patent as reward' [less special returns on investments]) does not prevent collegial oligarchies from creating anormative procedural rules (about assessing inventive steps, determination of scope of protection, involvement of technical experts, etc.) that will allow a small elite of national judges to operate a transnational institution that is created nevertheless – and perhaps to prevent deeper political challenges to the patent system altogether. This highlights an under-examined set of processes in the dynamics of transnational institutionalization, revolving around the identification of anormative rules and leaders in elitist settings, as well as future alignments on these norms and leaders as part of the institutionalization process. Their discussions are meant to guide their lobbying efforts in the elitist process of constructing a judicial institution dealing with patent litigation. Patents are specific types of protections against competition and the conditions under which they should be awarded to entrepreneurs and the ways in which they should be defined when adjudicating patent-related litigation are discussed by judges who, in such transnational institutions, represent themselves but also inevitably their national public authorities and the kind of capitalism that dominates in their respective country. This documents and analyses the extent to which they will play a crucial role in the joint regulatory regime set up by this European court. Important problems emerge in the progressive construction of the future Uniform European position (if any) with respect to patents. This chapter shows how Northern European forms of capitalism dominate this process at the expense of the Southern European forms of capitalism by looking at several dimensions of patents as construed by these judges and corporate lawyers.

This empirical case shows that transnational institution building is the work of collegial networks of elite institutional entrepreneurs who meet in such field-configuring events and negotiate new rules for the organizations that they represent or in which they are affiliated. In this multilevel context, individuals in personalized inter-individual networks operate with or without mandates to promote the interests of organizations in inter-organizational networks and processes of institution building (Lazega et al. 2008). In particular, professionals in transnational institution building negotiate the 'distributed agency' in how organizing occurs (Quack 2007) by thinking in multilevel network terms to make their moves and implement their strategies. They define the tasks and exercise control over their enforcement. I used network analysis to look into how such entrepreneurs interact to build institutions and try to create what I call epistemic convergence towards a common ground of anormative rules so as to control the heterogeneity of positions across borders.

In many ways the capacity of collegial oligarchies including political leaders, business executives, professionals or experts, and high level civil servants to join forces and to play the same tragi-comical game of building/buying bureau-professional legitimacy from inconsistent forms of status shows how strong national and international elites are in producing anormative rules. It also shows how weak they are in producing substantive and interpretive political compromises, i.e. to foster truly social regulation at national and international levels. In fact I would argue that social regulation does not really exist at the international level yet. Underneath every kind of rule, there is a conventional representation of the collective to which this rule is intended to apply (Favereau and Lazega 2002). Analyzing the structural basis of the normative order shows where the 'democratic deficit' comes from. Whether at the national or international level, anormative rules are the recipe for such a deficit, if not a threat to democracy itself (Mair 2013). In shaping the law of the future, the risk is that only powerful States and powerful private actors will have a voice in the regulatory process, reaching agreements in which the law is too distant from customs and social norms, and thus too costly to enforce in societies that wish to remain democratic. This is especially the case with joint regulation that comes from the private sector, spreads in societies and is never legitimized by the electoral system.

References

Amable, B. (2003). *The diversity of modern capitalism*. Oxford: Oxford University Press.

Archer, M. S. (1982). Morphogenesis versus structuration: On combining structure and action. *British Journal of Sociology, 35*, 455–483.

Archer, M. S. (1995). *Realist social theory: The morphogenetic approach*. Cambridge: Cambridge University Press.

Archer, M. S. (Ed.). (2013). *Late modernity: Trajectories towards morphogenic society* (Vol. II). Dordrecht: Springer.

Archer, M. S. (Ed.). (2014). *The generative mechanisms transforming late modernity*. Dordrecht: Springer.

Archer, M. S. (2016). Anormative social regulation: An attempt to cope with social morphogenesis. In M. Archer (Ed.), *Morphogenesis and the crisis of normativity*. Dordrecht: Springer.

Berends, H., Van Burg, E., & van Raaij, E. M. (2011). Contacts and contracts: Cross-level network dynamics in the development of an aircraft material. *Organization Science, 22*, 940–960.

Brailly, J., & Lazega, E. (2012). Diversité des approches de la modélisation multiniveaux en analyses de réseaux sociaux et organisationnels. *Mathématiques et Sciences Humaines, 198*, 5–32.

Braithwaite, J. (2005, October). *Neoliberalism or regulatory capitalism*. RegNet Occasional Paper N° 5, Australian National University: Regulatory Institutions Network.
Braithwaite, J. (2008). *Regulatory capitalism*. Cheltenham: Edward Elgar.
Breiger, R. L. (1974). The duality of persons and groups. *Social Forces, 53*, 181–190.
Breiger, R. L. (2010). Dualities of culture and structure: Seeing through cultural holes. In J. Fuhse & S. Mützel (Eds.), *Relationale Soziologie: Zur kulturellen Wende der Netzwerkforschung* (pp. 37–47). Berlin: VS Verlag.
Edelman, L. B., & Suchman, M. C. (2007). *The legal lives of private organizations*. Ashgate: The International Library of Essays in Law and Society.
Favereau, O., & Lazega, E. (Eds.). (2002). *Conventions and structures in economic organization: Markets, networks and hierarchies*. Cheltenham: Edward Elgar.
Flemming, R. B. (1998). Contested terrains and regime politics: Thinking about America's trial courts and institutional change. *Law & Social Inquiry, 23*, 941–965.
Flood, J. (2002). Capital markets, globalisation and global elites. In M. Likosky (Ed.), *Transnational legal processes – globalisation and power disparities*. London: Butterworths.
Flood, J. (2007). Lawyers as sanctifiers of value creation. *Indiana Journal of Global Legal Studies, 14*, 35–66.
Frank, R. H. (1985). *Choosing the right pond: Human behavior and the quest for status*. Oxford: Oxford University Press.
Franzosi, M. (1997). Worldwide patent litigation and the Italian Torpedo. *European Intellectual Property Review, 19*, 382–385.
Grossetti, M. (2011). 'L'espace à trois dimensions des phénomènes sociaux. Echelles d'action et d'analyse'. *Sociologies*.http://sociologies.revues.org/index3466.html
Hellman, J., Jones, G., & Kaufmann, D. (2000). Seize the state, seize the day: State capture, corruption and influence in transition. *World Bank Policy Research Working Paper* N° 2444.
Jettinghoff, A. (2011). The quest for a transnational patent system in Europe: A preliminary reconstruction. *Recht der Werkelijkheid (Journal of Socio-Legal Studies), 32*(3), 52–65.
Katz, J. (1977). Cover-up and collective integrity. *Social Problems, 25*, 1–25.
Lazega, E. (1994). Les conflits d'intérêts dans les cabinets américains d'avocats d'affaires: Concurrence et auto-régulation. *Sociologie du Travail, 35*, 315–336.
Lazega, E. (2001). *The collegial phenomenon: The social mechanisms of cooperation among peers in a corporate law partnership*. Oxford: Oxford University Press.
Lazega, E. (2009). Theory of cooperation among competitors: A neo-structural approach'. *Sociologica*. http://www.sociologica.mulino.it/main [*Italian Journal of Sociology Online*, N° 1/2009. With Comments by Luigi Burroni, Sophie Mützel and Harrison White and a "Short response to Luigi Burroni, Sophie Mützel and Harrison White", same URL.]
Lazega, E. (2011). Pertinence et structure. *Swiss Sociological Review, 37*, 127–149.
Lazega, E. (2012). Time to shrink to greatness? Networks and conflicts of interests in large professional firms. *Revue für post-heroisches Management, 10*, 68–77.
Lazega, E., & Favereau, O. (2002). Introduction. In O. Favereau & E. Lazega (Eds.), *Conventions and structures in economic organization: Markets, networks and hierarchies*. Cheltenham: Edward Elgar.
Lazega, E., & Mounier, L. (2002). Interdependent entrepreneurs and the social discipline of their cooperation: A research program for structural economic sociology in a society of organizations. In O. Favereau & E. Lazega (Eds.), *Conventions and structures in economic organization: Markets, networks and hierarchies* (pp. 147–199). Cheltenham: Edward Elgar.
Lazega, E., & Mounier, L. (2012). Networks of institutional capture. In B. Vedres & M. Scotti (Eds.), *Networks in social policy problems* (pp. 124–137). Cambridge: Cambridge University Press.
Lazega, E., Lemercier, C., & Mounier, L. (2006). A spinning top model of formal structure and informal behaviour: Dynamics of advice networks in a commercial court. *European Management Review, 3*, 113–122.

Lazega, E., Jourda, M., Mounier, L., & Stofer, R. (2008). Catching up with big fish in the big pond? Multi-level network analysis through linked design. *Social Networks, 30*, 157–176.

Lazega, E., Jourda, M.-T., & Mounier, L. (2013). Network lift from dual alters: Extended opportunity structures from a multilevel and structural perspective. *European Sociological Review, 29*, 1226–1238.

Mair, P. (2013). *Ruling the void: The hollowing of western democracy*. London: Verso.

McIntosh, W. V., & Cates, C. L. (1997). *Judicial entrepreneurship: The role of the judge in the marketplace of ideas*. Westport: Greenwood Press.

Merton, R. K. (1959). *Social theory and social structure*. Glencoe: The Free Press.

Quack, S. (2007). Legal professionals and transnational law-making: A case of distributed agency. *Organization, 14*(5), 643–666.

Reynaud, J.-D., & Reynaud, E. (1996). La régulation des marchés internes du travail. *Revue Française de Sociologie, 37*, 337–368.

Sellers, C. (1991). *The market revolution: Jacksonian America 1815–1846*. New York: Cambridge University Press.

Selznick, P. (1957). *Leadership in administration*. Evanston: Row, Peterson & Co.

Vedres, B., & Stark, D. (2010). Structural folds: Generative disruption in overlapping groups. *American Journal of Sociology, 115*, 1150–1190.

White, H. C. (1970). *Chains of opportunity: System models of mobility in organizations*. Cambridge: Harvard University Press.

Chapter 9
The Fragile Movements of Late Modernity

Mark Carrigan

Introduction

In his contribution to the present volume, Porpora (2016) analyses the 'great normative transformations' of the twentieth century and the mechanisms responsible for bringing them about. Through a series of 'capsule narratives' he discerns some "general elements of normative change": their causal complexity, the role of agency and the contributions of multiple agents at different levels of the social order. This chapter shares similar concerns but in a *prospective* mode. While Porpora (2016) looks back to see how what "may begin as isolated individuals [...] combine forces to form social movement organizations" and perhaps achieve success through a process that "involve[s] changes in formal rules that come from the higher placed agency of government officials", this chapter will look forward to consider how the present conditions under which motivated persons 'combine forces' might contribute towards the possible transition to a morphogenic social order of which the present project is an extended investigation.

Open systems being what they are, no attempt will be made to predict future outcomes. I will instead seek to identify mechanisms operative upon the transition from *personal* reflexivity to *collective* reflexivity in order to better understand the role of agency in contributing to social morphogenesis (or failing to do so). Donati and Archer (2015) offer couples, families, voluntary associations, cooperatives, labour unions, political parties, foundations, local communities and social movements as examples of those entities capable of exercising collective reflexivity i.e. "constituting a collectivity that evaluates objectives (discernment), deliberates about realizing its common concerns (deliberation) and commits itself

M. Carrigan (✉)
Centre for Social Ontology, University of Warwick, Coventry, UK
e-mail: mark@markcarrigan.net

M.S. Archer (eds.), *Morphogenesis and the Crisis of Normativity*,
Social Morphogenesis, DOI 10.1007/978-3-319-28439-2_9

to achieving them (dedication)" (Donati and Archer 2015: 62). The focus in this chapter will be upon *social movements* rather than any of the other collectivities identified above. This is because "the defining characteristic of all movements, big and small, is that they move history along, sometimes in significant ways" (Johnston 2014: 1). The cases in which, as Porpora (2016: 18) puts it, transformative change "was agentically motored intentionally from below by grassroots social movements" may be the exception rather than the rule but the *attempt* to do precisely this was a crucial factor in all the changes described in his chapter. While social movements are only one form of collective, they are significant for present purposes given their *potential* implications for social normativity at the macroscopic level.

This leaves us with an obvious question: what *is* a social movement? For present purposes, the capacity of movements for *collective reflexivity* is crucial but stressing this does nothing to help us define what movements themselves are and how they differ from other kinds of relational subject. The voluminous literature on social movements offers many potential answers to the question (Crossley 2002: 1–16). The notion that movements are in some sense *collective* invites widespread agreement but this only raises the more primitive question of what constitutes collectivity. For many, collectivity would encompass nothing more than aggregation, with the challenge of social explanation being a matter of elucidating the 'aggregation dynamics' through which microscopic action leads to macroscopic outcomes (Little 2012). Such effects are important and they will play a crucial role in the argument developed in this chapter but an exhaustive focus upon them leaves us unable to ask questions about the *emergent* characteristics of movements. The concern here is not just how people 'join forces' but how the manner of their coming together helps constitute a reality which influences their subsequent doings, individually *and* collectively, in a manner that exceeds the aggregate contributions of each individual. For instance we know that movements can have biographical consequences in both the short and long term (McAdam 1989). The contribution of social movements to morphogenesis can be as much a matter of changes undergone by those participating in them as the success or failure of their collective projects. In fact retaining these parallel categories of *biography* and *movement* not only helps us ask questions about the causal relation between them,[1] it also allows us to consider how extrinsic factors act upon each and how this may in turn generate second-order effects with consequences for the formation of future movements and the durability of present ones.

This is precisely what the present chapter attempts by asking how the diffusion of digital technology discussed by Archer (2014, 2015) acts causally upon biographies and upon social movements, as well as identifying second-order effects operative through the relation between the two. Social movements have *always* relied upon communications technology but the distinctive affordances of digital communica-

[1] For instance *what effect a particular movement had upon the lives of the activists who participated in it* or *how the movement was shaped by the particular route of these activists into it.*

tions have increasingly preoccupied both lay and academic commentators (Couldry 2014). The first section of this chapter aims to get beyond this at times hyperbolic discourse by identifying precisely what *has* changed in the sphere of digital communications and what is at stake in these changes. The second section considers the implications of these changes for *personal reflexivity*. Though their effects are uneven, three mechanisms are ventured which produce a *first-order* tendency towards people struggling to cope in the face of spiralling demands upon their attention and a *second-order* tendency towards a constrained practice of reflexivity inimical to considerations beyond the narrow confines of personal life. The third section turns to the reliance of social movements upon digital communications. The relative ease with which it is now possible to assemble a group for a protest is argued to have fatal ramifications for the capacity of that crowd to grow into a durable movement. The final section considers what happens when *distracted people* meet *fragile movements*: a growing susceptibility to manipulation by those other agents capable of exercising collective reflexivity who, unlike social movements, thrive in a social order in which digital data has become a new positional good of incomparable importance.

The case made is that digital technology is operating, at the level of personal reflexivity and collective reflexivity, in a way which militates against the organised and sustained transition from the former to the latter. This does not entail a diminution of the social critique (personal reflexivity) or political protest (collective reflexivity) that registers at an *empirical* level. The change being postulated is occurring in the relationship between the former and the latter. There is no suppression of the capacity of subjects, as strong evaluators in Taylor's (1989) sense, to orientate themselves critically towards aspects of social reality in a way which leads them to be seen as *necessitating* change. Through such an orientation, subjects can come to adopt 'causes' which exercise a transformative influence upon their biographical trajectories due to the centrality which social transformations come to assume in their lives as personal concerns which give rise to social projects (Archer 2007). Movements emerge from personal reflexivity in this way because transformative projects of this kind can rarely be accomplished individually. But existent movements also encourage this orientation in subjects by acting as 'carriers' of potential personal causes, holding out possibilities of sustainable projects which allow personal concerns to give rise to shared projects.

This is where the change is occurring: by independently contributing towards 'distracted people' and 'fragile movements', digital technology is undermining the capacity of social movements to contribute in a sustained way towards the steering of social morphogenesis grounded upon normative evaluation of what *does* exist and a collective commitment to what *could* exist. This does not so much represent a failure of moral imagination as a diminishing of the generic capacity to sustain collective projects which have such an origin. The further risk lies in the mutual reinforcement of each, as increasingly fragile movements flicker intensely during their brief but effervescent life, calling for normative evaluation by distracted people[2] who become less able to *sustain trajectories of engagement* with collective projects of transformation, even as their evaluative capacity and political activity register an empirical intensification. Meanwhile the same infrastructural transformation being brought about by digital technology brings us closer to a future which many would reject while facilitating new forms of intervention by collective agents who seek to bring such a future to pass. The gloomy conclusion of this paper is that durable movements are becoming less likely at precisely the time when we most need them.

Digital Capitalism and Digital Technology

In recent years a view of the emancipatory potential of digital technology has become widespread, such that it is assumed new (digitally mediated) social movements will increasingly emerge as the costs of organization decrease, subsequently providing democratic steering over a digital capitalism seen to be increasingly unstable in an age where history has returned with a vengeance (Zizek 2009). Though the technology is still in its infancy, we can already see how the putatively ameliorative force of digital technology provides a reassuring but chimerical answer to the question of who will control our 'runaway world' (Giddens 2002). In short, it is proposed that 'we' will do this, with digital technology (particularly social media[3]) being seen to bring to the fore "what 'we' do naturally, when we have the chance to keep in touch with each other, as of course we want to do": platforms like Facebook and Twitter are seen to herald the birth of collectivities more natural than those which were possible in the pre-web 2.0 age of centralised media and pervasive bureaucracy (Couldry 2014).

Best expressed in the work of cyber optimists like Clay Shirkey (2008, 2010) such a view – which Couldry (2014) suggests can usefully be treated anthropologically as a newly dominant myth – place great normative weight on the possibilities for discussion, sharing and creation afforded by digital technology. This emerging mythology serves to obscure the underlying interests at work, with digital corporations affecting the stance of neutral platform providers while being reliant on the monetization of the crowd they have assembled within their enclosed spaces.

It is helpful here to consider the metaphors which currently abound within discussions of digital technology. The imagery of 'the cloud' is a case in point: this marketing rhetoric regularly enters into the vocabulary of lay actors, reflecting its experiential plausibility vis-à-vis the lack of spatial-temporal constraint facilitated by contemporary digital infrastructure. But the weightlessness and placelessness

[2]Who can of course seek to evade such a call by retreating from the complexity of political questions.

[3]This popular phrase is being avoided for reasons which will hopefully become clear as the chapter progresses.

of 'the cloud' conceals a striking degree of centralisation which belies those who stress the liquidity of contemporary capitalism. The cloud is dependent upon increasingly vast data centres through which the operational requirements of ever increasing swathes of everyday technology are met, reflecting a growing tendency for computational capacity to be cloud-based rather than located in local devices. The mobile computing so central to 'the cloud' is dependent upon a production network which is more reminiscent of Blake's "dark satanic mills" then anything seen for decades in the countries within which these mobile devices are most widely diffused.

The putative weightlessness of the cloud disguises an extensive transformation in contemporary capitalism that has tended to manifest itself in popular consciousness in a heretofore limited way.[4] Consider the contrast offered by Lanchester (2015) between the most profitable corporations in the US in 1960 and in 2015: General Motors made $7.6 billion and employed 600,000 people while Apple made $89.9 billion and employed 92,600.[5] The trend is even more pronounced when we consider market capitalisation. For instance as Lanier (2014: 2) points out, Kodak employed more than 140,000 people and was worth $28 billion dollars at its peak while Instagram, which many would see as its replacement in the digital economy, was sold to Facebook for a billion dollars in 2012 when it employed only thirteen people. This takes place against a background where, as Lanchester (2015) notes, the link between productivity and wages has been broken and mass unemployment produced by new advances in robotics and computational technologies are widely seen as inexorable.

The 'credit-based consumerism' which served to buttress the perceived legitimacy of capitalism after the mutual regulation of the post-WW2 golden age broke down has begun to prove increasingly unsustainable at precisely the point when it would seem to be most needed. The gloomy analysis of Streeck (2014) suggests that the relation of complementarity between social democracy and the liberal economy in the post war period described by Archer (2015) has given rise to a relation of contradiction in which the stability of the liberal economy depends upon the subordination of social democracy.[6] Streeck's (2014: 172) discussion of the "instruments for the ideological marginalization, political disorganization and physical restraint" is likely to be directed at those committed to 'keeping democracy responsive' and 'keeping elites attentive' (Johnston 2014: 160). This immediately calls to mind Lazega's (2014) grim though plausible analysis of how digitised social control might lead to the inhibition of collective reflexivity: through the granularity with which 'big data' allows hierarchical influence to be exercised within organisations coupled with the wilful complicity of individual consumers

[4]For instance in concerns over tax avoidance or in outcries over the most egregious cases of oppression against those workers producing mobile consumer technology.

[5]General Motor's profits are adjusted for 2015s money and Apple's profits are projected by Lanchester on the basis of their first quarter results.

[6]See also Crouch (2004).

who embrace these devices in a way that expands the scope of digitised control. We are currently witnessing the infancy of a synergy between the data-driven behavioural science discussed by Lazega (2014) and anormative regulation of the sort Archer (2016) identifies: radically granular forms of data produced in real time by unobtrusive measurement (instead of being produced as a by-product of other forms of activity) enable types of calculated intervention,[7] licensed by a growing sense of 'big data' as imbued with unprecedented objectivity, to pursue the outcomes of those agents in a data-rich and therefore dominant position within the social order.

In this sense, the same affordances which are drawn upon by social movements for mobilisation also provide other groups with the capacity to monitor and intervene using the very data produced in the process (Tufekci 2014a). The unfortunate extension of this is the tendency of the former to be weakened by digital technology while the capacity for influence of the latter only grows. However such a claim would benefit from a more precise delineation of the multiple changes which are being subsumed under the category of 'digital technology'.

From 'Cyberspace' to the 'Semantic Web' and the 'Internet of Things'

Though any sequential typology has its limitations, the changes in digital technology that are the concern of this chapter can be conveyed in a manner that is analytically useful through the notion of subsequent iterations of end user experience.[8] The experience of *web 1.0* necessitated a desktop computer or laptop computer, with a cable connection to a modem, facilitating the consumption of predominately static content using a web browser. This interface enabled a range of experiences in which the vocabulary of cyberspace and virtual worlds still held intuitive plausibility. The spatial fixity of the access point, as well as the routines involved in creating the connection prior to broadband, served to buttress a sense of the interface as facilitating access to a virtual world in which one 'surfed the net' or traversed the 'information superhighway'.[9]

The experience of *web 2.0* was enabled by the growth of mobile computing, initially through internet enabled mobile phones before the growth of smart phones and

[7]See Crawford and Schultz (2014) for a conceptual discussion of the harms produced through such interventions.

[8]We should not be satisfied with an account of the user experience of digital technology but such a taxonomy can prove a useful starting point for elaborating a sociological account of the mechanisms underpinning these changing experiences.

[9]That these metaphors, which were so vividly represented within a popular culture that they permeated for some time, now seem so jarringly anachronistic illustrates the necessity of getting beyond empiricism in the study of Digitalization. See Lupton (2014: 168–175) for a perceptive discussion of digital technology and the phenomenology of embodiment.

tablet computers, as well as by wireless internet access that brought a new dimension to the inherent mobility of the laptop. Increasingly this was a personalised web in which users contributed to dynamic content as 'prosumers' rather than consuming static content that had been produced by distant others (Beer and Burrows 2007). The archetypical applications of web 2.0 are the Wiki and the Social Networking Service. Latterly, the expansion of cloud computing has facilitated new forms of behaviour, as the spatial-temporal fixity of computing purports to tend towards non-existence, with increasingly complex applications running from web servers (and relying on the computational power of the cloud to minimise lag) and software running on the client side tending increasingly towards high-end specialisation as both the ubiquitous and the niche are rearticulated as web based applications. The nascent *web 3.0*, referred to as the semantic web within the scholarly literature, is one "*no longer built on links between documents – as it is today – but, rather, operates by linking heterogeneous data, quantitative and qualitative, to particular entities: things, concepts, people, or places*" (Halford et al. 2013: 2). If *web 1.0* involved the consumption of fixed documents and *web 2.0* expanded the scope of these documents to incorporate content that was partially or wholly generated by users, *web 3.0* moves beyond the document as the fundamental unit of networked information technology: interlinked documents with discrete contents give way to interconnections between the data entities themselves.

If web 3.0 fulfils its promise, *linked data* will become part of the infrastructure of everyday life, with *technical* barriers to the consolidation of records between databases removed, as well as considerable commercial incentives for the exploitation of linked data for front-end user products (some of which may serve to make daily life much easier and prove extremely popular) and more obviously sinister back-end uses for data mining and targeted analytics. When seen against the backdrop of a putative *internet of things*, perhaps as part of (much hyped) *smart cities* in which data capture is built into the infrastructure of urban space rather than simply being a matter of personal consumption choices, we begin to see the lineaments of a socio-technical environment radically different from anything that has come before; potentially even a tipping point.[10]

This has been a brief sketch of a complex transformation. Two aspects are crucial for the ensuing argument: *the multiplication of communication channels* and the rise of the *filter bubble*. Each was incipient within web 1.0, emerged fully with web 2.0 and will increasingly be designed into the fabric of everyday life with web 3.0.[11]

[10]This technological possibilities opened up by web 3.0 raise important questions about intellectual property: Lanier's (2014) pessimistic analysis could be combined with Archer's (2015) account from the previous volume to forecast that this 'computationalization of everyday life' will intensify the advantages accrued through computational superiority, offering both motive and means to pursue further closure.

[11]For sake of brevity, a substantial discussion of the diffusion dynamics of these technologies was removed from this chapter. Suffice to say, it is not being assumed that these technological changes impact evenly upon all users (or for the matter that people respond to them in the same ways). The framework offered in this section will be developed at a later date into an empirically richer account of these changes as temporally *and* spatially sequenced.

The conceptual and practical challenge they pose for the social sciences has come to be widely recognised but without a stratified ontology that distinguishes between their potential effects at the individual and collective levels, it remains difficult to elucidate their full implications for a complex topic such as social normativity and movement formation.

Multiplication of Communications Channels

In recent years we have seen a proliferation of digital phenomena so rapid that it has led some to suggest that the primary focus of the social sciences should now be descriptive rather than explanatory (Beer and Burrows 2007). Part of the motivation here lies in the obvious challenge presented by their intensely morphogenic character i.e. they generate further novelty at the macro, meso and micro levels. They arise from a confluence of circumstances which is itself intensely morphogenic: the diffusion of new technology (smart phones, tablet computer, broadband access, WiFi, 3G/4G mobile networks etc), the availability of venture capital when profitability is only a distant aspiration and a broader conjuncture within market capitalism in which each of these conditions has come to obtain.

While we may see the rise and fall of particular services (e.g. MYSPACE) this takes place against a background of multiplying channels of communication. This is not simply aggregative because new innovations can serve to reinforce existing channels which were in decline (e.g. the app driven resurgence of text messaging) and contribute towards a socio-technical environment in which an expanding array of communicative possibilities exist and the reasons for their use in any particular instance cannot be assumed in advance. This pluralisation of communication channels, a state which Miller (2011) and Miller and Sinanan (2014) describe as *polymedia*, emerges alongside a glaring lack up to this point of any established norms governing their use. As Miller and Sinanan (2014: 135) put it, "if the grounds for choosing a media or the way people configured their combination of media was no longer based upon access or cost, then the reasons people choose, and even more importantly, the reasons others would impute to their choices were now presumed by others to be social and moral". This leads to a *quantitative* escalation in communication but also a *qualitative* change following from the expanded range of communicative activity and the greater necessity for personal reflexivity entailed by this range.

The Filter Bubble

The qualitative change in communication brought about by web 2.0 results in part from the mobile computing which ensures communication is always possible while incentivising innovation to take account of this expanding user base. Leaving aside the complex question of the relationship between consumption and communication under such circumstances, we can identify a comparable transformation in consumption behaviour under conditions of web 2.0 driven by strategic interest in seeking competitive advantage within a data-driven marketplace (Lanier 2014).

Algorithms built into online services for accessing cultural products (music, video, books etc) increasingly filter the items available, often using sophisticated strategies, that rely on a combination of human coding with data analytics and machine learning. For instance, music streaming services like Spotify aim to build 'radio stations' in which extremely simple feedback mechanisms (a thumbs up or thumbs down for an individual track) are leveraged at scale, along with data about *who* listens to *what* and *where* and *when*, in order to produce a listening experience which better retains users. Furthermore, matching algorithms facilitate searching of a catalogue sufficiently vast that it would outstrip the capacity of any one listener even if they were to devote themselves to it full time.

The Amazon recommendation engine serves a similar purpose, combining its data on past consumption by a particular user with patterns identified at scale, in order to recommend new products on the basis of past purchases. However the value of this depends on the particular model that has been constructed in each instance. To use my own purchases as an example, the recommendations made on the basis of a recent work of social theory are vastly more relevant than those made on the basis of purchasing a men's electric head shaver, presumably because the category of men who shave their heads is vastly more diffuse than that of readers of social theory. Another influential case can be seen in the streaming video service Netflix which uses 76,897 distinct categories, conducive to combination through an elaborate syntax generated by the synthesis of initial rounds of human coding with the vast datasets gathered by the company from its users, in essence constituting a form of micro-genre that (fallibly) finds emergent categories within cultural products beyond those that causally entered into their production. In fact the categorical structure actually outstrips the available offerings, indicating latent possibilities in terms of which new content acquisitions could be placed or new work developed, with these data analytical considerations increasingly guiding the corporation's (much acclaimed) in house commissioning of new television.

However the algorithmic filtering undertaken by such services is, at least quantitatively, dwarfed by the continuous filtering that takes place on Google (with a vast industry having been spawned by attempts to game the PageRank algorithm and accrue the competitive benefits which come with a higher google ranking) as well as on social networking services such as Facebook and Twitter. Certainly, there is a concern for the end user experience at work here but particularly with social networking services, filtering plays a role in their (until recently unsuccessful) attempts to monetize the gathered crowds. For instance, Facebook pages show posts on them only to a small fraction of those who have 'liked' the post if the page administrator has not paid for advertising. Furthermore, the sheer quantity of traffic generated for other websites (in many cases commercially dependent upon it) mean that small algorithmic changes can have profound ramifications for a whole online ecosystem that has built up around these channels of attention.

The significance of this trend lies in how ubiquitous this algorithmic mediation of cultural variety is. Google deploys past search data to prioritise those results it deems most relevant. Facebook uses its own data to prioritise updates from those friends with whom a user interacts with most frequently. This 'filter bubble' creates a potentially powerful tendency for our present horizons to be constrained by our past activity, particularly if users are unaware of the extent of the mediation involved in producing their end user experience (Pariser 2011). It can be evaded technically with relative ease but doing so requires a form of reflexivity which not all users will exhibit: some will not know; some will not care. Furthermore, the possibilities to opt out are limited because this tendency is not strictly speaking one into which people have opted-in. Websites regularly run experiments to refine user experience, using relatively crude metrics to track the duration and extent of engagement, while 'dynamic pricing' pushes against established boundaries of acceptable commercial behaviour. Algorithms in particular, as well as software more generally, increasingly constitute a 'software layer' incorporated within "control, communication, representation, simulation, analysis, decision-making, memory, vision, writing, and interaction" in late modernity (Manovich 2013: 369). In most cases, the mechanics of their operation is obscured behind corporate confidentiality, leaving this constructed environment jarringly opaque as its influence grows.

Distracted People

It has become a common observation that digital technology is in some sense rendering social life more distracted and superficial, provoking an equally common retort that similar observations have been made about every other comparable technological innovation that we might care to name. This chapter takes the notion of 'distracted people' seriously but argues that the mechanisms underlying it have been comprehensively misunderstood. Instead, the socio-technical innovations which were discussed in the previous section are suggested here to be creating two tendencies operative at the level of personal reflexivity: a *first-order* increase in the amount of claims upon the attention of subjects and a *second-order* reduction in the capacity for sustained reflexivity as a consequence of the varied strategies through which subjects attempt to cope with these demands.

Our neurophysiological inability to multitask in spite of the pervasiveness with which it is discussed (Levitin 2014; Wacjman 2015: 104) means that task-interruption should be taken seriously as a cognitive phenomenon with implications for social activity (Altmann and Trafton 2007; Ratwani et al. 2008). However, the claim being developed here is not the straight-forward one that we are more prone to distraction in an environment of 'constant connectivity'. While agreeing with Archer (2015) that digital communications need to be seen alongside mobile phones and television as subtracting from the time available for internal conversation, it is argued that the implications of this extend beyond the *expressive reflexives* for whom life becomes pervasively episodic as they increasingly forego reflexivity. The same mechanisms contributing, *amongst others*, to the generation of expressive reflexivity (cultural abundance and the intensification of labour) are inculcating tendencies amongst practitioners of the other modes which produce an unintended truncation of reflexivity through the 'triaging' necessary to cope with the ratcheting up of situational demands upon their attention.

Digitalization and Cultural Abundance

It is estimated that only a quarter of the stored information in the world was digital by the turn of the millennium, in contrast to a 2013 estimate of less than 2 % as non-digital (Mayer-Schönberger and Cukier 2013: 151). These estimates reflect a transition from a political economy of (cultural) scarcity, in which talent is scarce and difficult to locate and distribute, to one of *abundance*: instant availability of entire catalogues of content mean that the attention of consumers becomes the key to commercial success. However this poses a general challenge of there always being more to read, listen to and to watch: infrastructural constraints upon the mediation of cultural variety have diminished to the point of triviality in many cases, a change which can be located in the zero marginal cost of reproducing digital commodities. The implications of this might initially seem trivial but they will tend to contribute to an open-ended expansion of matters for reflexive discernment because constraints upon access to cultural variety have radically diminished alongside a corresponding increase in the channels available to discuss that variety with others.

To put it crudely: there is more for us to miss, what we are missing is more likely to be accessible to us and we are more likely than ever to know what it is we are missing through our communications with others. Each individual instance which might fleetingly be of concern will likely be trivial but the aggregate effect has significant implications for the exercise of reflexivity. We only have so much capacity to deliberate about the opportunity costs entailed by cultural abundance: if we cannot read *all* the books, read *all* the papers, listen to *all* the music and *see* all the films which we have reason to believe we would find value in, then which ones should we choose? It is easy to see how responses to this challenge might vary between modes of reflexivity: relying on trusted interlocutors (communicative), making choices that are useful to our existing projects and/or relying on the filter bubble to avoid wasting time on decisions (autonomous), elaborating upon what really matters to us and/or seeking to work on the conditions within which we choose (meta-reflexivity)[12] or simply to be overwhelmed by the whole situation (fractured). Each of these would entail specific costs for reflexivity that potentially have broader implications than the personal lives of any given individual.

[12]The potential costs of this approach for reflexivity are considered in the final part of this section.

The Intensification of Work

The literature on social acceleration has been preoccupied by the role of technology in bringing about radical change in the conditions of working life (see for example Agger 2004; Crary 2014) but it has done so in a way that is immensely problematic. The role of agency is either ignored entirely or conceptualised at a level of generality that ignores the quotidian exercise of reflexivity through which we negotiate the world on a day-to-day basis (Archer 2007). This reinforces a tendency towards technological determinism that sees the social unfolding of technological effects as an inexorable process: people become cyphers to be moulded by technological change. This literature comprehensively misses what Wacjman (2015) describes as "the detailed manner and circumstances in which time is organized into daily routines by gendered individuals within households" as this abstracted individualism obscures "the vicissitudes of scheduling and the intricacy with which our lives are tied to others" (Wacjman 2015: 65).

Nonetheless, it correctly identifies a crucial empirical question, even if its answer tends to be entirely inadequate: why has there emerged a widespread experience of intensive time pressure, despite the diffusion of labour saving technological artefacts[13] and without any corresponding diminution in the objective availability of free time? Wacjman's (2015) insightful study offers a number of plausible answers: individualised time-use data obscures asymmetries within households,[14] norms co-evolve with technology in a way that mitigates against time-saving devices actually saving time[15] and people respond to an experience of time-pressure by increasing the temporal density of their activities through multi-tasking which in turn intensifies the time pressure experienced.[16] The changing temporal structure of everyday life tends to mitigate against reflexivity by increasing susceptibility to task-switching with the cognitive costs which this entails. Sustained deliberation becomes increasingly unlikely to *begin* as the temporal density of a particular tract of time increases and it is unlikely to *resume* until that density diminishes.

The same mechanism operates within working life *under certain* conditions. The multiplication of communication channels play a crucial role in this through a tendency to ratchet up the expectations inherent in an occupational role without any corresponding increase in the time available for this work.[17] This follows from

[13]As Wajcman (2015) notes, aspects of our mundane domestic apparatus tend to be overlooked by theorists of technologically driven acceleration.

[14]All the available data suggests that the "working woman is much busier than either her male colleagues or her housewife counterpart" (Wajcman 2015: 68).

[15]For instance the diffusion of washing machines accompanied an increasing expectation about how regularly clothes were washed (Wajcman 2015: 119–120).

[16]See Wajcman (2015: 78–82).

[17]There is nothing inevitable about this failure to make additional time available for new responsibilities. However, it is less likely under conditions when roles expand through innovation-led drift. It will also be less likely when, as discussed later in the section, the novelty in turn

the morphogenic character of the new channels themselves: each is potentially relevant to existing responsibilities encoded within an occupational role and, in so far as these latent ***complementarities*** are activated then we see a tendency for the role to expand. For instance, as Carrigan (2016) discusses, we are seeing a growing expectation that early career researchers engage with social media. Such a trend will inevitably be empirically complex but the mechanism itself is not: existing occupational responsibilities (e.g. disseminating the results of research) can be enacted using a new technology (e.g. tweeting links to one's published research) in a way that is potentially open-ended because the efficacy of the practice necessitates increasing engagement (e.g. building up a follower base).[18] This trend is felt most sharply in sectors where mastery of these new communication channels has been tacitly incorporated into an expanded job specification and restricted career pathways increasingly reliant upon free labour (whether in the form of internships or provision of free content that can later be monetised in the hope that one is 'discovered'). For instance, we can see this in journalism where building a personal brand through continued engagement across a variety of platforms is integral to negotiating an increasingly ossified career structure in which high profile by-line figures thrive at the expense of the broader industry. But the generic tendency towards the *morphogenesis of occupational roles* will be operative anywhere new communications channels offer potential expansions of existing practices that are evaluated as worthwhile by those capable of initial innovation and those capable of supporting this innovation.

Furthermore, the growing reliance on crude metrics as the lingua franca of success[19] is reinforced by this process because the fact these new occupational responsibilities are digitally mediated renders them inherently susceptible to the digitalised social control described by Lazega (2014). The relative position of workers vis-à-vis management within the organisation is weakened at the same time as technological novelty creates incentives towards the gaming of figures and strategic arms races, in which strategies that are individually successful (e.g. tweeting more frequently than comparable accounts) lead to a general escalation of best practice, buttressed by innovative utilities to streamline this activity which collectively lead to a further escalation. Under such conditions, success[20] comes to be a function of visibility which in turn is largely a matter of shouting more loudly and frequently than one's competitors. As Beer (2012: 480) puts it, "Academics who are able to viral-market themselves are likely to be the winners in this situation".

weakens the position of employees vis-à-vis employers under circumstances where labour unions which might organize to pursue such a goal are already weak.

[18]To be clear, digital technology is far from the only factor leading to employees in many sectors being asked 'to do more with less'.

[19]This is likely to reach its apotheosis with entirely metricised research assessment within the UK, reflecting a broader tendency towards the metricisation of the academy that has been building for many years (Burrows 2012).

[20]At least in the sense of external goods.

But in the absence of an equal starting point, we instead see a further ossification, reflecting what Dean (2013) points out is a power law distribution to be found pervasively across digital networks: a small number get almost all rewards while most get little to nothing. To continue with the aforementioned examples, we can see this tendency at work already in the proliferation of 'unread and unloved' scholarly publications (Back 2008) and the vast numbers of largely unrecognized recording artists who publish music online and dream of commercial success (Beer 2012). Not only are occupational roles being changed by the new communications channels, they are becoming greedier in Archer's (2000) sense because the logic of visibility entails personal strategies involving open-ended commitments (there are no intrinsic limits upon possibilities for self-promotion) which in turn escalate the demands placed upon those seeking visibility in an environment which will reward only small numbers.

This constitutes a mechanism in its own right which leaves certain categories of knowledge work locked into the algorithmic filter bubble as *producers* rather than just as *consumers*. As Beer (2012) points out with the example of the music industry, the decentralisation of musical production and dissemination has actually fragmented the attention space in a way that has empowered the tiny cadre of artists who have achieved sufficient cultural prominence that they can be heard above the din. Rather than a democratisation of culture, we increasingly see the consolidation of hierarchies more pronounced than anything that came before, with careers ('jobbing' or otherwise) increasingly unsustainable for those outside the elite (Lanier 2014). Crucially, the opacity of the algorithmic mechanisms which increasingly shape distribution and promotion helps naturalise this state of affairs and contribute to the myth of a radical cultural levelling which is in reality anything but. Escape from the filter bubble is possible but it imposes its own costs upon the exercise of reflexivity and it leaves those who do not or cannot do so ensnared within a digitised environment in which they are ever more susceptible to manipulation by those corporate agents who thrive under these circumstances.

Cognitive Triage

Increasingly we find that the popular discourse of 'information overload' has generated all manner of tools and techniques intended to help the overwhelmed cope with the demands placed upon them. For instance the next generation of social media platforms (perhaps reflecting the hyperactivity of venture capital at a time of diminished economic expectations) is concerned with providing tools for better organising and retrieving information. These *curation* tools work in a variety of ways but they build upon the folksonomies (user generated taxonomies employing tags and categories) that have always been a part of web 2.0 (Beer and Burrows 2007) and elevate them into a medium in their own right, allowing users quickly and easily to compile collections of diverse items (links, texts, images, audio, video etc) which can then be packaged and shared on social networking services. The microblogging service twitter is often advocated, at least in professional circles, as a means by which to facilitate discovery by carefully cultivating a network of relevant contacts so as to rely on a kind of aggregated serendipity. As Ranie and Wellman (2014: 18) observe "[t]he explosion of information and information sources has the paradoxical impact of pushing people on the path of greater reliance on their networks". In this sense the escalation of *consumption* and *communication* under web 2.0 are mutually reinforcing.

We can see the problems people experience under these conditions illustrated by the increasingly popular notion of an *information diet* that seeks to avoid intellectual 'empty calories' through the development of conscious cultural consumption (Johnson 2011). The occasionally clumsy vein of metaphors that cuts through this developing discourse reflects the lack of a language heretofore for elaborated selectivity of this sort about the quality and configuration of sources of cultural variety that enter into everyday life: the problem simply did not exist in any significant way in a pre-web environment and only underwent generalisation with web 2.0. Productivity culture thrives amidst the blogosphere as a small number make sustained careers as gurus and consultants on topics such as *life hacking*, *bio-hacking* and *lifestyle minimalism*. Inevitably the power-law tendency discussed earlier in the chapter means that for every one such guru there are countless others seeking to build such a career and contributing to a discursive explosion which merits much more sociological scrutiny than it has received as yet.

We must be careful not read back a uniform motivation from a converging practice: a strategic response to cultural escalation can also be orientated towards the reclamation of relational goods which have been eroded by demands external to the relations in question e.g. a digital detox intended to ensure a better quality of time with family or an information diet which aims to ensure intellectually valuable news sources. We could suggest an ideal typical autonomous use of such strategies (seeking to minimise distraction and maximise focus) and a corresponding meta-reflexive use (seeking the expansion of cultural horizons and regular access to cultural items that matter) but such suggestions are speculative in the absence of empirical research which recognises the variability of personal reflexivity.

However the question remains about the viability of such strategies and their relation to cultural escalation: while the notion of the information diet is explicitly orientated towards a long term change in habits, as opposed to ad hoc palliatives, this says nothing about its likely success. More importantly, all these strategic responses involve a preoccupation with negotiating first-order responses in terms of situational demands (i.e. how immediate reactions help or hinder necessary tasks) at the cost of second-order responses in terms of trans-situational concerns (i.e. the contents of reflexivity). This entails a slide into situationalism but one which we misconstrue if we regard it as an epochal shift in the constitution of subjectivity, as can be seen in Rosa (2013). Instead, it is a conditional response to a process of cultural escalation which impacts divergently across the social order. It is a form of coping which can only be understood adequately in terms of the reasons why the subject seeks to cope (why do they persist under these conditions, why do they respond to them in the way that they do, why do they take strategic action to overcome the difficulties they encounter etc.).

The notion of *cognitive triage* was offered by Roose (2014)[21] to describe the 'compartmentalization phenomenon' he witnessed amongst the young stock brokers who were the object of his study. Having already offered their graduate recruits the possibility of temporising, providing substantial material rewards at a time when the job market for millennials was then uniquely inhospitable and helping them forgo the necessity of selection for a fixed term commitment, the finance houses sought dominion over the everyday lives of the young financiers: cutting them off from the non-financial world, demanding their presence for 18 hours a day, soliciting a continuous stream of often trivial busy work and socialising them into the precise social norms which govern the financial world. The result was a form of crisis-management divergent from the expressive reflexivity described by Archer (2012). Rather than living episodically by gut feelings, cognitive triage entails living episodically by instrumental rationality[22]: attending to only the most immediate priorities because of the intensity of situational demands upon the self. It might be temporarily bounded in a predictable way (e.g. a junior year at a finance house or academics with heavy teaching loads during term time) or a response to a contingent confluence of demands that diminish upon completion. The result of consciously attending to only the most urgent features of the situation diminishes the scope of reflexivity (particularly though not exclusively in its temporal horizons) and particularly a tendency for the *important* (what matters to subjects) to be crowded out by the *urgent* (what is demanded of subjects).

Fragile Movements

Social movements have always relied upon communications technologies. As Gerbaudo (2012) points out, "[s]ocial media can be seen as the contemporary equivalent of what the newspaper, the poster, the leaflet or direct mail were for the labour movement". Rather than "an essentialist vision of social media as being automatically either suitable or unsuitable as a means of mobilisation" we need to consider the material affordances of these technologies and how they shape the development of movements which utilise them for mobilisation (Gerbaudo 2012: 4–5). The stratified ontology of social realism proves extremely useful for addressing such questions because it allows us to distinguish analytically between movements as emergent collectives capable of exercising collective reflexivity, the technologies drawn upon in their operations and the biographical trajectories of

[21]In a work of journalism which nonetheless compares well with much qualitative research by academic social scientists.

[22]Though the strain of living this way may very well lead to the development of expressive reflexivity over time.

participants *into*, *through* and *out of* movements. For sake of brevity, broader ontological questions have been exempted but see Brock and Carrigan (2014) for a consideration of these with a particular focus on how movements are symbolically constituted through specific protest events.

What is of concern for present purposes is the question of how the *characteristics of the collective* are shaped by the *role of communications technology* in bringing about *particular trajectories of participation* on the part of subjects. This section discusses how the multiplication of communications channels facilitates an *ease of assembly* which has the unintended consequence that movements will tend to fail to develop the organisational capacities to negotiate their changing environment and hence exhibit what will be characterised as 'fragility'. The following section discusses how *distracted people* will tend to compound this fragility, as well as how the tendency of social movements to draw on the affordances of polymedia inadvertently compounds the distractedness of the people they hope to mobilise.

Ease of Assembly

The enthusiasm that has come to surround the capacity of social media for the mobilisation of social movements finds it most emblematic expression in Shirky's (2008) *Here Comes Everybody*. At the heart of the book is a simple observation: social media reduce the transaction costs involved in organisation to near zero and hence effectively eliminate the logistical constraints upon mobilisation. The rhetoric surrounding this claim has since become entangled in a naïve faith that social media were undermining established systems of social control, particularly prominent as a reading of events in the Middle East during their early stages (Cockburn 2015: 116–133) but representing a broader trend of cyber utopianism (Morozov 2012). However underlying this intensely problematic discourse, which as Cockburn (2015) notes was utilised by rebel groups to frame their actions in a way expected to win support, we can nonetheless find an entirely plausible claim. Tufekci (2014b) insightfully observes how the logistical demands of mobilization have changed dramatically in our present socio-technical environment:

> Social media affordances have altered which capabilities underlie the ability to mount popular mobilizations. For example, in the past, the capability to organize a large-scale march on Washington, or a bus boycott in Montgomery, required extensive organization, coordinating everything from car pools to laboriously publishing pamphlets to setting up many meetings that in turn determine organizational and logistical issues. Similarly, battling for visibility through broadcast media often required investing in institutions that became familiar with the workings of media and power.

Under present conditions activists turn to social media to pursue tasks such as co-ordination and publicity and it is the sometimes spectacular achievements that result, with a small number of people bringing about mass action, which goes some way to explaining the enthusiasm for social media in certain circles. As Tufekci (2014b) points out, "There are countless examples of how social media allows mobilizations to carry out fairly impressive feats with little prior infrastructure". However when there is no pressing need for this infrastructure, it is unlikely to develop it: why expend the effort when ad hoc *co-ordination* seemingly suffices? The possibility that many protestors might be intoxicated by the experienced spontaneity of their actions in a cultural environment affirming the epochal significance of such networked action risks further compounding this problem by mitigating against any shared project of developing these capacities.

What Tufekci describes as 'sediments' which remain after a practical activity has been acted out, can perhaps better be characterised as emergent causal powers within relationally constituted movements. It is through these that the capacity of a movement to retain its form through change is underwritten. It might be true that, as Johnston (2014: 139) puts it, social media lead to a "shrinking [of] the time required for coordinating protest tactics to a flash" but the important question is what the reliance upon these affordances means for the emergent character of the movement. This is of course a substantial empirical question in its own right and the argument developed here does not pretend to be a comprehensive answer. The claim being made is a more limited one: a reliance upon social media for assembly will mitigate against the development of collective reflexivity. The ensuing movements may be symbolically rich but their capacity for deliberation about their ends or how to pursue them will be limited if assembly rarely amounts to anything more than drawing a crowd or inciting a swarm. The relational density of the movement, which tends to be much lower than would otherwise be the case and the organisational capacities upon which assembly would have depended formerly will tend to be absent: there is a greater risk that such a movement will 'fizzle out' and lack the logistical capacity which might otherwise mitigate against this. They can be said to be 'fragile' because without collective reflexivity, what unity exists will be distinctively brittle in the face of new circumstances that complicate existing plans or challenge prevailing assumptions because there will be little capacity for 'us' to decide how 'we' should respond to these changes. If the 'we' is wholly or largely symbolic, resting on an image of the movement conveyed culturally rather than as an experienced orientation towards a shared project, it is unlikely to survive in the face of change because it lacks the converging commitments which incentivise reciprocal action after the taken-for-grantedness of what 'we' are doing has collapsed.

The Morphogenesis of Movements

In the previous section, it was argued that social movements reliant upon social media for mobilisation will tend to be characterised by a latent fragility in spite of what may be a superficially impressive capacity for assembly. The logistical challenges posed by assembly using earlier communications' technologies led inevitably to the development of organisational capacities which supported the development of collective reflexivity: the emergence of a shared project in relation to which individual commitment motivated sustained action. In their absence, the 'we' experienced by participations will, if it exists at all,[23] be entirely or predominately symbolic[24] and thus ill equipped to respond to changing circumstances or sustain the movement in the face of challenges. Participants may very well have been changed through their participation (McAdam 1989), but the 'we' through whom individual grievances[25] might take the form of collective projects fails to acquire the durability necessary for the normative transformations explicitly or tacitly sought to stand much chance of achieving fruition. Participants in fragile movements may have undergone transformation through their engagement, in turn potentially disposing them towards participation in cognate movements at future points in time, but recognising this does nothing to mitigate against the constitutive instability which will likely characterise a potential future movement if formed from similar 'parts' within a similar environment.

Unfortunately the same factors which generate *fragile movements* operate concurrently to produce *distracted people*. One set of mechanisms operates at the level of personal reflexivity (*cultural abundance* and the *intensification of work*) and the other operates at the level of collective reflexivity (*digitally driven assemblies mitigate against the development of organisational capacities*) but the same socio-technical transformations discussed in section two are at work in each case. Not only are the ranks of expressive reflexives likely to swell (Archer 2012) but the tracts of lived time in which those who might otherwise be inclined towards becoming movement participants find themselves in a state of *cognitive triage* that is expanding under digital capitalism. If we struggle to see beyond the next month, week or day then it is hard to commit ourselves to sustained participation in movements. It is too easy to forego a demonstration we might otherwise attend because of an impending deadline or, in the event we did make it, to follow up and actively participate in a way we might otherwise do if only we had the time. Further triaging strategies only compound this problem by encouraging the scrutiny

[23]The fact it is possible to participate in social movement events without feeling in any way part of the social movement in question is an interesting phenomenon that it would be valuable to explore empirically.

[24]Obviously, any 'we' will necessarily have a symbolic component in so far as that there is a reciprocal recognition of being known to one another as a minimum condition of being a 'we' rather than a disconnected aggregate of anonymous strangers. The point is that a sense of who 'we' are and what 'we' are doing is much more durable when a genuinely collective project has emerged to which individuals orientate themselves as evaluative beings. Participants in an online crowd action, or even strangers coming together for a flash mob, might recognize themselves as one of a (temporary) collective in which they are fallibly aware of others having a corresponding recognition but an absent relational history means any such collective is fragile, as well as fleeting, even if the collective project might be a meaningful accomplishment for those concerned. This experience would likely contrast to that of the non-governmental organization team who planned and enacted such a successful online campaign. The familiar rhetoric of openness is belied by a surreptitious privatism when collective activity is reliant upon existing closed networks to co-ordinate the action of strangers.

[25]This phrase is used as a place holder for the diverse range of personal motivations which contribute to social movement participation. This chapter necessarily proceeds at a level of generality which does a disservice to the empirical variability of the topic. Hopefully this is justified because of the potential utility of the account developed for later empirical work into this topic.

of first-order responses (e.g. tracking quantity of sleep, recording food consumption, interrogating the quality of one's 'information diet') which, along with the time spent mastering and using such tactics, inclines us further away from extended consideration of second-order responses i.e. what matters to us (Sayer 2012). The multiplicity of human doings are subsumed under the generic category of tasks, as potentially rewarding projects increasingly become obstacles to be negotiated in way that can be (self) quantified with a view to improving future performance. Furthermore, even those triaging strategies which do not have this effect, such as 'digital detoxing', represent a form of temporising: relying upon sustained periods of voluntary disconnection in order to cope with the involuntariness of constant connectivity elsewhere in life.

The point is not that cognitive triage means people cease to be critical or to take action. It rather means they will tend to prioritise that action because of the intensity of the situational demands to which they are subject. However as any of the more intelligent advocates of productivity culture will make clear, to feel one does not have the time for something in fact simply means that it is not being prioritized. But prioritization in this sense is strong evaluation of precisely the form that cognitive triage mitigates against (Taylor 1989; Sayer 2012). Looking to productivity culture for guidance in solving an experienced problem obviously constitutes an exercise of reflexivity but it is reflexivity of a particular sort, representing a resurgent conventionalism in which subjects look to expertise, rather than relying upon deliberation, in order to address what are straight forwardly matters of reflexivity[26]: exercise choice but relying on expertise to ensure we make the *right* choice (Mäkinen 2014; Salecl 2011). This is something encouraged by an increasingly pervasive management philosophy concerned with 'wellness' as a project of cultivating human capital and actualizing discretionary effort while also demanding excellence and threatening intervention in its absence (Cederstrom and Spicer 2015). The ratcheting up of situational demands upon employees of which cognitive triage is an outcome has to be considered in terms of the broader context of market capitalism discussed in the second section. Digital communications contribute to the intensification of work through the morphogenesis of occupational roles *and* through facilitating new technologies of measurement and intervention upon which contemporary management increasingly depend.

Conclusion

The notion of cognitive triage helps us explain how the adaptations which may be necessary at the level of *personal reflexivity* work against potential attempts at the level of *collective reflexivity* to take action intended to ameliorate shared conditions, let alone sustain a trajectory of participation in a social movement that has a wider

[26]That is to say these are questions about how to organize one's life, how to prioritize one's work and establish 'productive' routines as opposed to matters of psychopathology, putative or otherwise.

purpose. The reliance of those movements upon mediated assembly further hinders that possibility by effectively making it harder for someone to get involved and contribute to what 'we' are doing because there is inevitably much less of a network in terms of which one can participate, let alone a durable organization with clearly defined roles and responsibilities. But even if that were not the case, people who triage are much less likely to engage in this way, even if they might otherwise wish to do so. This is the sense in which it is being argued that *distracted people* and *fragile movements* are mutually reinforcing at a *second-order* level even though the causal mechanisms responsible for each at a *first-order* level operate independently.

It is possible that other forms of action thrive under these circumstances so inimical to the emergence of durable social movements. The issue of electronic activism can be useful recast in these terms. Such actions are asynchronous, symbolically meaningful and easily diffused through social media. Rather than classifying such activity as intrinsically worthy or otherwise, it can be usefully considered in terms of the biographical context within which people take such action. While as Tufekci (2014b) notes such "semi-public symbolic micro-actions can slowly reshape how people make sense of their values and their politics", it is equally likely that they can act as a salve to those triaging, providing symbolic satisfaction to those for whom a second-order commitment to some transformative project persistently finds itself crowded-out by all manner of first-order imperatives. This problem is compounded by the corporate agents making claims upon the attention of an increasingly distracted public being mired in the logic of competition by virtue of this distraction. There are only so many moral claims to which we can attend, only so many petitions we can sign and only so many donations we can make. The difficulty of gaining traction under such circumstances incentivises communicative innovation which raises the standards for others corporate agents and contributes to the intensification of work within them by acting to increasingly preclude routine action. Unfortunately making messages bigger and louder, while distributing them across more channels, in turn intensifies the social distraction to which it is a strategic response.

Recognising the symbolic richness of such online politics helps illuminate the broader question of future normative transformation which this chapter has sought to address. This issue can best be raised by way of an example. The initial version of this chapter was given as a paper at the Social Morphogenesis workshop in Cardiff in January 2015, the morning after gun men had massacred the journalists at the satirical magazine *Charlie Hebdo* in Paris. That night many thousands of Parisians took to the streets in a spontaneous show of solidarity, marked by defiant displays of raised pencils (as they are mightier than the sword), and signs proclaiming "I am *Charlie Hebdo*". Images of this assembly circulated on social media, with 1.8 million tweets by midnight GMT on the most prominent solidarity hashtag amongst a number which had emerged through which the events of the day were being discussed.[27] These displays were matched by similar demonstrations in over 30 cities around France, as well as many cities around the world. What was notable is how readily certain themes spread, particularly that of the raised pencil, as well as the outpouring of satirical cartoons that soon circulated around social media, presumably acting as encouragement to other artists inclined to address the day's events through this form.

The outpouring of activity was immense but it has not, as yet, led to anything which may be described as a movement. If the argument of this chapter is correct then any movement that *had* emerged would very likely soon have soon 'fizzled out' and before this point been characterized more by expressive action than reflective goals. But could participation in such assemblies and online displays of solidarity have primed subjects for mobilization by corporate agents less prone to fragility than any nascent movements? The precise empirical question here (the implication of the *Charlie Hebdo* attacks for the far-right in France) is of much less importance than the issue it illustrates. If social movements are becoming fragile then we need to ask *what effects they are having upon their fleeting participants* and how these might influence the activities of corporate agents who lack this fragility. In this sense, effects upon individuals should be seen as *present actions* seeding latent potentialities which might be drawn upon in future. If movement participation changes people in non-random ways then considering how the *character of movements* and *participation trajectories* produce particular biographical effects[28] comes to seem a key question for understanding the great normative changes which may characterize the twenty-first century to parallel those that Porpora (2016) analyses in the 20th.

Asking the question in this way implies no prediction about this under-recognized biographical contribution being anything we could characterize in general terms as positive or negative. It might seed the ground for future progressive movements that overcome their latent fragility. It might prime participants for mobilization by a resurgent far-right that gives cultural form to longstanding grievances. It might engender a retreat into the protective micro-climate of personal life licensed by experienced failure of movements. All of these effects and many more are possible because the causal powers we are talking about here are ones which operate with a finite set of subjects who participated in a particular movement for a discreet period of time.[29]

However one further issue needs to be considered that will factor into the potential normative transformations of the twenty-first century: the asymmetrical impact

[27]For those unfamiliar with Twitter, a hashtag is a stamp that indexes individual messages as sharing a topic. By affixing a hashtag (e.g. #JeSuisCharlieHebdo) a user signifies that their tweet relates to a broader trend. The most popular hashtags are displayed prominently as 'trending' and this encourages users to adopt them when sending messages. The contents of a hashtag can be read in real time by any user, as I found myself doing obsessively late on the evening of the attacks.

[28]That is to say leads to *personal morphogenesis*. See Alford (1995) and Carrigan (2014).

[29]Rather than the familiar dichotomy of individual action and collective action, we are talking about how *present* collective action might shape *future* individual action and, in turn, contribute to *future* collective action. The fact the category itself is impossible to sustain without a stratified ontology makes it easy to see how this could be overlooked.

of the multiplication of communications' channels upon corporate agents. While social movements become prone to fragility and large scale collective reflexivity[30] becomes harder to sustain, the socio-technical transformation which has brought this about contributes to what Tufekci (2014a) describes as a "data–analytic environment that favours the powerful, data–rich incumbents". Digitalization creates new possibilities for monitoring and control because of the digital data produced as a by-product of transactions which existing corporate agents are uniquely poised to exploit. This creates a situation which turns "political communication into an increasingly personalized, private transaction" driven, it should be noted, by the situational logic of competition[31] into which organized political parties are locked more than any deliberate project to privatize the public sphere. Advances in behavioral science coupled with the psychometric modeling, increasingly being generated using large propriety data-sets generated by social media platforms, create new possibilities for manipulative mobilization, drawing upon precisely those established grievances which might lead someone to join a 'fragile movement', in a way that serves a purpose opaque to the subject. Crucially, "such messages are not visible to broad publics and thus cannot be countered, fact–checked or otherwise engaged in the shared public sphere the way a provocative or false political advertisement might have been" (Tufekci 2014a). In an online environment increasingly prone to generating 'shaming' campaigns in which micro-harassment by hundreds of thousands or even millions via social media leads to jobs being lost, people being hounded by the media, death threats and even suicides (Ronson 2015) the somewhat dystopic suggestions made by analysts like Tufekci (2014a) and Couldry (2014) need to be taken seriously. The account of *distracted people* and *fragile movements* offered in this chapter provides a framework within which we might begin to investigate the conditions under which such opaque strategies might thrive: the absence of durable movements to articulate grievances and the capacity of fleeting participation to prime subjects for subsequent 'shadow mobilisations'.

References

Agger, B. (2004). *Speeding up fast capitalism: Internet culture, work, families, food, bodies.* Boulder: Paradigm.

Alford, J. D. (1995). *Journeys: Personal morphogenesis: A study of the interplay between structural, cultural, familial and biographical factors affecting mature students' decisions to undertake an Open Access course for possible entry to university.* Doctoral dissertation, University of Warwick.

Altmann, E. M., & Trafton, J. G. (2007). Timecourse of recovery from task interruption: Data and a model. *Psychonomic Bulletin & Review, 14*(6), 1079–1084.

[30]Under these conditions, it is possible that collective reflexivity at the micro level might thrive. In fact this might be something deliberately sought by those who wish to preserve the evacuation of the political sphere.

[31]Compounding the communicative escalation to which, as discussed at the start of the conclusion, the logic of competition in which 'good causes' are enmeshed gives rise.

Archer, M. S. (2000). *Being human: The problem of agency*. Cambridge: Cambridge University Press.

Archer, M. S. (2007). *Making our way through the world*. Cambridge: Cambridge University Press.

Archer, M. S. (2012). *The reflexive imperative in late modernity*. Cambridge: Cambridge University Press.

Archer, M. S. (2014). The generative mechanism re-configuring late modernity. In M. S. Archer (Ed.), *Late modernity* (pp. 93–117). Cham: Springer.

Archer, M. S. (2015). How agency is transformed in the course of social transformation: Don't forget the double morphogenesis. In M. S. Archer (Ed.), *Generative mechanisms transforming the social order* (pp. 135–157). Cham: Springer.

Archer, M. S. (2016). *How social regulation becomes anormative with morphogenesis*. In M. S. Archer (Ed.), *Morphogenesis and the crisis of normativity*. Springer.

Back, L. (2008). Sociologists talking. *Sociological Research Online, 13*(6), 3.

Beer, D. (2012). Open access and academic publishing: Some lessons from music culture. *Political Geography, 31*(8), 479–480.

Beer, D., & Burrows, R. (2007). Sociology and, of and in Web 2.0: Some initial considerations. *Sociological Research Online, 12*(5), 17.

Brock, T., & Carrigan, M. (2014). Realism and contingency. *Journal for the Theory of Social Behaviour, 45*(3), 377–396.

Burrows, R. (2012). Living with the h-index? Metric assemblages in the contemporary academy. *The Sociological Review, 60*(2), 355–372.

Carrigan, M. (2014). *Becoming who we are: Theorising personal morphogenesis*. Doctoral dissertation, University of Warwick.

Carrigan, M. (2016). *Social media for academics*. London: Sage.

Cedertröm, C., & Spicer, A. (2015). *The wellness syndrome*. Cambridge: Polity.

Cockburn, P. (2015). *The rise of Islamic state: ISIS and the New Sunni revolution*. London: Verso.

Couldry, N. (2014). A necessary disenchantment: Myth, agency and injustice in a digital world. *The Sociological Review, 62*(4), 1–18.

Crary, J. (2014). *24/7: Late capitalism and the ends of sleep*. London: Verso.

Crawford, K., & Schultz, J. (2014). *Big data and due process: Towards a framework to redress predictive privacy harms*. 55 B.C.L. Rev. 93.

Crossley, N. (2002). *Making sense of social movements*. Buckingham: Open University Press.

Crouch, C. (2004). *Post-democracy*. Cambridge: Polity.

Dean, J. (2013). *Blog theory: Feedback and capture in the circuits of drive*. Cambridge: Polity.

Donati, P., & Archer, M. S. (2015). *The relational subject*. Cambridge: Cambridge University Press.

Gerbaudo, P. (2012). *Tweets and the streets: Social media and contemporary activism*. London: Pluto.

Giddens, A. (2002). *Runaway world: How globalisation is reshaping our lives*. London: Profile.

Halford, S., Pope, C., & Weal, M. (2013). Digital futures? Sociological challenges and opportunities in the emergent Semantic Web. *Sociology, 47*(1), 173–189.

Johnson, C. A. (2011). *The information diet: A case for conscious consumption*. Sebastopol: O'Reilly Media.

Johnston, H. (2014). *What is a social movement?* Cambridge: Polity.

Lanchester, J. (2015). The robots are coming. *London Review of Books, 37*(5), 3–8.

Lanier, J. (2014). *Who owns the future?* London: Allen Lane.

Lazega, E. (2014). Body captors and network profiles: A neo-structural note on digitalized social control and morphogenesis. In M. Archer (Ed.), *Generative mechanisms transforming late modernity*. New York: Springer.

Levitin, D. J. (2014). *The organized mind: Thinking straight in the age of information overload*. London: Viking.

Little, D. (2012). Analytical sociology and the rest of sociology. *Sociologica, 6*(1), 0–0.

Lupton, D. (2014). *Digital sociology*. London: Routledge.

Mäkinen, K. (2014). The individualization of class: A case of working life coaching. *The Sociological Review, 62*(4), 821–842.
Manovich, L. (2013). *Software takes command*. London: Bloomsbury.
Mayer-Schönberger, V., & Cukier, K. (2013). *Big data: A revolution that will transform how we live, work, and think*. London: John Murray.
McAdam, D. (1989). The biographical consequences of activism. *American Sociological Review, 54*(4), 744–760.
Miller, D. (2011). *Tales from facebook*. Cambridge: Polity.
Miller, D., & Sinanan, J. (2014). *Webcam*. Cambridge: Polity.
Morozov, E. (2012). *The net delusion: The dark side of internet freedom*. London: Penguin.
Pariser, E. (2011). *The filter bubble: What the internet is hiding from you*. London: Viking.
Porpora, D. (2016). *The great normative changes of the twentieth century*. In M. S. Archer (Ed.), *Morphogenesis and the crisis of normativity*. Springer.
Ranie, L., & Wellman, B. (2014). *Networked: The new social operating system*. Cambridge, MA: MIT Press.
Ratwani, R. M., Trafton, J. G., & Boehm-Davis, D. A. (2008). Thinking graphically: Connecting vision and cognition during graph comprehension. *Journal of Experimental Psychology: Applied, 14*(1), 36.
Ronson, J. (2015). *So you've been publically shamed*. London: Pan Macmillan.
Roose, K. (2014). *Young money: Inside the hidden world of wall Street's post-crash recruits*. London: Hachette UK.
Rosa, H. (2013). *Social acceleration: A new theory of modernity*. New York: Columbia University Press.
Salecl, R. (2011). *The tyranny of choice*. London: Profile.
Sayer, A. (2012). *Why things matter to people*. Cambridge: Cambridge University Press.
Shirky, C. (2008). *Here comes everybody: The power of organizing without organizations*. New York: Penguin Press.
Shirky, C. (2010). *Cognitive surplus: Creativity and generosity in a connected age*. London: Allen Lane.
Streeck, W. (2014). *Buying time: The delayed crisis of democratic capitalism*. London: Verso.
Taylor, C. (1989). *Sources of the self*. Cambridge: Cambridge University Press.
Tufekci, Z. (2014a). Engineering the public: Big data, surveillance and computational politics. *First Monday, 19*(7).
Tufekci, Z. (2014b). Capabilities of movements and affordances of digital media: Paradoxes of empowerment. *DML Central*.http://dmlcentral.net/blog/zeynep-tufekci/capabilities-movements-and-affordances-digital-media-paradoxes-empowerment
Wajcman, J. (2015). *Pressed for time: The acceleration of life in digital capitalism*. Chicago: University of Chicago Press.
Žižek, S. (2009). *First as tragedy, then as farce*. London: Verso.

Part III
Morphogenesis and What Makes for Changes in Normativity

Chapter 10
The Relational Understanding of the Origin and Morphogenetic Change of Social Morality

Pierpaolo Donati

The Issue and the Main Arguments

What is it that comes to be socially defined as 'morally good' or at least acceptable? And by whom? Who defines which moral norms are accepted and which are excluded? For example, the morality of 'politically correctitude' imposes the norm of not expressing any judgement (implying a *negative* judgement) on other people's behaviours and life styles, which they believe to be positive, given that, according to post-modern public morality, a universal truth does not exist: only partial truths exist, all debatable and private. Who defines and imposes this new universal morality? Is it so-called 'public opinion', that is, the normative orientation of a supposed majority? Or is it certain social groups (lobbies) that are acquiring greater power in society? Or does this morality spread because it is imposed by laws enacted by the political system, making it legally binding?

Possibly all these explanations (public opinion, lobbies, laws) play a role in changing social morality. It always remains to be seen what specific combination of them is working in a particular case.

What I intend to argue is that with the processes of globalisation, a dynamic of morality is emerging that, alongside the processes of privatization and collectivization of moral norms, is opening up spaces for moral norms that are the expression of autonomous social networks acting as mediators between individual morality and system morality. This dynamic is what characterises the different pathways in changing social morality through a peculiar combination of public opinion, lobbies and legislation.

P. Donati (✉)
Department of Sociology and Business Law, University of Bologna, Strada Maggiore 45, 40125 Bologna, Italy
e-mail: pierpaolo.donati@unibo.it

M.S. Archer (eds.), *Morphogenesis and the Crisis of Normativity*, Social Morphogenesis, DOI 10.1007/978-3-319-28439-2_10

This thesis implies that changes in social morality originate in the birth of a type of morality that is neither private (where the moral norm is defined or interpreted from a self-referential point of view) nor public (the moral norm is defined by some sort of 'public opinion'). The new morality becomes 'public' only at a later time.

This argument is prompted in the first place by two considerations. On the one hand, impersonal morality is losing ground because socio-cultural systems are becoming increasingly pluralised, social networks are elaborating their own normativity with different types and degrees of individual and social reflexivity, and, therefore, the normative cement constituted by shared values and norms is breaking down. Society is expressing itself in many different social networks, which are working out their own morality.

On the other hand, individual (private) morality turns out to be too weak to influence collective processes. There certainly exist phenomena representing the privatisation of moral norms (for example, in the area of human reproduction), just as there are phenomena that represent the forced collectivisation of moral norms, which are imposed on individuals without their consent (for example, the evaluations of teachers in schools and universities). From the point of view of relational sociology, these phenomena are also relational in that moral norms are constituted on the basis of a specific structure of relations between the subjects involved (for example, between individuals engaged in a process of artificial insemination or between government bureaucracies and teachers in the school system). In all cases, the norms express the power relationships between the actors involved.

Post-modern society is highly ambivalent, contradictory, and paradoxical because in it we see dynamics and mechanisms at work that attempt to assert universal values and moral norms while, at the same time, social groups are emerging in which individuals attempt to elaborate a new, 'group' morality, different from the tendencies that they perceive to be predominant.

All of these processes point to different paths of morphogenesis. I am interested here in elucidating those processes in which morality is changing because human subjects feel the need to relate to one another according to a moral sense that is neither strictly public (because it is not generalizable in a universalistic way) nor strictly private (because it does not correspond to particularistic interests), but is *social* [1] in that it must satisfy the needs, interests, and rights of social groups or communities that want to characterise themselves according to their specific relational qualities and properties. I am referring to those spheres of society in which moral norms are elaborated because they have to meet the relational needs of sociality of an associative type, which is not finding adequate answers in society's institutional arrangements.

---

[1] H. Arendt (1958) delineated the historical development of this *social* sphere distinct from the private sphere and from the public sphere, starting in classical Greece, judging it negatively (which I do not share).

I will advance the thesis according to which the crisis of modern morality is manifested through various forms of morphogenesis. We can certainly observe forms of *sequential* (in series) and *concurrent* (in parallel) morphogenesis, as Al-Amoudi[2] has maintained. It is a matter of analysing in which fields these processes take place, that is, wherever one moral norm replaces a prior norm (as when a more refined consumer product replaces the previous one), in contrast to a new moral norm simply taking its place alongside another in the framework of a morality that allows various types and degrees of pluralism (as in the doctrine of multiculturalism: Donati 2009). However, here I am interested in focusing on those processes of morphogenesis that – *on a meso level* – create new moral norms through the establishment of social networks that, by altering the interdependencies between acting subjects and social systems, as expressed by societal (associational or corporate) agents, become carriers of a new morality. The question of the scale at which moral changes take place is crucial, since I maintain that the norms of social morality have different dynamics at the levels of individuals (*lib*, markets), within networks (informal groups, civil associations, more or less organized corporate agents) and in systems (*lab*, structural 'wholes').

In short, the fundamental argument is that an emergent form of social morality exists, which constitutes a (morphogenetic) response to the need to create a new relationality between (individual and collective) subjects, in as much as such a relationality expresses an autonomous reality on a meso level, which becomes all the more important the more relationships between the micro and macro levels of the social dynamic slacken, fragment, and, in many cases, collapse.

Alongside those processes of the morphogenesis of morality that are sequential or concurrent compared with the typically modern morality (which follows a binary private/public logic), we can see the rise of a *relational morphogenesis* that is characterised by meta-reflexivity. This defines morality as the need to enter into relationship with oneself, others, and the world as a consequence of the uniqueness and particularity of the outputs that derive from a certain kind of social relation rather than from other types of relations. Changes of social morality are advancing in parallel with the crisis in the *lib/lab* arrangements that characterised the socio-political systems of modernity, which are guided by a morality of compromise between private and collective interests.

The framework that I am about to delineate asserts that today's rapid changes of morality can be explained as a variety of responses to the 'double binds' that are inherent in the modern dialectic between agency and structure (that is, *lib/lab*). The fundamental double bind is that which consists in the fact that the moral imperative dictated by post-modern socio-cultural structures seeking a remedy for the oppression of individuals, works exactly like a mechanism for

[2] Ismael Al-Amoudi (2014) has proposed the interesting distinction between *sequential morphogenesis* (which consists in the displacement of one institution by the next) and *concomitant morphogenesis* (which consists in the multiplication of concomitant institutions, without necessarily entailing the disappearance of earlier ones).

their oppression. The slogans, "You must be free," "You must fulfil yourself by rejecting all constraints," and "You must take care of yourself without depending on others" today represent the prevailing moral norm which, while it promises to free individuals, in reality oppresses and estranges them from themselves in as much as one's identity is formed, exists, and operates in the context of relations with others and cannot be completely cut off from them.

Responses to these double binds can take various forms. Some individuals remain stuck in the double bind and feel constrained within the *bound morality* of the double bind (communicative reflexives). Others try to maintain an autonomous reflexivity, but with great difficulty and frequent failures. Still others try to exit from the double bind by taking paths that avoid all constraints and adopt an *unbound* morality, such that their reflexivity becomes fractured or hindered; a popular song addressed to youngsters today tells us: 'I do not want to go to school, I want to break the rules'. Still others try to exit from the double bind via various strategies that are based on recognizing the double bind for what it is and on the separation of the two binds ('you must' and 'be free'), where freedom is understood as the ability to choose from whom or on what one depends and the capacity to pursue one's own concerns ethically by overcoming contingent failures. These are meta-reflexives. Moral norms are then elaborated through a *steered morality* that is realised whenever reflexivity becomes relational. On the empirical level, it is a matter of identifying those social phenomena in which we can detect these different processes of morphogenesis in elaborating upon social morality.

Where the Agency/Structure Debate Has Failed

The Mainstream View of Social Morality

According to the scheme I believe to be prevalent in sociology today,[3] morality consists in the attribution of meaning to the action taken by individual humans who, in aggregating with one another, arrive at a consensus that constitutes collective morality. The latter is then reflected back to single individuals, directing their actions toward a social order in which the moral distinction between good and bad corresponds to that between normality and deviance.

The two processes ranging, respectively, (a) from the system to the individual and (b) from the individual to the system are often thought of as *circular* and somehow *reversible*. Positive feedbacks regulate an 'order from contingency'. In such a case, we have the slide, found in certain theories, that Archer (1995) rightly calls 'central conflation' between agency and structure. The notion of a 'pure relation' proposed

[3]The list of authors who use this scheme is quite long, and I thus avoid citing them. Just to give an idea, I shall limit myself to naming a few emblematic authors: Coleman (1990), Bourdieu and Coleman (1991), and Hechter et al. (1990).

by Giddens (1992) is a paradigmatic example: the morality of Ego and that of Alter consist in the fact that they live their relationship on the basis of the moral norm of self-realisation; in other words, they believe that the relation is good if and in as much as it is useful to each of them in order to realise their own Self. The things that Ego and Alter exchange must be gratifying to each one's 'I'. The relation is neither emergent nor generative; it has only to confirm their individuality. The relation is formed by the actions of the partners, who use it to satisfy their own 'I's. The 'pure relationship' theorised by Giddens is a form of aggregation and is not properly relational since the relation is not emergent and does not carry any intrinsic good in itself.

What I want to emphasise is that, in the mainstream view of social morality, the circularity (conflation) between agency and (cultural and social) structure glosses over two problems: (i) the issue of the relational constitution of agency/Self[4] and (ii) the issue of the relational constitution of cultural and social structures.[5]

In my opinion, much of the debate over *agency and structure* is flawed by these ways of reducing morality to a game between individuals and social structures. What they seriously undervalue and distort is the theme of morality as a relational phenomenon. The morality of social relations is attributed to the individuals *as such*, who feel uncertain, anxious, insecure. The relatively autonomous role of social relations in forging morality is overlooked or relegated to the shadows.

As an alternative, I propose the framework of Fig. 10.1, which will have to be explained specifically in terms of morphostasis/morphogenesis. My intention is to understand the origin and change of morality, not as the result of aggregations of individuals in a context defined by certain (social, cultural, and communicative) structures or, vice versa, as the influence of structures on individuals' agency, but as the product of the relationality that develops in networks of social relations that connect social agents/actors. The problem needs to be brought into focus. It is a matter of understanding if – and if so, how – one can speak of an intervening variable, i.e. *the morality of social relations as such*, which constitutes a *sui generis* order of reality in as much as relations have simultaneously to meet individuals' needs, on the one hand, and the needs of the governability of institutions, on the other. The question is: does a morality of networks of relations exist that is distinct from the morality of individuals and from that of socio-cultural systems? Put another way: can we speak of morally good social relations/networks and morally bad social relations/networks? Can we do this without falling into the holistic fallacy of believing that social relations/networks can themselves think (morally)?

In my view, the morality of a social relation (or network of relations) is due to the fact that it can produce relational goods or relational evils. In order to produce relational goods, a social relation should meet the following requisites: (i) be an emergent phenomenon; (ii) be morally good in itself and not merely a matter of subjectively being deemed so; (iii) be such as to give the subjects individual goods

[4]Stetsenko and Arievitch (2004).

[5]Porpora (1987).

that they could not obtain otherwise (the achievement of a common or collective good may be present or not, in any case it is not utterly necessary as Uhlaner thinks).

Solidarity, subsidiarity, or friendship are social relations – and not only individual feelings – that are morally good, obviously on certain conditions (the structuring of the relation must have an ethically good end). Contempt, the refusal to help, aggression, and violence are morally bad social relations, and not only individual feelings. Certainly, the moral qualities of social relations have correspondences in the properties of individuals, but they are not the same thing because these are two different orders of reality. The morality of reciprocity on the part of the individual (as a feeling, attitude, or act) is not the same thing as the morality inherent in the social relation of reciprocity. I will now try to explain these assertions.

An Alternative View

In Fig. 10.1, morality can be analysed from three points of view, which correspond to three different paths for the formation of moral agency.

– Path [1] explains social morality by the conditioning of social and cultural systems which, through their normativity, impose themselves on individuals' agency. Here are situated theories of the 'collective conscience' (for example, Durkheim and Mary Douglas) and of cultural traditions (for example, Putnam and Fukuyama). The morphostasis/morphogenesis of morality is explained there as the product of normative systems that reproduce themselves or transform themselves on the basis of a logic that is inherent in the same social and cultural institutions, in functional and/or communicative terms. As Mary Douglas (1986) would say, morphogenesis happens when institutions, which are supposed to be thinking entities, change 'their way of thinking'. As Luhmann would have it, the morphogenesis of moral norms is the product of the change of semantic codes

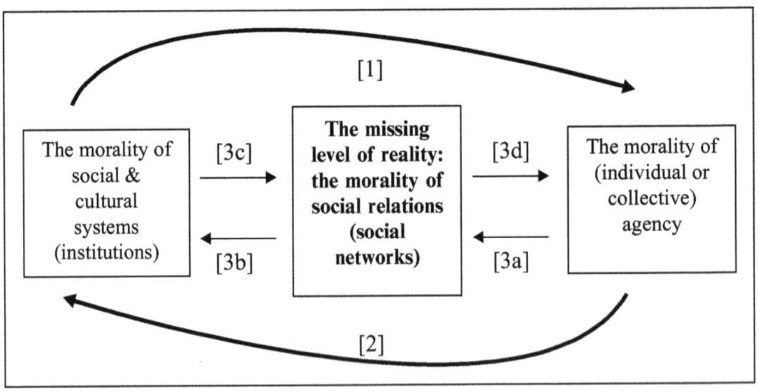

Fig. 10.1 The three 'layers' of morality (agential, relational, and systemic) and the different paths through which they contribute to the moral fabric of society

due to the effects of mechanisms of communication (it is assumed that the process of communication depends on the inherent laws of the communication system itself, which is ironically expressed in the aphorism, "*Only communication can communicate*").[6]

– Path [2], which is opposite and complementary to the first one, explains social morality as the product of individual actions that generate a collective system of values and norms *by aggregation*. A number of individuals, driven by mechanisms of an aggregative type, participate in processes of identification with a shared set of symbolic and normative values that replace other, existing values. Here are situated the collective movement theories of Smelser (1963), Pizzorno (1966), and others. Examples are radical feminist movements, anti-global, LGBT, protest and revolutionary movements, such as the so-called 'Arab Springs'. The collective movement replaces certain values and moral norms with others. It is a matter of understanding what this path's specific morphostatic/morphogenetic process is. In general, it consists in the fact that, given certain forms of systemic conditioning, large groups (or even masses) of individuals set themselves up in reaction to them and radicalise certain values: these groups can be of a conservative type (for example, fundamentalist religious or racial movements) or of a transgressive or rebellious type (for example, when gender difference or market competition is radically rejected).

As I have already said, the majority of theories explain social morality as the product of a combination between these two paths. The most emblematic example is the morality that I call *lib/lab*. This consists in the fact that, on the one hand, the morality of individual freedom and of free aggregations of individuals (*lib* morality) is invoked while, on the other hand, morality is instead considered as an institutionalised entity that has the task of guaranteeing equality of opportunities in the relationships between individuals (*lab* morality).

In the language of Fig. 10.1 (paths [1]–[2]), it is assumed that: (i) on the one hand, free individuals can adhere (or not) to a shared system of values and moral norms (the *lib* dimension of moral agency) and (ii) on the other hand, the system of shared moral values works in such a way as to guarantee its own effective realisation through systemic mechanisms of a 'mechanical' type (the *lab* dimension of moral agency), which end up strengthening individual orientations. Morphogenesis happens only if aggregations of free individuals change the moral system; otherwise, the system continues to be reproductive.

A macroscopic example of the *lib/lab* view is the idea of the European Union's master plan as supported by the former President of the European Commission,

[6]Luhmann defines morality as a special form of communication that carries with it indications of approval or disapproval. "The moral is not something good. Of course, that should not lead us to say that the moral is something bad. [...] The moral functions only as a distinction" (Luhmann 1993: 996). Trust itself, which for Parsons arose from the normative order of the open society, in Luhmann can no longer count on norms that disappear and must be entrusted to communication (Jalava 2003).

Romano Prodi (2002: 20): "The integration of free market forces and competition, on the one hand, with equality of opportunity for all citizens, on the other, is the master plan of the new European construction." This is a vision of society that has its roots in early modernity and in recent times has found expression in such authors as Ralf Dahrendorf (1994) and Anthony Giddens (1998). It was relaunched by Tony Blair in his speech to the British Parliament in July, 2014, when he proposed the co-penetration of state and the market because neither of them can resolve social problems by itself. *Lib/lab* theorists care little that actual reality demonstrates that this model produces more problems than it solves. They do not see that its failures are due to the fact that it forces social subjects to act within the double bind between state and market.

Figure 10.1 indicates there is also a rather more complex path. In this path [3/a,b,c,d] morality certainly depends on moral (primary and corporate) agents, but it has its own relational dynamic. If we agree that individuals necessarily find themselves confronting already existing institutional structures, the morphogenetic process starts from individuals who create networks of social relations (line [3a]) which, *on certain conditions*, confirm or alter moral institutions (social and cultural systems) (line [3b]). Institutions, in turn, and always on certain conditions, strengthen or alter the morality of networks of social relations (line [3c]) and, thus, influence individuals (line [3d]). In this path the explanation of morality must come to terms with what happens in the intermediate space between individuals and institutions (normative systems). The ways in which (intersubjective and/or impersonal) social relations structure social networks become crucial. The understanding of the social morphogenesis of morality becomes much more problematic because the intermediate transitions are subject to great variability.

What I want to elucidate is the difference between the morphogenesis described through paths {[1]-[2]}, which correspond to the morality of *lib/lab* arrangements, and the morphogenesis that passes through social networks (path [3]), which corresponds to new relational configurations.[7]

In the circular path between [1] and [2], the T2–T3 phase of the morphostatic/morphogenetic diagram is regarded as an aggregation of individual behaviours that identify themselves – positively or negatively (through positive or negative feedbacks) – with the same symbols/values that, if they are institutionalised, reflect on the aggregations of individuals and can be confirmed (morphostasis) or altered (morphogenesis) by new aggregations of individuals. The keystone of this interpretation of social morality lies in individual agency's adhering to one or another 'group consciousness' (corporate actors), which can be of the majority or specific to minority groups (as is called for by the doctrine of multiculturalism). According to this view, the participation of individuals happens through their identification with a shared symbolic 'focal point' (a social class, a cultural or religious tradition, or a social movement) that does not necessarily require specific interpersonal and network relations among the participants.

[7] See Donati (2011: 221–315).

In path [3], instead, we can observe changes of morality in much more detail through four moments (a, b, c, d) because a 'relational logic' operates in phase T2–T3, which is overlooked or underestimated by explanations based on the {[1]–[2]} paths. I propose that we analyse these processes in greater detail and with several examples.

The Morphogenesis of Morality According to the Relational Paradigm

The Obsolescence of Classic Paradigms

The *lib/lab* paradigms of social morphostasis/morphogenesis (M/M) can generally be traced back to a framework in which the conditioning structure at the initial time T1 dictates the moral norms with respect to which individuals must take a position in their interactions in phase T2-T3.[8] This is true whether the conditioning structure privileges moral norms of a libertarian and individualistic type (as happens in the U.S. since the *lib* side prevails over the *lab* side there), or whether the opposite happens, as in Europe, where the *lab* side of political regulation prevails over the *lib* side of the free market. In this paradigm it is claimed that individuals can conform, or not, to the conditioning structure according to modalities that Merton (1938) synthesised in his famous five types of adaptation to legitimate ends and means (among which are moral norms) that characterise the conditioning structure.

Merton's typology is built on positive (+) and negative (−) feedbacks on the part of individuals vis-à-vis the conditioning structure's ends and norms. These are first order feedbacks. The scheme assumes that the formation of collective actors in phase T2–T3 consists in the adherence of a certain number of individuals to each of these modalities (this is an example of the use of the binary agency/structure, micro/macro scheme). The aim of this theory is to discover "how some social structures exert a definite pressure upon certain persons in the society to engage in nonconformist rather than conformist conduct." Merton's answer is that "certain phases of social structure generate circumstances in which infringement of social codes constitutes a 'normal' response" (Merton 1938: 672).

With reference to change in morality, it is assumed that: (i) conformity and ritualism produce morphostasis, (ii) renunciation leads one to stay out of the social arena, while (iii) innovation, in as much as it alters norms but not ends, seems to constitute the modality of internal development of the same system according to the

[8] I am referring here to the M/M scheme elaborated by Archer (1979, 1995, 2013) and discussed by other authors (contributions to Archer 2014, 2015).

Parsonian model of modernisation (the Parsonian model of up-grading modernity and successful modernity).[9]

Where Is Morphogenesis?

My thesis is that the Mertonian type of scheme (which follows the [1]–[2] path of Fig. 10.1) commits a series of fallacies. The first fallacy is that it explains morphogenesis through positive and negative feedbacks alone. The second fallacy, in parallel, is to assume that morphogenesis is produced by automatic mechanisms. For example, Cartocci (2007) assumes that buying newspapers, donating blood or participating in sport or cultural associations automatically indicates that these individuals share a civic culture and have relations of trust, cooperation, and reciprocity with one another. Such a correlation, much less a causal connection, does not have any empirical foundation.

In other words, these theories overlook the feedbacks activated both by individuals and institutions on social relations, and they think that adherence to certain norms produces social change in and of itself. To my way of thinking, it is not so. Adherence alone to the change of a moral norm (via positive feedback) is not sufficient for explaining the changes in the relations that individuals have with one another and with the object of their actions. If we want to understand the current morphogenesis of morality, it is necessary to introduce a relational view on the ways in which moral norms form and change society.

Why Relationality Matters in Generating Different Morals

In previous contributions (Donati 2014a, 2015a) I have argued that feedbacks to social relations follow a different logic compared to the logic inherent in feedbacks to single actions.[10] In this contribution I want to develop this argument and make the claim that feedbacks to social relations (relational feedbacks), rather than feedbacks to simple actions, change the normativity of the generative mechanisms that produce social morphogenesis through positive and negative feedbacks.

The argument's key point is that reactions (feedbacks) to the single actions of Ego and Alter and reactions to the relation between them are different orders of reality. It is possible that Ego rejects (or accepts) Alter's action and accepts (or rejects) the relationship with her/him, and vice versa, if and only if the feedback exercised

[9]On the empirical plane, it is a matter of knowing the size of groups that adopt each adaptive modality, their structural characteristics (age, gender, socio-economic status, etc.), and their power relations.

[10]'Logic' here means principles, or rules, of reasoning.

toward the single action is of a different order of reality with respect to the feedback toward the reciprocal relationship. The different order of reality implies a different normativity (logical rules)[11] in as much as agents refer to single actions or, instead, to social relationships.

Table 10.1 synthesises the differences between conceiving M/M processes on the basis of mechanical mechanisms (MecMec) and on the basis of relational mechanisms (RelMec). In the case of MecMec, moral norms arise from the adherence/deviation of individuals' actions vis-à-vis systemic morality. In the case of RelMec, moral norms arise as a consequence of taking into account the autonomous relationality between agents. Let us look at this in more detail.

(I) In the case of *mechanical mechanisms* (*MecMec*): moral norms are expected to operate independently of the social inter-relations among actors, and therefore:

- the normative order depends on conformity/deviance of individuals' actions toward the system (this is the logic of the 'agency and structure' debate);
- the feedbacks can be positive and negative, but not relational;
- the black box of the mechanism works with a trivial causality (operating with internal functional constraints and given boundary conditions);
- the normativity of social mechanisms is supposed to be 'automatic' in so far as the interactions in the mediating social network (phase T2–T3 of the morphogenetic process) are bound by standard norms;
- the outcomes are aggregative social phenomena or functional performances, i.e., the outcome is determined by the mechanisms inherent in the social network conforming to structural constraints;
- as examples we can think of: social systems/institutions working as goal-seeking machines (e.g. traffic norms); organisations relying upon belief-formation mechanisms, bandwagon effects, snowball effects, etc. (e.g. advertising agencies or election campaigns); procedural justice; procedural democracy; adiaphoric normativity in facing social issues; bureaucratic anormative regulations.

(II) In the case of *relational mechanisms* (*RelMec*): norms are expected to emerge and operate through the dynamics of sociability/relationality among agents, and therefore:

- the normative order depends on social relations generated by agents and their networks;
- the feedbacks are positive and negative at the first order, and relational at the second order of the interactions in the network;

[11] As I have asserted in previous papers (e.g. Donati 2014a, 2015a), properly speaking, 'logic', in its classical (Aristotelian) sense, is the set of rules (normativity) used to achieve valid knowledge. By extension, I understand logic as the set of rules that connect – in various ways – the components of any social relation (its goal, means, value-pattern). Knowledge is a particular social relation, one that connects the knower with the object to be known.

Table 10.1 Two different types of social mechanisms working with different kinds of normativity and producing a different normative order

	Mechanical mechanisms (MecMec)	Relational mechanisms (RelMec)
Types of mechanisms	(Norms are expected to operate independently of the social inter-relations among actors)	(Norms are expected to emerge and operate through the dynamics of sociability/relationality among agents)
The normative order	Depends on individuals and systems (agency and structure)	Depends on social relations
Positive and negative feedbacks	Yes	Yes
Relational feedbacks	No	Yes
Black box	Trivial causality (operating with internal functional constraints and given boundary conditions)	Non-trivial causality (whose workings depend on internal complexity and in interaction with the environment)
Normativity of the social mechanisms	The interactions in the mediating social network (phase T2–T3 of the morphogenetic process) are bound by established norms	The interactions in the mediating social network (phase T2–T3 of the morphogenetic process) are *nomos-building*
Outcomes	Aggregative social phenomena or functional performances where the outcome is determined by the mechanisms inherent in the social network under structural constraints	Emergence of a relational subject (We-relation, including corporate agents) whose normativity is an expression of an underlying interacting social network
Examples	Social systems/Institutions working as goal-seeking machines (e.g. traffic laws)	Relational couples (e.g. the higher the commonality of the couple's external network, the greater is the sharing of conjugal roles),
	Organisations relying upon belief-formation mechanisms, bandwagon effects, snowball effects, etc. (e.g. advertising agencies or election campaigns)	Civic associations
	Procedural justice	Peer production, co-production
	Procedural democracy	Relational goods
	Adiaphoric normativity in facing social issues	'Beyond GDP' indicators (e.g. economic well-being depends on the quantity and quality of bonding and bridging social capital – see the Stiglitz report)
	Bureaucratic anormative regulations	Justice based upon norms of social (relational) equity
	etc.	Fair trade
		Deliberative democracy
		Associative democracy
		Community foundations
		Social streets
		etc

- the black box of the mechanism works with a non-trivial causality (whose workings depend on internal complexity and in interaction with the environment);
- the normativity of the social mechanisms is sensitive to the interactions in the mediating social network (phase T2–T3 of the morphogenetic process) and, for that reason, is *nomos-building*;
- the outcomes consist in the emergence of relational subjects (primary and corporate agents) whose normativity is an expression of an underlying interacting social network;
- as examples we can think of: relational couples (e.g. the higher the commonality of the couple's external network, the greater is the sharing of conjugal roles)[12]; civic associations; community foundations; social streets; peer production and co-production; relational goods; 'Beyond GDP' indicators (where economic well-being depends on the quantity and quality of bonding and bridging social capital – see the Stiglitz Report); justice based upon norms of social (relational) equity; fair trade; deliberative democracy; associative democracy.

Relational mechanisms are generative in as much as they are relational operations. They are so when the normative dimension of the mechanism corresponds to a 'logic' (in the sense of a rule or set of rules) that combines the elements of the relationship between the agents (Ego and Alter) in such a way as to ensure some validity and efficacy in what emerges from their relationship. Otherwise, it is a mechanical mechanism.

For example, the basic mechanism of Western political democracy is the rule that after a contest between the majority and minority, one votes yes or no on a proposal. This logic (normativity) is not relational. The morality is inherent in the logic of numbers: the political decision is taken on the basis of the majority of votes. This is the moral norm leading to political decisions. In this case, voters vote through the mechanism of positive and negative feedbacks. Therefore, morality (the logic) is mechanical: what the majority vote decides is considered as good, what gets fewer votes is considered as bad. The democratic process is regulated by power relations, and therefore its morality is based on power, not on truth or on certainty regarding consequences. If, instead, democracy proceeded on the basis of a reflexivity having as its goal the activation of a certain type of relations and a certain societal context (and not to do 'something'), then democracy would use not only positive and negative feedbacks (which still decide the final vote), but also relational feedbacks. Their use makes it possible to understand better which type of society one is thinking of generating, and not only what one decides to accept or reject. Democratic procedures would become mechanisms of a relational, rather than a mechanical type.

[12]As Elisabeth Bott has demonstrated, the connectedness or the density of a husband's and wife's separate social networks is positively associated with marital role segregation, and vice versa.

The activation of relational mechanisms does not happen in the current political system of parties because they operate with a binary morality and do not allow consensus building to happen through the establishment of networks of relations among the political decision makers who are members of the different political parties. If this were possible, it would also be possible to form democratic networks of decision makers in political bodies that reflect the networks of civil society. This possibility is available in the decision making sphere of certain Third Sector organisations (such as in true social cooperatives) in so far as they give priority to the value of the relations of civil society, which their decisions create. It could also happen in the political system if a 'relational state' model was adopted, which would operate through relational inclusion rather than through a compromise between market and state, i.e., *lib/lab* inclusion.[13] 'Relational inclusion' means that a full participation of people in society (or a social subsystem) is realised by providing citizens with the opportunities to act as relational subjects in relation to other social subjects – with the same rights and obligations – and not on the ground of adhering to market competition ruled by the political power.

Put schematically, the reason that the individualism/holism mix (in other words, *lib/lab*) does not work and generates moral evils is that it does not take into account the fact that the individual, with his/her action, alters or interprets in his/her own way the moral norm (*lib*), but it is not a given that the actual relation that ensues from this will change the system in a morally good direction (*lab*) because a network of relations operates between the individual and the system. The *lib/lab* system is built precisely in such a way as to make the system immune to this network of social relations.

Conversely, if the system alters its own normativity, it is not the case that social relations are automatically altered in the same direction and, then, that individual actions conform to systemic change of norms. In between there is the normativity of relational networks. Luhmann's a-relational functionalism[14] leads to erroneous conclusions because it assumes that the functional mechanisms of social differentiation can separate what is human from what is non-human in moral

---

[13]On the 'relational state' see Donati (2002/2003, 2015b) and Cooke and Muir (2012).

[14]I call Luhmann's theory 'a-relational' not because he ignores the relation – indeed, it permeates his thinking – but because he refuses to base sociology on the social relation. Specifically, it is a-relational for two reasons. The first is that he uses a binary code, which is notoriously ill adapted to deal with relations: "Communication is correspondingly coded as a (positively or negatively interpreted) proposal of meaning, which can be understood or not understood, accepted or rejected. The control of this doubling and especially this negativity of not understanding or rejecting unfolds recursively and thus already determines the selection of the proposal – whether the proposal aims at agreement or conflict. Thus a knowledge of how to estimate what can be understood emerges" (Luhmann 1995: 445). The second reason is that the system as such (specifically: biological, psychic, and social) is for him immune to the social relations of the living world. I am perfectly aware, instead, that Luhmann uses the concept of relation in a logical (cybernetic) sense to the point of theorising a sort of ontological and epistemological relation*ism*.

norms, given that the moral norm becomes a pure, functional communication,[15] whereas communications are non-human when operated by the social system and human when they are enacted by humans in the system's environment. His slogan is: "Everything that is possible becomes morally licit." In such a way, *paradoxically* with respect to its premises, the Luhmannian theory ends up by converging with the relatonal*ism* of neo-constructivists (for example, McFarlane 2013), who assume that the human and the non-human can merge with each other, giving rise to moral norms which are identical for human beings, animals, and other non-human living beings. In this way, the human-social and non-human moral norms are 'fused' (conflated) with each other, while experience and empirical research tell us that they remain ontologically and practically distinct from each other, precisely due to the substantive differences in their inner relational constitution. For instance, animals do not have relations of sophisticated mutual envy or long term strategies in their behaviour, while humans do.

To illustrate, let us think about the new human reproductive technologies and how they require the creation of new moral norms that could not have previously existed because certain bio-medical methods were not available. These technologies can give a baby to anybody through surrogate motherhood (by means of a uterus for rent), alter the embryo's genes to produce a made-to-order child as regards eye colour or other anatomical features, or clone a human being. These technical possibilities create unprecedented social relations (between the child's surrogate mother and social parents, between the parent who has the responsibility for having wanted a made-to-order child and that child, between individuals who are clones). Can we separate the human aspects of these relations from the technical aspects of the same relations? Or can we fuse them? Empirical research tells us that neither of these two possibilities is really feasible because the relations created by technology present human problems to which technology is unable to provide answers. Human social relations exist at a *sui generis* level of reality. Many examples can be given to show that this autonomous level of reality exists.

First example: Reciprocating a gift cannot be explained by an automatic functional mechanism, nor as a mere individual response that Ego gives to Alter, who

[15]According to Luhmann (1996), morality is becoming a self-referential system that is specialised in responding to the problem of esteem and lack of esteem in communication. He defines morality as an ability to sustain the self-referential reproduction of communication: "Neither life as such, nor the functions of the brain, nor the conscious operations of perception and thinking have intrinsic moral quality. [...] The moral makes an important difference only in communication, namely, a difference in the communicative reaction to the expression of esteem or disesteem. [...] There are, in other words, no good people or bad people, but only the possibility of indicating people as good or bad" (Luhmann 1993: 1000). To him, recourse to the 'normativity of norms' or to 'values' proves to be untenable because all norms and values reveal themselves to be undecidable (Luhmann 2008b).

gave Ego the gift.[16] Reciprocation is a relation that has its own morality; it is the expression of a moral norm that does not depend either on the impersonal function of the gift or on the individual action of giving 'something' that is owed to one person in particular, but resides in the super-functional meaning of the gift relation as such, as a good in itself (which means for the goods it carries with it beyond the utility of a particular exchange of things and/or services).

Second example: The electoral vote follows a different moral norm (logic) if it is given as a relation to a person or to an ideology in the contest between political parties. The reason resides in the fact that the morality of interpersonal relations is different from the morality that is applied to impersonal relations.

Third example. In a hierarchical network where the founding relation stipulates obedience, the ordinary dynamics are mostly productive of conformity to norms, while a network that works with a 'be different' norm[17] is more likely to produce anomie. An example of the former is Horstink's (2011) research on a group of soldiers in the military.[18] An example of the latter type is provided by studies on those social networks on the internet that aggregate individuals who act as hackers without having anything or very little else in common (Haythornthwaite 2002, 2005). In both cases, a crucial explanatory factor of the different outcomes lies in the properties and powers inherent in the specific relational morality of the networks.

In all of these examples, the morality of agency follows one 'logic' rather than another because the reference to the relations entailed by the agency (i.e., the moral good or bad inherent in the relation) changes. If the relations are virtual, the morality also can become 'virtual', meaning that the moral norms lose some of the constraints characterizing and binding interpersonal relationships (it is empirically verified that, in the environment of virtual communications on the internet, users are often encouraged to simulate or suspend certain rules of responsibility that they cannot avoid in real relationships). By changing reference to different kinds of relationality, morality can follow a different logic (e.g., in the anonymous matrix of communication provided by the internet, morality becomes more impersonal, and, by virtue of the means of communication, the rules combining goals and value-patterns may disregard the distinction good/bad which would be necessary in a non-virtual environment). On the empirical plane we see that the normativity of being 'ethical' toward individual persons or impersonal institutions (impersonal

[16]The idea that moral responsibility consists in the infinite debt of whoever has received the gift, as Bauman (1998) maintains, is clearly individualistic. And it is because of this that Bauman considers morality as a poisoned gift (Junge 2001).

[17]The international film festival aimed at adolescents held in Griffoni (Italy) adopted as its motto, 'Be different', which clearly indicated a moral imperative aimed at the young people.

[18]This study investigates the influence of relationship density and relationship power on moral reasoning. Findings show that social network properties influence moral reasoning by creating similarity within groups. No support was found for the influence of informal leaders or of group development.

discourses, systems, distant others) is actually different precisely because of the different morality (tighter or looser, more expressive or more utilitarian, etc.) implied in these relational references.

It is for this reason that it is necessary to take into account unexpected, indirect, and perverse effects. The following seems to me to be an interesting example. If we accept that in late modernity the socio-cultural structure imposes the moral imperative to 'be different' (i.e., 'choose your own option of what is good and bad'), we can ask: why is moral indifference the unexpected and unintentional outcome? A possible explanation in terms of the M/M paradigm is the following. The morality of institutions pushes toward moral individualism, but the network of individuals has a structure and moral dynamic that are such as to nullify the value of personal choices. The network's moral reflexivity is hindered or fractured (as is the post-modern public sphere in general) so that indifference (non-differentiation) predominates in moral choices. This process is obviously favoured by those ICTs (not all of them, e.g. not Wikipedia) which work by cancelling out the value of moral differences due to the composition effect (choices elide with one another), so that the medium becomes the moral norm ('the medium is the message'), as those who use Facebook, twitter, or other social media as their exclusive or principle means of communication illustrate.

How the Relational Framework Can Be Applied: The Morality of Welfare and Its Morphogenesis

From its inception, the welfare state has been the object of endless discussions regarding its moral foundations and its consequences for the morality of society as a whole. It is not possible to discuss this issue extensively. I will come to the point.

The point is that over the course of its development, the welfare state has adopted an increasingly impersonal morality. The moral responsibility for social problems (poverty, unemployment, health needs, pensions, social assistance, as well as education and housing, etc.) was handed over to the 'system'. The welfare package (inclusive of all basic needs that must be satisfied to have a decent standard of living) has become an automatic social right (a right of citizenship), in the sense that it does not take into consideration the beneficiaries' conduct. The morality of this welfare resides in the principle of solidarity (that is, of inclusion and social cohesion) realised through state redistribution.

With reference to Fig. 10.2, we can say that moral responsibility passed from individuals to the system (from [1] to [2]), completely skipping over social networks (path 3/a, b, c, d). The system has thus proceeded to protect single individuals, relieving the social networks (families, informal networks, associations and institutions of civil society) of obligations toward the collective well-being.

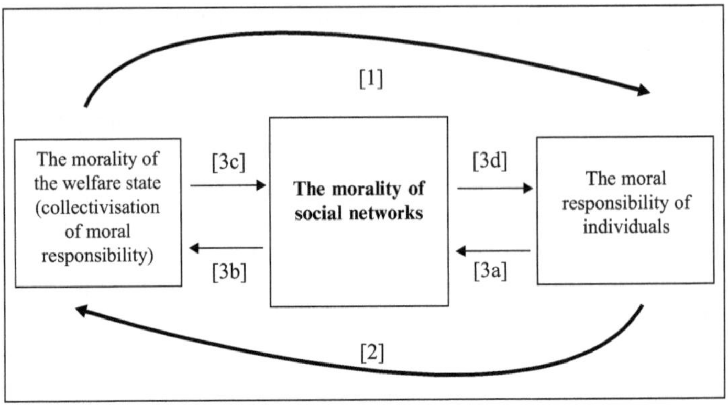

Fig. 10.2 The three 'layers' of welfare morality (agential, relational, and systemic)

In recent decades a vast literature has shown the negative effects that this course of action has had on the forms of primary solidarity (informal networks) and secondary solidarity (networks organised in associative forms). The outcome of this story has been, and is increasingly, the crisis of the welfare state, which derives from not only the State's inability to address social problems (the fiscal crisis, the inadequacy of public bureaucracies, etc.), but also, and especially to the fact that it generates perverse effects, among which are the progressive lack of responsibility of individuals and the fragmentation of social integration. Undoubtedly, the rhetoric of conservatives and parties on the right when they speak about this issue is overblown.[19] Nevertheless, beyond the rhetoric of conservatives, the problem is real.

The morphogenesis of the moral norms that justify the welfare state is thus in a radical crisis. My thesis is that the morphogenetic process of the moral norms that must give a moral meaning to welfare is blocked today because the existing model of the welfare state is propped up by the reproduction of *lib/lab* morality: the *lib* side calls for a return to individual responsibility (autonomous individual reflexivity) while the *lab* side relaunches public intervention with Keynesian types of adjustments, reaffirming the primacy of collective responsibility. The proposal of a 'third way' that introduces a new mix between moral *lib* principles and *lab* principles (Giddens 1998) has not yielded significant results. Proposals of this type cannot work because *lib/lab* morality is blocked; it does not produce a creative morphogenesis, but only a bound morphogenesis.

In the past there were those who attempted to propose a typology of the welfare state according to its differing constitutive moralities. For example, Zijdervel (1986)

[19]'Moral Atrophy in the Welfare State' (Robert E. Goodin, in *Policy Science*, 26, 1993, pp. 63–78). 'Moral Inferiority of the Welfare State' (by Rev. Robert Sirico, Acton Institute); 'The Rise of Government and the Decline of Morality: the growth of government has politicized life and weakened the nation's moral fabric' (by James A. Dorn, Cato Institute, 1996); 'How the Welfare State Corrupted Sweden' (*Mises Daily*: Wednesday, May 31, 2006 by Per Bylund).

has observed that welfare systems are rarely moral (with the important exceptions of the United States and Japan), but more often are a-moral (like Italy's) or immoral (like Holland's).[20] The moral ones take into account the moral responsibilities of single individuals. The amoral ones consider the person's conduct as morally indifferent when it comes to enjoying the rights and benefits of welfare. The immoral ones offer unconditional compensation, thus rewarding – directly or indirectly – morally irresponsible behaviour. In my view, only moral welfare systems can adequately deal with the social challenges that result from a constant and progressive inclusion of the population in the politics of welfare.

It is evident that Zijdervel's moral argument, and the moral typology of the welfare state that he elaborated, is carried out from the point of view of individual morality. He overlooks the problem of solidarity and redistributive justice as elements of morality. On the other hand, however, one could ask: can the moral norm of solidarity (and redistributive justice) nullify the moral responsibility of individuals?

It is here that the argument about the morality of social relations makes its entrance. Individuals must be morally free, and the social system must guarantee social solidarity, but how can we proceed so that by choosing one we do not eliminate the other term?

Figure 10.2 suggests that we look at how individuals and systems interface through social networks: in other words, whether or not they invest the relationality of the networks with morality and how they consider the morality of interpersonal and communitarian relations as such. Freedom must make reference to the concrete relations that individuals create and in which they live. And the system must take care of relations by evaluating whether they produce relational goods or evils (this is the 'relational state'). The goodness or badness of social relations comes into play, in and of themselves and in their effects. It is here that a new morality of welfare comes into being. Alongside other morphogenetic processes, another type of morphogenesis is taking shape, which I call 'relational'.

On the theoretical plane, the sequence of change that the morality of welfare has undergone can follow different paths of morphogenesis in the cycle T1–T4. I offer three as examples (Fig. 10.2).

- T1: the 'starting' situation is given by the systemic crisis of the welfare state's morality: the welfare state enters into crisis perhaps because it nullifies individuals' moral responsibility by completely impersonal principles of responsibility, or perhaps because – vice versa – it appeals to individual responsibility while overlooking the norms of solidarity;

[20] Zijderveld's favourable assessment of the morality of welfare in the United States is merely comparative. His affirmation that the welfare state in the U.S. is more moral is not meant to imply that it is always ethical, but merely that in the U.S. debate regarding the ethical criteria of welfare is more explicit and carries more weight than in other countries. For further evidence of Zijderveld's comparative claim, see Mead (1986).

- in the intermediate T2-T3 phase: the interactions between agents represent the search for moral norms in response to the systemic crisis; these interactions can follow, roughly, three paths:

  (I) interactions are guided by an action model that tries to adjust the norms of negotiation between state actors and market actors, leaving aside other actors; this modality (of communicative reflexivity within the *lib/lab* system) represents a search for internal adaptations to the 'system', which are generally of an opportunistic type;

  (II) interactions are predicated on action models characterised by an autonomous reflexivity, so that the social networks, lacking any shared moral constraints, become chaotic;

  (III) interactions adopt action models supported by a meta-reflexivity that is oriented toward building social networks in which there is an important effect of 'open coordination'[21] between the parties, valorising the morality of reciprocal relations (relational steering);

- T4: the structure of emergent morality depends on how the normativity of phase T2-T3 was elaborated; according to the three above paths and three types of morphogenesis are possible:

  (I) a morphogenesis of *lib/lab* morality (the *lib/lab* is not in and of itself morphostatic); the emergent norms are a combination of criteria of efficiency and efficacy in the definition of welfare morality;

  (II) an unbound morphogenesis of *lib/lab* morality, which means the appearance of moral norms of individual freedom and of collective constraints that proceed on their own, without significant connections between them, thus producing contradictions and perverse effects;

  (III) a morphogenesis of morality that amplifies, selects, and stabilises new opportunities on the basis of a normative criterion that valorises relationality between the parties as a primary good; for example, welfare measures come to be considered as morally good/bad depending on whether or not they lead to the flowering of interpersonal relations (in the positive case, one speaks of 'relational state', 'welfare society', etc.); here the moral norm of social structures is based on the qualities and causal properties of the social relations that are promoted.

---

[21]As an example, we can refer to the open method of coordination (OMC) adopted by the European Union. The OMC provides a new framework for cooperation between the Member States, whose national policies can thus be directed towards certain common objectives. Under this intergovernmental method, the Member States are evaluated by one another (peer pressure), with the Commission's role being limited to surveillance. The European Parliament and the Court of Justice play virtually no part in the OMC process. The open method of coordination takes place in areas which fall within the competence of the Member States, such as employment, social protection, social inclusion, education, youth and training.

The third alternative (III) indicates a morality characterised by the moral norms of equitable and sustainable welfare as the product of *sui generis* relational networks. As examples one could cite: co-production (Pestoff 2009),[22] public-private partnerships generating new networks at the local level (Evers 2015); social cooperatives able to be counter-cyclical instead of having only a buffering role on the impact that the systemic crisis has on citizens (Vidal 2015); and, in general, the so called 'relational turn' in social innovation (Fløysand and Jakobsen 2011).[23]

Every society has to come to terms with an intrinsic ambivalence: on the one hand, it must make individuals understand that they *depend on the collectivity* and that, therefore, the altruistic orientation must prevail over an individualistic orientation but, at the same time, it has to encourage individuals to maintain a certain *distance from the prevalent norms* so as always to be able to develop their own evaluations and thus guarantee a certain degree of *creativity*, innovation, and pursuit of change on the part of the individual.

The problem of *lib/lab* is that its moral norms do not provide a solution to this ambivalence. We can take the case of bibliometric evaluations of scientific research. Leydesdorff (2014) considered the ethical and cultural consequences of relying on metrics to assess the quality of scholarship, and reached the conclusion that the present system, centred on individual production, penalises the research of groups, networks, and between cooperating individuals. The answer to the problem of how to combine individual creativity and collective subjectivity can only come from a relational approach that highlights that innovation is a product of networks that share norms formed in an autonomous manner by the sociability of participants without being imposed by a superordinate structure. The problem is whether the network is able to avoid the absence of or lack of clarity in the norms. The answer is the relational subject, the morality of the we-relation (Donati and Archer 2015). Lacking this, networks fail.[24]

---

[22]"Co-production of social services offers new opportunities as well as challenges for collective solutions to growing problems facing the public provision of social services in Europe. It gives citizens both more choice and more voice, as well as a more active role in the provision of public services. But, greater citizen participation and more third sector provision of social services can meet with resistance both from traditional public administration and New Public Management (NPM), each based on a separate logic. However, New Public Governance (NPG) is based on network governance and relies on greater citizen participation, co-production, and more third sector provision of public financed social services." (Pestoff 2015).

[23]Fløysand and Jakobsen (2011) argue that recent contributions within the system of innovation approach are marked by an instrumentalism that views innovation as a predictable and standardised process that in most aspects counters theories and empirical observations stressing the multilevel, spontaneous, and complex features of innovation. Informed by the relational turn within economic geography these scholars develop an alternative analytical framework. They do this stepwise: first, by elaborating on how innovation was originally defined within the systems of innovation approach; second, by outlining a relational based analytical framework based on the concept of social fields; and, finally, by demonstrating how it has been applied.

[24]Schrank and Whitford (2011) have shown that network failures are not due to the simple absence of network governance, but rather to a situation in which transactional conditions for network desirability obtain but network governance is impeded either by ignorance or opportunism, or by a

Let me recapitulate the fundamental argument. The social and cultural structure given at T1 enters into a systemic crisis as regards the moral norms that it contains, explicitly or implicitly. The crisis leads to the commencement of interplay in phase T2–T3, from which derive effects to which, de facto, society responds, depending on the case in question, with three types of morphogenesis that have three types of outcomes: (a) circularity of the morality between subjective norms and institutional forms (Beck et al. 2003); (b) widespread anomie and morality of the 'hit the bottom' type (Teubner 2011); (c) morality generated through new forms of relational steering (Donati 2013, 2015a). This is the moral scenario of society as it makes the transition beyond modernity, which I would like to now briefly to delineate.

The Morphogenesis of the Societal Moral Fabric in the Era of Globalisation

The scenario that we have before us is that of *lib/lab* systems continuing to operate while encountering growing failures and perverse effects. Their morality is self-defeating. The rapidity of failures depends on the accelerating erosion of certain values and traditional norms that early modernity had preserved in the past. The immediate consequence of such failures is perceived as unbound morphogenesis, which means growing widespread anomie.

If we generalise the scheme in Fig. 10.2, we can hypothesise that morality in the era of globalisation will proceed according to three *concomitant* types of morphogenetic changes (Fig. 10.3). The processes can be described through the morphogenesis of the basic structure of social relations (see the framework in Donati 2014a: 144–159), or what we can call the 'founding relation' – or the 'relational pattern' – that characterises a social network.[25] Such a structure (CTMN) consists in the emergence of interplay among the following components: (C) the value attributed to the relation's concern/interest; (T) the concrete and situated target/goal selected or selectable for the implementation of the relation on the ground of the relation's value; (M) the means available to pursue the relation's concern/interest; (N) the logic of relating C, T, and M (through distinctions and connections).

combination of the two. Network failures are depicted as continuous rather than discrete outcomes. They have more than one cause. Two undertheorised – if not undiscovered – types of network failure (i.e., involution and contested collaboration) are analysed.

[25]Every social network has a 'relational pattern'. We could think of any organisational or associative form describable as a network that is inspired by a certain relational modality among participants: a company can be hierarchical or not, a voluntary association or a rehabilitation community for drug addicts identifies with (and uses) a certain relational pattern of help, a cooperative has a relational pattern among members, a sport or cultural association contemplates a certain modality by which the members relate to one another, a network of families think about their relations as 'family' relations, a social network on the internet comes into being from a relation-type among people who communicate, etc.

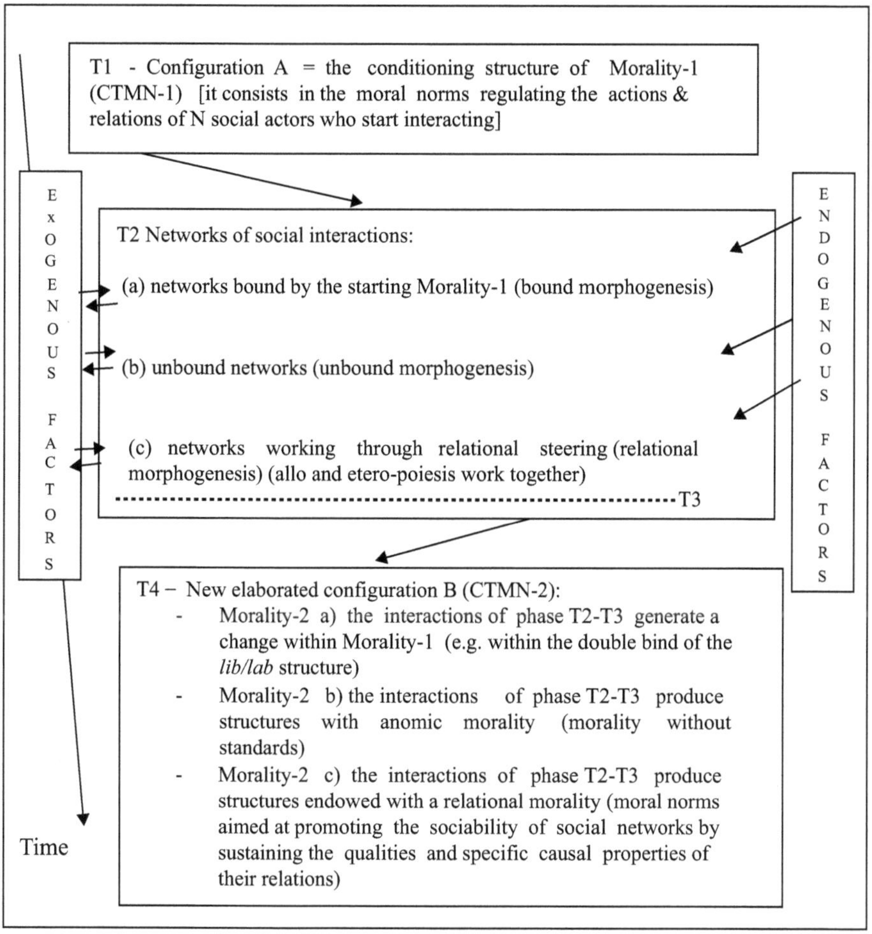

Fig. 10.3 The different paths of the social morphogenesis of morality from a relational perspective (as it emerges in late modernity) (in a cycle T1–T4) [For the more general theory, see: Donati (2013: 216)]

At time T1 we find a structure that contains its own Morality-1, which conditions agents when they begin to interact with one another.

In phase T2–T3 three scenarios are possible:

(a) the network of agents operates on the basis of Morality-1, which at time T4 can produce both morphostasis (communicative reflexivity) or a *bound* morphogenesis (autonomous reflexivity); for example, within the double bind of *lib/lab* morality, CTMN-2 reproduces CTMN-1 or is a variation of CTMN-1 that maintains the *lib/lab* morality.

(b) The network of agents breaks the structure of Morality-1 and at time T4 generates an *unbound* morphogenesis, that is, an anomic morality. Here the CTMN-2 structure is characterised by a relational logic that is unable or refuses to draw distinctions (thought to be discrimination)[26] and, thus, does not valorise connections, but fosters reflexivity in a fragmented or impeded way.
(c) the network of agents operates with strategies of a relational steering type and produces *relational* morphogenesis. The structure of CTMN-2 is characterised by a meta-reflexive logic that indicates ends and means as a function of relations' value. This is the case of morality that is generated in those social spheres where relationality is taken seriously as a source of moral norms. In other words, interactions are guided by the morality of the relation as such, which is based on relational feedbacks. New opportunities are created by means of relational steering: the network, in interaction with the exterior, introduces variations in resources, actors, power relations, and norms that legitimate the variations that stabilise relational feedbacks.

The framework of Fig. 10.3 underscores the fact that the structure of the relation that establishes and characterises the social network contains the moral norm that organises the means and ends of agency – both individual and collective – as a function of the value of the relation itself.

In case (a), a norm of collective utility prevails that maximises the criteria of efficiency and efficacy. An example is found in organisations that operate with a managerial style (business morality).

In case (b), a norm that maximises criteria of contingent preference prevails. It could be of an expressive or opportunistic type, in the sense of seizing the most attractive opportunities of the moment: for example, the morality of Facebook networks.

In case (c), a norm prevails that gives priority to the criterion of the moral value (the dignity) of the relation that characterises the social network. Civic networks, such as '*social streets*' (http://www.socialstreet.it/), are an example of this type if and when the relation that inspires associative agency is the value to be pursued, independently of its utility, efficacy, or efficiency. In these social practices, what matters is not the material goal that can be achieved (for instance, the maintenance of a common good like a public garden in the neighbourhood) as such, but 'the sociality behind it', i.e., the sociality among the neighbours who produce it.

The third solution at time T4 (Morality-2 c in Fig. 10.3) entails the primacy of the *moral value* over the relation's other components.[27] Moreh (1986) has shown that the economic theory of utility does not take into account moral behaviour, that is, behaviour in which an individual faced with two courses of action may choose

[26]For example, in his essay *On Being Morally Considerable*, the American ethical philosopher Kenneth E. Goodpaster (1978) maintains that any distinction between organisms thought to be in some way "worthy" of moral consideration and others that are not is clearly a case of discrimination.

[27]I provided a relational theory of 'value' in Donati (2009, 2014b: Fig. 10.2).

the one that is *less* profitable to him or her. According to relational theory, when the goals that the individual has to achieve consist of peculiar social relations (e.g. personal care, education, friendship, etc.) then the morphogenesis has to be steered toward the achievement of higher relational goods. My thesis is that this behaviour has greater probabilities of being chosen when the individual is in a relational context endowed with certain properties and powers rather than in another one. The context is not only a constraint, but also a resource, a pool of opportunities offered by the network formed with others.

Luhmann (2008b) wonders: 'Are there indispensable norms in our society?' His answer is negative. In his view, it is impossible reasonably to expect that any given moral or legal norm is normatively indispensable. This answer is in line with the ontological and epistemological premises of his approach, which is decidedly sceptical and amoral. I think that he should be challenged with an even more paradoxical question: 'Are there still indispensable social relations in our society?' The latter issue is strictly linked to the former. Let us take the example of work relations. No doubt work is increasingly considered an indispensable social relation, not only from the standpoint of economic support, but also of the person's emancipation/humanisation, and in this sense it is a moral imperative, which of course admits of exemptions in special circumstances (such as chronic or severe illness).

To understand the argument according to which there are social relations that are morally indispensable, it is necessary to consider the fact that social relations always involve morality. The *practical* moral norm (not the ethical principle, which is located on another level of reality, i.e., in the cultural system) is redefined and changes the moment that the agent *reflects on relations* with others *in a context*, and not when he/she reflects internally on his/her own 'I'. The individual's internal reflexivity considers the moral norm in order to define his/her moral agency in terms of the aspect of his/her subjective determinations (the process of discernment, deliberation, dedication is analysed in depth by Archer 2003), but the moral norm has a dynamic that does not depend only on individual agency, whether of a single individual or of a multiplicity of N individuals (aggregated or interacting with one another) – just as it does not depend entirely on the dynamic of structures (social and cultural institutions). The practical moral norm is formed and created in the relational process among agents. The problem is how we can analyse the contribution given to the formation of the moral norm inherent in the social relation (for example, that of work and family) by, respectively, the single agents, institutions, and the relation itself.

The present *moral imperative* in Western culture, which has been absorbed into social theory, is that individuals *should be* active, intentional, autonomous, independent, reflexive, capable, and constantly able and willing to make rational choices in their lives. Behind this moral imperative for agency, other aspects of what it is to be human remain in the shadows. In terms of actions, the human aspects consist in the fact that agents 'always and as such have *patients*, beings which the action affects' (Reader 2007: 588). Whoever teaches influences the student necessarily, but the student retroacts upon the teacher. Whoever sells necessarily conditions the buyer, but is also conditioned by him/her. Whoever cares for a sick person has an impact on him/her, but is also influenced by him/her. To put this more sociologically, every action entails a relationship. No single person is ever completely an agent or a patient during any one moment of interaction. The Self is called, like it or not, to acknowledge itself as a relational subject (Donati and Archer 2015). This reality is grasped if one understands that, from the moral point of view, what is at stake resides in the relation; indeed, what is at stake is the relation *itself*, considered for its moral properties and powers, because it is in the relation that what is good/bad, right/wrong is defined in (and is relevant to) the identity of being an actor or a patient, an active or a passive subject. When the relation presents itself as ambivalent, the ambivalence can be dissolved by determining what type and degree of reciprocity exists between *Ego* and *Alter*, given the fact that it is the properties and causal powers of reciprocity that define what is good or bad.

Conclusions

Morality is a social fact, but it is treated as being a problem of the individual or the system, or a mix of the two. Current mainstream sociologies explain changes of morality in terms of opposing accounts. For some, morality evolves by 'systemic emergence'. For others, morality evolves through an 'emergence of subjectivity'. If, until a few years ago, these two versions were seen as antithetical (Durkheim's 'collective conscience' vs. Weber's 'individual subjectivity': in particular, 'charisma'), today structure and agency seem to operate in a synergic manner. My explanation is that this happens because a *lib/lab* configuration of morality prevails, which intrinsically contains a double bind (the double bind of the systemic constraint on individuals to be morally 'free').

(a) The theses arguing for morality as 'systemic emergence' maintain that morality becomes a product of functional systems that, in as much as they proceed only through communications and are (ontologically) only communication, *de-normativise society*, including human beings, in a system that includes animals, plants, and every other entity, obviously including the entire artificial world of technology.

This thesis claims that in the differential and complex modern societies, the true protagonists of such events and processes are no longer humans or groups of humans with their material needs and their 'values', but roles and functions, systems and environments: a whole world of givenness and systemic relations in which human individuals operate as mere interchangeable and perfectly fungible elements. According to Luhmann (2008a), this fact leads to a new style of *morality* that is founded on the shared interest in reducing fear, and no longer on norms.

It is in this way that the era of globalisation presents itself, according to some, as morally 'adiaphoric'. Decisions that need to be taken can no longer and should no longer be regulated based on a substantive distinction between good/bad that appeals to some 'nature', 'reality', or 'objectivity' because decisions on good and bad become 'technical', ethically indifferent, adiaphoric.

In this contribution I have tried to show that this vision commits a macroscopic error of perspective because it does not see the human character of the social as a *nomos-building* activity. The type of morphogenesis that it recognises is only that of the de-humanisation of social morality.

(b) In contrast, the theses arguing that morality is becoming completely subjective (morality as the 'emergence of subjectivity') commit an error of perspective that is symmetrically opposed to the previous one because they make the morality of institutions (structures) coincide with that of individuals. Those who support this thesis (including many academic scholars and even many magistrates in courts) argue that morphogenesis takes place through those cultural movements that claim that people, as pure individuals, *have the right to define their identities and their relations as they like*. The distinction between social relations (as structures) and subjective consciousness is no longer productive. What individualisation of social relations essentially means is that *the perceived relation is the social structure*, and that, consequently, both the individual perception and the social structure might vary at people's will. In their opinion *culture becomes an experiment* whose aim is to discover how we can live together as equal but different; the aim of normativity is less and less to prescribe a certain way of living and more and more to clear the institutional conditions for a multiplicity of lifestyles to be recognised. This means that *any collectively shared definition of relationships and individual positions has gone*.

My opinion is that these two broad currents are, at the same time, antithetical and complementary (the moral norm refers to two polarities that are simultaneously opposite and complementary) because they entrust impersonal morality to the system and locate the morality of free individuals in the system's environment where it can fluctuate at will. Systemic morality guarantees subjective morality, which can create the most disparate social forms. On the basis of this perspective, the morphogenesis of morality would be destined to play out this game between individuals and the social system (the circular and conflationary path between 1 and 2, skipping path 3, in Fig. 10.1).

In this contribution, I have tried to show that this scenario identifies the processes of morphogenesis inside *lib/lab* that leads to the dissolution of *lib/lab*. If we manage to see that morphogenesis happens through complex social networks, in which specifically human relationality takes on increasing importance – which is different from that of animals and other living beings – we can glimpse other forms of morphogenesis. These forms are not simply the crisis of morality *tout court* or the replacement of modern morality by the synergy between systemic a-morality and subjective a-morality, but rather the birth of a new morality that valorises the good/bad of social relations upon which human flourishing depends, as well as the morality of human persons.

Once upon a time, society was believed to rest on a morality. When a foundation could no longer be found in religious beliefs, it had to be sought either through reinterpreting these beliefs or looking elsewhere. Contemporary society does not prevent morality from still existing. Rather, it renders morality morphogenetic by continually generating and destroying moral norms through the reduction of what is moral to pure communication, understood as the transfer of information and images. Moral norms seem to become purely communicative. This kind of morphogenesis configures a society riddled with paradoxes. There are those who play on these tendencies to gain advantages. Others become their victims. Still others react, creating other ways of making society, and are carriers of a new morality. In any case, in the long run, the key to solving the problem lies in the fact that a sustainable morality must come to terms with the normativity that is intrinsic in the properties and causal powers of each kind of social relation and, specifically, of the 'founding relation' that characterises the social network in which individuals define their personal identity at a given time among the manifold networks to which they choose to belong.

References

Al-Amoudi, I. (2014). Morphogenesis and normativity: Problems the former creates for the latter. In M. S. Archer (Ed.), *Late modernity. Trajectories towards morphogenic society* (pp. 193–219). New York: Springer.

Archer, M.S. (1979). Social origins of educational system. London: Sage (second edition 2013).

Archer, M. S. (1995). *Realist social theory: The morphogenetic approach*. Cambridge: Cambridge University Press.

Archer, M. S. (2003). *Structure, agency and the internal conversation*. Cambridge: Cambridge University Press.

Archer, M. S. (2013). Social morphogenesis and the prospects of morphogenic society. In M. S. Archer (Ed.), *Social morphogenesis* (pp. 1–22). New York: Springer.

Archer, M. S. (Ed.). (2014). *Late modernity. Trajectories towards morphogenic society*. New York: Springer.

Archer, M. S. (Ed.). (2015). *Generative mechanisms transforming the social order*. New York: Springer.

Arendt, H. (1958). *The human condition*. Chicago: The University of Chicago Press.

Bauman, Z. (1998). What prospects of morality in times of uncertainty? *Theory Culture & Society, 15*(1), 11–22.

Beck, U., Bonss, W., & Lau, C. (2003). The theory of reflexive modernization. Problematic, hypotheses and research program. *Theory, Culture & Society, 20*(2), 1–33.

Bourdieu, P., & Coleman, J. (Eds.). (1991). *Social theory for a changing society*. Oxford: Westview Press.

Cartocci, R. (2007). *Mappe del tesoro. Atlante del capitale sociale in Italia*. Bologna: Il Mulino.

Coleman, J. (1990). The emergence of norms. In M. Hechter, K.-D. Opp, & R. Wippler (Eds.), *Social institutions. Their emergence, maintenance, and effects* (pp. 13–33). New York: Walter de Gruyter.

Cooke, G., & Muir, R. (Eds.). (2012). *The relational state*. London: IPPR.

Dahrendorf, R. (1994). The changing quality of citizenship. In B. van Steenberger (Ed.), *The condition of citizenship* (pp. 10–19). London: Sage.

Donati, P. (2002/2003). Welche soziale Inklusion? «Lib/lab'sches Neo-Panopticon» und sozietale Staatsbürgerschaft: zwei verschiedene sozialpolitische Strategien. *Soziologisches Jahrbuch*, 16, 392–426.

Donati, P. (2009). Beyond the dilemmas of multiculturalism: Recognition through 'relational reason'. *International Review of Sociology, 19*(1), 55–82.
Donati, P. (2011). *Sociologia della riflessività*. Bologna: il Mulino.
Donati, P. (2013). Morphogenesis and social networks: Relational steering not mechanical feedback. In M. S. Archer (Ed.), *Social morphogenesis* (pp. 205–231). New York: Springer.
Donati, P. (2014a). Morphogenic society and the structure of social relations. In M. S. Archer (Ed.), *Late modernity. Trajectories towards morphogenic society* (pp. 143–172). New York: Springer.
Donati, P. (2014b). Social capital and the added value of social relations. *International Review of Sociology, 24*(2), 1–18.
Donati, P. (2015a). Social mechanisms and their feedbacks: Mechanical vs relational emergence of new social formations. In M. S. Archer (Ed.), *Generative mechanisms transforming the social order*. New York: Springer. ch. 4.
Donati, P. (2015b). Beyond the welfare state: Trajectories towards the relational state. In G. Bertin & S. Campostrini (Eds.), *Equiwelfare and social innovation*. Milan: FrancoAngeli.
Donati, P., & Archer, M. S. (2015). *The relational subject*. Cambridge: Cambridge University Press.
Douglas, M. (1986). *How institutions think*. Syracuse: Syracuse University Press.
Evers, A. (2015). Social innovations on the local level. Approaches, instruments and different ways of dealing with them. In P. Donati & L. Martignani (Eds.), *Towards a new local welfare. Best practices and networks of social inclusion*. Bologna: Bononia University Press.
Fløysand, A., & Jakobsen, S. E. (2011). The complexity of innovation: A relational turn. *Progress in Human Geography, 35*(3), 328–344.
Giddens, A. (1992). *The transformation of intimacy. Sexuality, love and eroticism in modern societies*. Cambridge: Polity Press.
Giddens, A. (1998). *The third way. The renewal of social democracy*. Cambridge: Polity Press.
Goodpaster, K. E. (1978). On being morally considerable. *Journal of Philosophy, 75*(6), 308–325.
Haythornthwaite, C. (2002). Strong, weak, and latent ties and the impact of new media. *The Information Society: An International Journal, 18*(5), 385–401.
Haythornthwaite, C. (2005). Social networks and internet connectivity effects. *Information, Communication & Society, 8*(2), 125–147.
Hechter, M., Opp, K.-D., & Wippler, R. (Eds.). (1990). *Social institutions. Their emergence, maintenance, and effects*. New York: Walter de Gruyter.
Horstink, T. (2011). *The effects of social networks on group moral reasoning in the Royal Netherlands Army*, Masterthesis, Communication studies, Universiteit Twente.
Jalava, J. (2003). From norms to trust: The luhmannian connections between trust and system. *European Journal of Social Theory, 6*, 173–190.
Junge, M. (2001). Zygmunt Bauman's poisoned gift of morality. *British Journal of Sociology, 52*(1), 105–119.
Leydesdorff, L. (2014). Advances in science visualization: Social networks, semantic maps, and discursive knowledge. In B. Cronin & C. Sugimoto (Eds.), *Beyond bibliometrics: Harnessing multidimensional indicators of scholarly impact*. Cambridge, MA: MIT Press.
Luhmann, N. (1993). The code of the moral. *Cardozo Law Review, 14*(3–4), 995–1009.
Luhmann, N. (1995). *Social systems*. Stanford: Stanford University Press.
Luhmann, N. (1996). The sociology of the moral and ethics. *International Sociology, 11*(1), 27–36.
Luhmann, N. (2008a). *Die Moral der Gesellschaft*. Frankfurt am Main: Suhrkamp.
Luhmann, N. (2008b). Are there still indispensable norms in our society? *Soziale Systeme, 14*(1), 18–37.
McFarlane, C. (2013). Relational sociology, theoretical inhumanism, and the problem of the nonhuman. In C. Powell & F. Dépelteau (Eds.), *Relational sociology. Ontological and theoretical issues* (pp. 45–66). New York: Palgrave Macmillan.
Mead, G. (1986). *Beyond entitlement. The social obligations of citizenship*. New York: The Free Press.
Merton, R. K. (1938). Social structure and anomie. *American Sociological Review, 3*(5), 672–682.
Moreh, J. (1986). Morality and welfare. *Theory and Decision, 21*, 209–230.

Pestoff, V. (2009). *A democratic architecture for the welfare state*. London: Routledge.

Pestoff, V. (2015). Co-production as social innovation in public services. In P. Donati & L. Martignani (Eds.), *Towards a new local welfare. Best practices and networks of social inclusion*. Bologna: Bononia University Press.

Pizzorno, A. (1966). Introduzione allo studio della partecipazione politica. *Quaderni di Sociologia, XV*(3–4), 235–287.

Porpora, D. (1987). *The concept of social structure*. New York: Greenwood Press.

Prodi, R., et al. (2002). La mia visione dell'Europa. In C. D'Adda (Ed.), *Per l'economia italiana. Scritti in onore di Nino Andreatta*. Bologna: il Mulino.

Reader, S. (2007). The other side of agency. *Philosophy, 82*, 579–604.

Schrank, A., & Whitford, J. (2011). The anatomy of network failure. *Sociological Theory, 29*(3), 152–177.

Smelser, N. J. (1963). *Theory of collective behavior*. New York: The Free Press of Glencoe.

Stetsenko, A., & Arievitch, I. M. (2004). The self in cultural-historical activity theory. *Theory and Psychology, 14*(4), 475–503.

Teubner, G. (2011). A constitutional moment. The logics of "hitting the bottom". In P. Kjaer, G. Teubner, & A. Febbrajo (Eds.), *The financial crisis in constitutional perspective: The dark side of functional differentiation* (pp. 3–42). Oxford: Hart.

Vidal, I. (2015). The role of third sector in local welfare. In P. Donati & L. Martignani (Eds.), *Towards a new local welfare. Best practices and networks of social inclusion*. Bologna: Bononia University Press.

Zijderveld, A. (1986). The ethos of the welfare state. *International Sociology, 1*(4), 443–457.

Chapter 11
Collective Practices and Norms

Tony Lawson

Social positioning is an essential and central feature in the production and reproduction of social reality. This is a thesis I have explored and defended in various previous papers. Specifically I have argued that through social positioning: (a) human beings are incorporated as components of (participants in) communities (Lawson 1997, 2003, 2012a, 2015c); (b) artefacts are harnessed as functional components of various sorts of social systems (Lawson 2012a, 2014, 2015c); and (c) whole communities are incorporated as functional components of the wider society (Lawson 2015a, b). Here I explore the seemingly less intuitive idea that practices too can be, and are, so positioned.

Society, currently, is undergoing particularly significant structural transformation. This is a view widely expressed. Thus a premise underpinning Margaret Archer's (2016) account of social morphogenesis is that the latter "is intensifying in late Modernity, meaning that it is currently transforming the contours of social stratification, altering the operative principles of all major social institutions, and impacting negatively upon societal integration" (Archer 2016).

Against the backdrop of this assessment by Archer and others, my question is: given the potential for, and ongoing experience of, turbulence that exists in the world, not least in the operative principles of various social institutions, how does relative fixity in institutional structure and practice survive as much as it does.[1] For

[1] I do not here explore the issue of why individuals seek stability and indeed routine as much as they do (an issue I have studied elsewhere, for example Lawson (2015d), though see footnote 9 below), but rather how it is achieved, or anyway arises, in conditions of turbulent change.

T. Lawson (✉)
Faculty of Economics, University of Cambridge, Cambridge, UK
e-mail: tony.lawson@econ.cam.ac.uk

M.S. Archer (eds.), *Morphogenesis and the Crisis of Normativity*,
Social Morphogenesis, DOI 10.1007/978-3-319-28439-2_11

against any intensification of morphogenesis and the seeming fragility of social life there remains a significant degree of structural stability in the social world, even in domains where change would appear to be beneficial to most if not all concerned (see below).

Of course, this chapter is in a book concerned primarily with morphogenesis, rather than morphostasis, which is my emphasis here. But little if anything in the social world is uniform, not least processes of rapid change; and change, at whatever speed, always involves elements of continuity (just as continuity always involves change). By investigating not just where, but how, relative fixity can remain even through processes of intense morphogenesis, we can be better understood the latter's possibilities and limits (on all this see also Lawson 1997; Archer 2015; Porpora 2015). This is the thinking motivating the focus I have taken in the context of a book on morphogenesis. The current chapter thus continues a project in fact initiated by Doug Porpora (2015)[2], also foregrounded by Andrea Maccarini (2015)[3], and explored somewhat further by Maccarini (2016).[4]

A central thesis I shall be exploring is that one very important reason that relative fixity can and does persist is that social reality is constituted to a significant degree by social positions, where these can work to bring stability to occupants. Previously I have explored the role of social positioning in the creation and (re)distribution of power. Here I want to look at it its contribution to maintaining social stability through facilitating the continuity of occupants *qua* position occupants. In doing so I will be examining the idea that practices too can be said to be positioned, with positioned practices interpreted as collective practices containing/carrying norms. It is the latter, in particular, that underpin those features of societal stability we continue to observe.

In order to indicate that and how aspects at least of positioned practices can be highly resilient even in the face of significant surrounding turbulence I focus on an example where fundamental changes in response to the kinds of societal upheavals that are underway might have been expected to be especially significant and yet are almost non-existent. The case I have in mind is that of the continually reproduced

[2] And indeed my strategy is similar to that of Porpora (2015) in that I focus on factors that underpin relative stasis in situations "where we would expect change – or at least more change than observed" (Porpora 2015: 186).

[3] Thus after setting out his account of the emergence of morphogenetic environments, in his conclusion Maccarini suggests one of the central remaining tasks is to address the following questions: "What normative processes are still working, and what personal strategies are successful in the context of the areas and boundaries marking the structural and cultural landscape of the new world? In other words, how 'unbound' is 'unbound morphogenesis' going to be from normativity itself, its prompts and its restraints?" (Maccarini 2015: 179). On the idea of Morphogenesis unbound (or not) see also Emmanuel Lazega (2014).

[4] Maccarini (2016) raises the possibility that in scenarios of intensifying morphogenesis/morphostasis survives in situations of that he terms 'enclaves' and 'vortexes'. Perhaps the example used in the current paper is an example of an enclave.

(mathematical modelling) practices of modern economics. I think these practices do, as much any example I can think of, indicate the sort of staying power that can be achieved through the social positioning of practices.

Social Positioning

So what is social positioning? I mean by it any process wherein individuals or objects, etc. are harnessed to serve as components of wider social totalities. In the case of the positioning of human beings, the latter are constituted as components of communities (or sub-communities). In this process a status is allocated to an individual, say of university lecturer, judge or traffic warden, whereby the individual gains access to certain sets of positional rights and obligations, and thereby gets to serve a certain function in some community.

Other positions have artefacts as their occupants. Thus very specific bits of metal and paper become occupants of the social position cash, pieces of wood can be positioned as doors, or panes of glass as windows, and so forth. In being so positioned any object gains the identity of cash or a door or a window, etc., and thereby one [or more] of its causal properties becomes its [set of] system function[s] (see e.g., Lawson 2012a, 2013a).

Even whole communities can be positioned. In this way organised groups can become constituted as, for example, business partnerships, or as corporations (see Lawson 2015a, b). It is as positioned communities, I suggest, that we must understand the nature of all businesses, trade unions, local councils, football teams, and other forms of organised groupings of human individuals.

Positioning and Relative Fixity

Previously I have, as I say, drawn attention to the way that positioning affects the distribution of power (the matching sets of positioned rights and obligations, see e.g., Lawson 2012a, 2015c); that is I have focussed upon the social relational aspect. In the present paper I want instead to draw attention to the manner in which positioning serves to bestow a degree of permanence on the position occupants *qua* position occupants.

It is a familiar enough insight that any aspect of social structure can be only relatively enduring at best, and is always liable to change. For all social structure exists as a feature of a human-practice-dependent transformative process; this is its mode of being. Think of the structure of a language such as English. This is a (typically unacknowledged) feature of all our numerous speech acts in English, and the reproduction/transformation of the language structure is the (typically unrecognised) outcome of the sum total of all speech acts in the language.

But not all features of social reality are reproduced/transformed in the same way, with the result that some features are more stable than others. Here I want to draw attention in particular to an interesting feature of positioned items. Position occupancy, or the attachment to an individual of a status that goes with acceptance of being positioned in a specific way, lasts until an individual formally is removed, or exits, from the position. Whilst many aspects of social structure exist only through being continually actively reproduced through practice, positional occupancy, once achieved, persists rather more passively until a formal exiting takes place (assuming the position itself is continually reproduced).

Consider positions occupied by human beings. Once an individual is admitted to the position of, say, a partner in marriage, a member of parliament, a worker in company, a member of the board of directors of company X, the individual retains the position occupancy until he or she formally gets a divorce, retires or loses an election, is a sacked, or resigns. Thus, for example, if in the UK a married couple decide to go their separate ways and the two individuals never even see each other thereafter, they may well (i.e., unless they act positively to actively change things) remain married until one of the couple dies.

Artefacts of course tend to be positioned physically. Thus, they remain in place until they (e.g., windows, doors, curtains, tables, televisions, wedding rings, cash in the form of notes and coins) are physically removed/replaced or they materially collapse or decay, etc. The same sort of relative fixity tends to apply to communities positioned as schools, churches, universities, football clubs and (other) businesses, etc., at least until they fail.

In the case of positioning of human beings the positioned occupants can become so attached to their positions and positional identities that they develop personal identities to match. Thus some individuals may be recognised even after retirement as (having once been positioned as) teachers, police officers, taxi drivers, etc.

If positioning adds an extra degree of stability to positioned individuals and things *qua* positioned individuals and things, I now want to argue that this whole analysis carries over to practices, and that when so carried over serves to explain why so much continuity and stability can be observed in the midst of developments of the sort noted by Archer. Let me elaborate my notion of positioned practices.

Collective Practices

A central category here is that of *collective practice*. To be a *practice* I take it is to be a way of proceeding or going on that is actually pursued or followed. Here the emphasis is on both a *way* of proceeding as well as on the fact of it actually being followed. If I am engaged in the activity of eating an apple or running for a train, such activities may not yet be practices. If I regularly peel an apple before eating it, this may constitute a practice, a way of eating the apple, or at least for preparing it for eating.

What though is a *collective* practice? Let me quickly stress that I do *not* intend the term to express something that will somehow be carried through other than by individuals (or groups of individuals). It is collective *not* in relation to who, or to the unit that, performs it, but in that within the community it is an *accepted* or done way for an individual or a group to proceed to reach a particular end in a given context. As such it a practice that in effect has the status of being accepted as legitimate for the circumstances within the community.

Let me also emphasise that the notion of acceptance involved here does *not* mean necessarily agreed with or liked particularly by all community members in all its aspects. Nor even need an accepted way of proceeding be universally adhered to. Rather a collective practice is an accepted practice in the sense of being recognised or acknowledged as a currently done way within a specific community. Particular individuals may actually very much dislike aspects of queuing, or paying certain taxes, or even following practices that derive from the fact of private property. Nevertheless, to get by in a particular community, individuals generally adhere to relevant collective practices in order to participate at all.

So acceptance is essentially a form of collective or community recognition (in contrast to the more evaluative notion of individual acceptance that I consider elsewhere – Lawson 2012a). The idea of individual practices being accepted in the relevant sense is in effect, as I say, a status. A collective practice carries, and rests upon, community-wide recognition, and serves in turn to signal a way of proceeding as being a done way of proceeding within a community.

Examples of collective practices so understood for, say, the modern UK are (ways of) motorway driving, eating in public restaurants, attending church services of a specific denomination, holding seminars, shopping, queuing at food stands, and so on. They are sets of ways of doing these things that are considered to be community-accepted.

A collective practice then, being an accepted way of proceeding within a community, is way of proceeding with which each community participant typically complies recognising that this is in effect a condition of community participation.

Collective Practice as Positioned Practice

I have already noted that a collective practice is a practice that in effect carries the status of being accepted in a particular sense within a particular community. In this it is accepted as being proper or legitimate in some way. But this is just another way of saying that a various individual practices have been socially positioned; they have in this case been positioned as (versions of) a specific collective practice.

Being so positioned or accepted as 'done' ways, collective practices are of course copied or taken up by newcomers wishing to be proficient and accepted as viable community participants. In this manner the collective practices are replicated. There is more to be said on this matter, but I will return to this issue in due course.

Just as categories such as university lecturer, prisoner, or Queen are best used to designate both a position and an occupant, I suggest that categories like motorway driving, or restaurant eating behaviour are best used to designate both positions for an occupant and practices.

With specific names applied to specific positions for practices, I am also suggesting that the term collective practice stands to a community much in the way that university officer stands to the university, or a civil servant does to the civil service. It is a generalist term for any occupant of a position for practices within the relevant community.

Further, because a collective practice is an actual material practice it will always occur in a context. The space in which it occurs can be referred to as the collective practice *domain*. Typically it will relate to a sub community (e.g., of motorway drivers, diners in a restaurant, travellers on a plane or train) of a wider community (e.g., the UK) and so the domain of a collective practice will coincide perhaps with the boundaries of the specific sub-community. Thus, UK motorways will be the domain of the collective practice of motorway driving (in the UK).

Variability and Commonality, Relative Permanence, and Norms

Clearly if (certain ways of) motorway driving in the modern UK, or eating in restaurants, or queuing for food at, say, a rock concert, are positioned practices, that is, each is a specific form or type of collective practice for a determinate domain, numerous versions or manifestations of each type of collective practice will exist even in a given domain; each practice position (as with positions for humans, artefacts and communities) has numerous occupants. Thus, there will be many different examples of motorway driving that will be recognised as legitimate (as positioned), i.e., as ways of proceeding that are included within the practice position motorway driving, as carrying that relevant status (of a specific collective practice).

At the same time individuals can be involved in activities that might be loosely described as doing some X without their partaking in the collective practice X. Thus, an individual on the motorway in the modern UK who overtakes on the inside lane, fails to signal before manoeuvring, drives within inches of a car in front, repeatedly flashing headlights or using the car horn, under the influence perhaps of a large quantity of alcohol, would be engaged in an individual practice that is motorway based and oriented to completing a journey, but which would not constitute a collective practice, even if loosely describable as motorway driving.

So the emergence of a specific collective practice is consistent with some but not all variety at the level of individual practices in a domain. Making sense of this is where the notion of a *norm* enters the picture. A norm is any component or aspect of a collective practice that is (*ceteris paribus*) compulsory, that (normally[5])

[5]Individual practices may deviate from norms either unintentionally through error or intentionally if the perpetrator does not care about being found out or (more typically) believes he or she will not be. Examples of the latter in the modern UK would presumably include parking illegally after traffic wardens are thought to go off work, or, when it is dark or it is supposed that no one is looking who cares, not picking up dog (or any other kind of) litter, or cycling the wrong way up one-way

ought not to be deviated from. Thus in the modern UK this would include such aspects of the collective practice of driving on public roads as keeping to the left side of the lane, overtaking on the right, stopping at red traffic rights, and so on. It is any departure from the norm components of collective practices that is regarded as deviant behaviour.

So interpreted, a norm might be reformulated as a segment or an aspect of a collective practice that carries within itself (if typically implicitly) an obligation. But understood in this manner a norm remains a material component of a collective practice. And importantly, a norm can exist implicitly without notions of obligations being linguistically articulated.

That the latter is so is something I regard as a strength, certainly a requirement, of the conception. For a criterion of adequacy of any framework of interpretation, I take it, is that it can accommodate the fact that social structure serving to facilitate co-ordinated human interaction will have been in place prior to the emergence of language. If the emergence of language outside of a pre-existing community seems unlikely, so does the emergence of pre-linguistic community in the absence of (simultaneously emerging) organising structure. And collective practices, I am suggesting, are the most basic and elemental forms of organising structure, serving everywhere to help coordinate community interaction.

Of course, if accepted/positioned practices do indeed provide the basic structure to human interactions, there is, as I say, the possibility in linguistic communities for the primary structuring components of these practices to be analytically unpacked as implicit rights and obligations. And once analytically unpacked, rights and obligations can be assessed and manipulated etc. But the fact that this is so does not mean that the collective practice cannot function in the absence of this analytical activity. Some representations of collective practices including their norms must always be held by competent community participants of course. But all that is ultimately required is some awareness of their being 'done' or accepted (in the sense of reputedly adhered to) ways of proceeding in specific contexts, and some notion (perhaps determined just by following others) of at least one way of acting that is accepted as conforming in the current context.[6]

---

streets, or walking on Cambridge College lawns, etc.. Notice, in such examples there is no warrant for the conclusion that a norm is anything other than a feature of practice.

[6]More formally, perhaps, a component or feature of a collective practice constitutes a norm if within the relevant community most participants (or at least a significant proportion) have beliefs and/or judgements and/or expectations and/or attitudes, and so forth, that entail/presuppose that the component of the practice in question will be typically adhered to by most (at least a significant proportion of) participants, and *for that reason* at least (if amongst others) should be adhered to by each individual participant. Clearly the notion of the norm developed here (as a component of a collective practice) conflicts (despite many commonalities) with that both of Colin Wight (2016) who prefers to interpret norms as specific kinds of ideas, and Doug Porpora (2016) who mostly restricts the term norm to mean 'regulative rule'.

This is not to deny that the viability of any collective practice (certainly in the modern world) will depend on the participation of more than those who directly adhere to the given accepted way of proceeding by individually acting in accordance with it. It will depend also on the participation of others who act in connected ways that facilitate, presuppose or otherwise maintain the accepted practice, including avoiding intentionally impeding the actions of those more directly participating. But it is not difficult to imagine a set of (perhaps relatively simple and basic) mutually coherent collective practices emerging via a kind of evolutionary process even in pre-linguistic communities.

To repeat, it is clearly warranted that where a set of ways of proceeding are constituted as examples of a collective practice, as community-accepted ways of proceeding, this involves the participation of effectively all members of the community. For the most basic point or function of collective practices *qua* collective practices is the coordination of community life. They are an essential part of the organising structure of all totalities that are communities, serving to facilitate the coordination of the separate activities and goals of individual participants. The organising structure as such can work in this way only in so far as there is fairly generalised adherence to the community-accepted ways of proceeding. So collective practices in being constituted as ways in which things are in fact done in a community in specific contexts are by that token also normative in nature. In their signalling how things *are* done, they simultaneously signal to would-be community participants how things *should be* done. As I say, this is where norms enter the picture.

But significantly, or so I am suggesting, norms or implicit obligations are merely particular features of collective practices carried by individual instances; for any given occasion of participating in a collective practice involves much more than the adhering to norms. For example, participating in the collective practice of motorway driving in, say, the UK involves much more than driving on the left.

It is precisely because the collective practice is a positioned practice that its normative component gets carried forward over time. For, as with other forms of position occupancy, positioned practices stay in place until removed. Once particular ways of proceeding are accepted as the 'done' ways, they remain the 'done' ways until they lose the status of being the done ways. They remain positioned in this sense until they are formally removed from the position. In particular it is the obligatory aspects or norms that, being positioned objects, tend to have durability.

Social reproduction of collective practices, then, involves several aspects. In any give domain where a structure of coordination is required for human interaction there will tend to be collective practices in play. These will be manifest in various ways. However certain components, those corresponding to positioned norms will normally not be deviated from. Individuals whose practices in part do diverge from accepted norms will indeed find that their actions tend to be met at the very least by derision, disdain, resistance or opposition on some level. Once positioned then collective practices contain parts – aspects that indeed constitute individual practices as collective practices – that have a degree of durability.

I will need to say more in due course about how norms in particular are replicated. But before I do so let me indicate how the category of rules fits with the picture. The point I would make here is that rules are as much the (emergent) products of already emergent collective practices as they are constitutive of components of the latter.

Rules

In linguistic communities, of course, representations of norms can always (though they need not) be codified. It is such codes that are most usefully categorised as rules. As such, rules can be interpreted as expressions of the content of norms under their purely indicative aspect. They are thus stipulations of rights and more particularly obligations interpreted as generalised procedures bearing on forms of practice.

Rules can always be formulated along the lines of: In C, if X then Y. Here C is the relevant community or context, X is type of activity (for which there is a collective practice) and Y is a feature that is accepted as a norm or obligatory component for anyone participating in the relevant collective practice. For example, if in the relevant community C an individual wishes to drive on motorways (engage in the collective practice of motorway driving), participate competently in a particular event such as a funeral, or dine at high table in a particular Cambridge College, all being instances of X, then the content of some Y, such as drive on the left, etc., wear black or a tie, indicates an essential component of any accepted way of doing it.

I might acknowledge at this point that I am not wishing to suggest that rules are always *a posteriori* emergent features of spontaneously evolving collective practices. Clearly, in linguistic communities rules may equally be (and of course are regularly) introduced in an a priori fashion via a decision or declaration by a relevant body or subgrouping of the community and designed to modify, or even facilitate, new forms of collective practices or coordination, or to transform the manner in which forms of coordination have previously been achieved, etc.

But either way a rule is an expression or formulation of a normative aspect of a collective practice, whether as an emergent representation or by design. Thus, on this understanding, a rule is something that may be broken, or conformed to without acknowledgement, or misinterpreted, etc., and so is clearly ontologically distinct from the individual practices that actually occur.

Fundamentally, then, I am suggesting that collective practices can operate without the explicit articulation of accounts of rules, rights and obligations, and such like. Social reality, so conceived, is essentially practical, so that all problems of interpretation, conflicts of co-ordination, and other mysteries of human interaction, can ultimately be best resolved in practice.

Central and essential to it all are (often implicit) processes of (i.e., that can be described as) social positioning, and these impart to social life a degree of stability whatever else is going on.

Intra-community Emergent Collective Practices

If the positioning of practices serves to facilitate stability in the midst of flux, the most interesting cases to consider at this juncture are *not* those collective/positioned practices that are constituted in relation to other collective/positioned practices – say those of teachers to those of students, or of employers to employees, or landlords/ladies to tenants, etc. Rather, the more interesting collective practices in my view are those that *intra*-relate participants of the same position or community, i.e., that apply to all community members. The former *inter*-relational practices are less interesting only because they are well-researched and understood, and transformations in relevant social structures, including those bearing on position occupancy and associated positional practices, tend to come down to the explicit display of relative power.

The intra-community situation, in contrast, is I think less often recognised let alone systematically addressed. I contend that just about all human interaction in public spaces involves forms of collective practice, though I suspect too that such a suggestion may require some elaboration and defending. But if I am right, it is in this domain that questions of relative transience versus relative stability of collective practices are especially significant, least understood, and warranting systematic analysis. Before embarking on the latter, though, let me indicate why I suppose that intra-community collective practices do proliferate.

Think of the commonplace activity of walking down a street in any community, for example, in the modern UK. Perhaps this is a realm of human activity that *prima facie* promises not to be structured by the prevalence of collective practices. However, a little reflection reveals that even here there are restrictions on how one may go about things; each individual finds her- or himself to be subject to obligations to conform in so many ways. An individual would likely soon be in trouble if he or she wore no clothes (or perhaps clothes regarded as outrageous), used 'bad language', was especially noisy, walked to the front of queues, stood overly close to others, expressed moral or political generalisations regarded as offensive or disgraceful, discarded quantities of litter in the roadway, walked into people, and so forth.

But what follows for the perpetrators of such deviant forms of behaviour? What sort of trouble would someone be in if they did not participate appropriately?

Community participants by and large refrain from the forms of activities noted above, knowing that a failure to do so would likely be met by one or more of a variety of sanctions including ridicule, contempt, ostracism, aggression, social exclusion, and so on. Of course, what is acceptable in one community or sub-community may not be in another and vice versa. But we all live in communities where the rights of community participation are accompanied by obligations that apply to all, or most of, its members. These are always numerous, often non-formalised, yet widely understood and generally adhered to, and met with forms of sanction by other community members if/where not followed.

Who Has Power Over Whom in Such Cases and, When Exercised, What Is the Intentional Content?

To be a community participant is to enjoy the rights of participation as well as the obligations that go with it. Each participant expects all other participants to conform to the obligations implicit in accepted collective practices, and has the right to object to, display a form of negative sanction or disapproval towards, and so undermine, individual behaviour interpreted as deviant (relative to those collective practices). So the intentional content of any exercise of that power is in essence (albeit a concrete or particular version of) the community requirement to 'conform to the currently accepted collective practice(s)'. With (or to the extent that) social being (is) everywhere structured though accepted collective practices, social being is continuously subject to the wielding of social-systemic power by all of us over each other.

Put differently, where collective practices exist each participant is typically expected to conform and is accountable to all others if found to be deviating. That is, community participation involves the implicit granting by the community as a whole to each individual of a right to participate, whereupon the individual simultaneously accepts: (1) the obligation to do so in accordance with accepted or collective practices; and thereby (2) to be accountable to each and all others if found deviating. Notice that this aspect of accountability is not a feature that supplants the co-ordinating capacity of norms. Instead, it is an element of the process whereby norms work as vital components of co-ordinated community interaction.[7]

I repeat, though, that to participate in a community, to accept the relevant obligations and a degree of accountability, does not mean at all that every participant is particularly enamoured by the components of collective practices positioned as norms. Many such norms are even fairly easily revealed to be harmful of human flourishing. I think the norm that is my own focus below is an example, namely the insistence on methods of mathematical modelling that is a positioned feature of modern academic research practice in economics. More obvious examples to be

[7]There does appear to be a difference between presuppositions of the view expressed here and the view explicitly articulated by Archer (2016). A feature of my position is that compliance with community collective practices is a moral concern, that if we accept to participate in a particular community, then compliance with that community's collective practices is morally good *ceteris paribus* (or better transfactually), whatever the process whereby the practice comes into being (including through declaration by some community authority) and irrespective of how much we might seek to transform it. As such, I believe contra Archer, that regulations as with all other coordinating features of social structure, exert a causal force that is always in part a moral force, however weak may be the moral influence in certain contexts. This is not to say that we do not allow other considerations to dominate when necessary (or when we can get away with it and suppose no harm is done) in deciding how actually to act. I am thus not sure I go along with the thesis of anormativity that Archer advances. Indeed, I elsewhere argue the thesis that all action in human communities is, when and where affecting others, inevitably moral action (see Lawson 2015e).

found in the world include genital mutilation, routine reliance on guns and other weapons, cultures of corruption, and so on. The point, however, if to repeat, is that intra-community collective practices can, and very often do, consist in positioned components that, if always co-ordinating of human interaction, are from a broader perspective seen as obstacles to human flourishing.

Transforming Collective Practices by Adjusting the Norm Content

The interesting set of questions then, given my concerns as set out initially and immediately above, relate to how intra-community collective practices come into being and are sustained or overthrown. Or rather, because each case will no doubt have its own peculiarities, the question is really whether it is it possible to develop a realistic framework which allows these sorts of issues to be systematised.

Once more I think it appropriate to narrow down and focus on a subcase, and specifically on those (widespread, and perhaps the most typical) situations where the norms involved are not imposed or managed by some sub-group with the authority to do so, but emerge seemingly spontaneously. Thus, in the following I will not be concerned with cases involving authoritative declarations. Examples of the latter are widespread of course. Thus the relevant authorities of London underground have put in place signs that declare that on escalators commuters should 'stand on the right'. Though of interest such processes in themselves are not difficult to analyse, and indeed have been so extensively (see for example Searle 2010). My focus is on situations where no explicit declaration of any kind appears to be involved.

Given the apparent informality of the sorts of processes I have in mind, involving, as they do, the emergence of social order in the apparent absence of design, and given, too, that numerous emergent norms are frequently found to be obstacles to human flourishing, it is conceivable that mechanisms of this sort of spontaneous emergence, change and development are broadly Darwinian in nature. That is, given that the focus here is on features that are successful (in the sense of persisting) despite being (or even when they can be seen to be) harmful, an evolutionary explanatory framework seems *prima facie* particularly promising. For Darwinian evolution is not in essence a story of progress but one of 'survival' or *relative* propagation of certain members of (or traits within) a population without any necessary presupposition or implication as to the worth or standard of performance of that which happens to turn out to survive or propagate, etc.

If in fact an evolutionary framework of sorts is broadly appropriate here for systematizing the issues before us, then the evolutionary story is seemingly one in which individual practices in effect (albeit of course always through the agency of human participants in a community) compete to be selected first as occupants of a relevant practice position and second as aspects of accepted practices that constitute norms; the objective is for aspects of behaviour to become components of a collective practice, and perhaps obligatory components. I do believe such a framework to be quite relevant. Let me now briefly elaborate how.

The PVRS Model

By evolutionary in a Darwinian sense I mean first and foremost a process that can be described as descent with modification. Any feature or thing that in significant part reproduces, in the sense of being maintained though replication, through the making of new copies of its type, albeit sporadically incorporating 'mutations' or modifications in features along the way, can be said to evolve.

Of course the Darwinian natural-selection story is a specific case of a particular evolutionary conception that posits a population (P), with variety under some of its aspects (V), a process of copying or replicating certain features in the population (R), and a process of environmental selection amongst the aspects that vary (S). Notice that for this PVRS model to express a strictly 'natural selection' process of a Darwinian sort, the V and S mechanisms must be wholly, or at least largely, independent.

With any such PVRS model there will be features that can be identified as *interactors* and *replicators*. An interactor, following Hull (1981), is a feature that actually interacts with the environment. A replicator, following Dawkins (1976, 1978), is an entity that passes on its structure by replication. Usually the interactor and replicator will be different.

Clearly, a replicator and the process of replication are in themselves insufficient, typically, for natural selection to occur. Thus, if a mechanism of gene replication is essential for the reproduction of, say, finches with relatively large beaks, this is insufficient to explain the rise to prominence of finches with that trait in certain observed (isolated) locations (see Weiner 1994; Lawson 2003). The interaction of the whole organism with its environment (under conditions where larger beaks are more apt to emergent conditions than smaller ones) is an essential feature of the causal evolutionary process.

I repeat that for the account to be one of Darwinian natural selection there must be a degree of independence between the process whereby the variety of traits is produced (V) and the manner in which the environmental mechanism doing the selecting has come about (S). Such independence is essential if the model is to explain the appearance of order or 'fit' in the absence of design. Otherwise there is nothing that necessarily distinguishes the explanatory schema from any other as found in modern social theory including economics. Specifically, without independence it can be argued that either trait or environment is produced in order to match the other, so that the puzzle of order in the absence of design, the puzzle that Darwin helped solve, is not, after all, addressed.

Notice further that evolutionary change in line with natural selection can come about over a period of time because either (a) a new trait emerges within a relevant population, one that is found to be favoured by the existing environment, or (b) the environment shifts in a way such as to favour a trait that has long been in existence (or through a combination of these two types of development). In each such scenario, however, the *possibilities* turn on the processes generating the traits or variety, and the contribution of the environment lies in its 'selecting' amongst the particular set of features in evidence.

Back to Collective Practices

So how do I suppose this framework fits with the discussion of norms and collective practices, above? I am suggesting, of course, that the obvious candidates for interactors, the features that interact with their environment, are individual practices in a given domain; the environment is the sum total of all competing and relating practices in the community operative in the domain in question; and the sort of thing or aspect that might be interpreted as a social replicator, the entity that passes on its structure in replication, is that feature of the collective practice that I am calling a norm.

So competition, at least concerning practices, is, as already noted, really competition to achieve positioning. Two forms of change can be distinguished in this regard. The first is where new traits or features or modifications emerge amongst the individual practices that are regarded as accepted, that come to be included amongst, or as comprise aspects of, collective practices. The second is where a set of features or segments of certain collective practices become not merely allowed or accepted, but newly interpreted as obligatory, as constituting norms. Thus, there may be a struggle initially for practices of electronic transfer to be counted amongst the forms of legitimate banking; to be considered an accepted way of proceeding for cancelling debts. But it seems likely that in the near future for at least certain forms of monetary transfer, electronic banking will be the norm. Similarly, just as electronic devices in the form of telephones were originally strongly resisted, so electronic forms of non-face-to-face communication eventually became not merely accepted but effectively the norm.

Of course every occupant of a practice position, though unique in many ways, will take on characteristics of existing occupants of any given position, even if the emergence of novel norms means a more significant transformation.

Just as for example, a new university lecturer assumes obligations borne by existing university lecturers, so a new variety of collective practice will carry existing norms. Norms of polite interaction for example are usually preserved within the extension of communication practices to include novel electronic forms. Where the norms themselves are transformed (novel obligations are included or others absented) then the situation will be more complex depending on the context.

This then, or so I am proposing, is the basis of a (and I suspect the most basic) process of social evolution. It concerns the evolution of collective practices. A feature of it all is a process of replication. As in biological replication the social process serves to make a copy of features that already exist. In the biological process of DNA replication, each of the two strands of the double helix acts as a template for the formation of a new DNA molecule. Somewhat in parallel, in social replication, or so I am suggesting, existing occupants of any given position act in effect as templates for new occupants. In the case of individual practices, specifically, one or more versions of a particular collective practice will serve as templates in the formation of new versions of the collective practice.[8]

A collective practice such as driving on the motorway or eating in a restaurant in the UK, does of course contain within itself numerous rights and obligations (in the former case driving on the left, keeping to a certain speed, overtaking in a certain way, etc.). The latter come packed within collective practices. Thus the relation of rights and obligations to collective practices, is somewhat similar that of DNA to a chromosome, with any specific stretch of practice-bearing obligation being equivalent to the gene or basic unit of DNA.

In any case, with social change of the type in question here, any novel individual practice that is coherent with existing norms may be regarded as a novel form of the prevailing collective practice, whilst significant change occurs with a transformation in the features that are regarded as norms of the collective practice.

So to sum up, I am proposing that the issues of concern here can be systematised by way of employing an evolutionary framework. According to it, the interactors of social life are, or include, the population of individual practices oriented to a given end in an identifiable community context – like driving on a UK motorway, eating in a restaurant (or at high table in a Cambridge College), travelling on a train, attending a religious service of some denomination, conducting economic research, and so on. The environment includes all the community practices with which the individual practices interact.

Transformation can take one or other (or both) of two forms. First there may be a change in the recognised variety of individual practices that are accepted as versions of a particular collective practice in a given domain. Second there may be a change in the features of the collective practice that are considered in effect as obligatory, as essential features of all instances of the collective practice in question. So modifications affecting the range of individual practices that are accepted may occur, just as there may be adjustments regarding features that are selected as dominant, as indicating those aspects that in effect are obligatory. In short, there can be a change in the variety of positioned practices as well in the components that serve as norms.

The variety or range of accepted practices may change due to a number of factors, but when individuals are instructed or trained to drive on motorways, eat in public

[8]In the case of DNA replication, copying occurs at a localized region called the replication fork (a Y shaped structure) where new DNA strands are synthesised by a multi-enzyme complex. In the case of collective practice replication, copying occurs at a localized region I am calling the collective practice *domain* where new versions of the practice are synthesised by appropriately positioned human participants.

or with others, speak a language, they are primarily taught how to follow collective practices comprising a varying number of existing norms.

Clearly, if qualifying for position occupancy takes place in the context of all other community practices then this is the context in which we will find the forces responsible for allowing features of practices into practice positions as well for determining which aspects get to count as norms.

Let me now seek to illustrate these brief remarks and the social evolutionary framework elaborated, by focussing on, and indeed seeking to explain the unreasonable persistence of, certain practices in modern economics.

Modern Economics as a Resistant Positioned/Collective Practice

I started the preceding discussion noting observations that ongoing social developments are everywhere 'transforming the contours of social stratification, altering the operative principles of all major social institutions, and impacting negatively upon societal integration' (Archer 2016). If this is so then prima facie one might have expected the practices of modern economics to have been radically revised in recent times. Most especially, the developments noted might have been expected to generate a challenge to the near exclusive emphasis on methods of mathematical modelling, and so to the hierarchical structure and group cohesion based on it. However, the developments in question have seemingly had no noticeable non-superficial impact on its operative principles, fortunes and internal cohesion whatsoever.

Why might matters have been expected to be otherwise? The first reason is the evolving nature of subject-matter of the discipline, at least at a level of significant concreteness. Of course methods of mathematical modelling carry presuppositions about the nature of social reality. In effect they presupposes closed systems of isolated atoms (see e.g. Lawson 1997, 2003, 2012b, 2013b). This ontology is easily shown to be inconsistent with the real social world in which we live (again see Lawson 1997, 2003, 2012b, 2013b). That said, where developments in the economy are found to be relatively smooth, then such methods, indeed any methods, can, at least retrospectively be shown or made to 'fit' to a degree, irrespective of any associated causal rhetoric.

If, perhaps after suitable data transformation, these sorts of conditions have sometimes been held (however dubiously) to characterise economic development up to about 2007, few have claimed that such a state of affairs has prevailed after this point. Indeed by all accounts in the last 8 years or so the set of aspects of social reality that most observers take to be (and traditionally has been) the object or focus of study in economics, has been undergoing (and continues to experience) significant and often turbulent change. Most graphically, these years have seen developments interpreted almost universally as an economic and/or financial crisis, while major developments in technology and corresponding changes in technological products affect how, where and what sorts of, things are done.

Yet far from all this resulting in a reorientation of the discipline to accommodate ongoing developments, topics like economic crises and the impact of changes in new technology rarely if ever figure on any faculty of economics curriculum even now; nor actually do concrete developments in the economy feature much at all. Rather the discipline sticks only to topics that mathematical modelling methods appear capable of accommodating. The crisis in the economy is essentially ignored.

If we focus instead on the methodological options, then the advances in digital technology over the same period and longer significantly expand the research procedures available to individual economists, bearing for example on ways of using evidential sources and of presenting results, on opportunities to collaborate with researchers in different disciples familiar with alternative approaches, of interdisciplinary work in general, and so on. Yet economics remains a relatively isolated enclave, a community focused more on preserving its mathematical orientation, and supressing alternative methodological approaches. To the extent it relates to other disciplines at all, it is mostly by way of seeking to colonise them, through rendering them (or the study of their subject matter) a branch of mathematical-economic modelling.

If we focus further on the performance of the discipline of economics itself, the latter is found on close inspection actually to be characterised by years of explanatory failure, unrealistic formulations, lack of clear direction, and a general sense of being detached from social reality. Moreover, it is easy enough to show that these failings stem largely from a misplaced emphasis on methods of mathematical modelling (see e.g. Lawson 1997, 2003, 2012b, 2013b). With the recent crisis in the economy, the failings of the discipline itself have now become widely appreciated and acknowledged, even by the British Queen. Indeed, the discipline has received significant admonition for its failures from a very broad spectrum of observers. In such a situation it might have been expected that the opportunities for improving the performance of the discipline that have arisen would grasped, or at least that the prevailing emphasis on methods of mathematical modelling would be seriously questioned. Yet, with very few exceptions, there is little evidence of this happening.

This example, I will shortly argue, does highlight the sort of contribution to relative fixity that embedded norms can make. Of course, one likely would not have expected that if an academic discipline is characterised by localised collective practices, these could carry such methodologically restrictive norms. In other, more successful, sciences, in contrast, research practices are clearly flexibly and continually adapted to the topic and nature of subject matter. If physicists want to seek out a Higgs boson particle in order to test aspects of the standard model of particle physics they build an electron accelerator as at CERN. If others want to explore distant planets they construct telescopes of a relevant sort with the capacity to detect signals, etc., or they construct a craft to go there, or at least to travel to a region where signals can be detected.

In economics, however, whatever the question or context, it is methods of mathematical modelling that are pursued. That is, although an academic discipline might be thought to be quintessentially a community oriented to adapting to all new knowledge and technological developments, the discipline of economics is instead one that strives to maintain its isolated way of being. It continues to focus almost all its resources on a particular project that illustrates well how collective practices with stubborn norms can work to facilitate continuity when all around (including the economy and other university departments) are in the throes of crises and uncertainty. Moreover, in the case of economics, the noted norm or set of norms persists even though it is so easy to demonstrate how adherence to it is the main cause of most of the discipline's (by now widely appreciated) explanatory problems.

I should acknowledge that my claim here that the modern emphasis on mathematical modelling per se is the problem is not something that is accepted/recognised by all observers, including many who refer to themselves as heterodox economists. In fact the most prominent diagnosis of the cause of the discipline's continuing failures puts it down to political-economic ideology; it is all due to neo-liberalism or neoclassical theorising oriented to maintaining the economic-political status quo.

But assessments of this sort are not sustainable (Lawson 2013b). Most economic modellers, in my experience, have not a clue what neo-liberalism is, and more to the point do not care (Lawson 2012b). At the same time it is doubtful that neoclassical theorising has a coherent meaning; certainly there is no neoclassical school (Lawson 2013b). More relevant still, most economists do not research topics that even have any appearance of bearing on the functioning of a capitalist system. In the one area that might be said to be otherwise, namely equilibrium theorising, the formulators of the theory, or at least the more careful ones (e.g., Frank Hahn[9]), openly acknowledge that their models have no relation to the real world at all.

The *only* feature that is common to *all* (or even to more than a small fraction of) the various contributions by (mainstream) economists regarded as serious, proper, worthwhile, scientific, deserving of promotion, or being awarded the Nobel Memorial Prize, etc., is the emphasis on mathematical modelling (see Lawson 2003). This I repeat is an emphasis that is easily shown to be misguided in the context of explaining social reality, given the nature of the latter.

Thus by any account, the emphasis of modern academic economists on mathematical modelling is one that warrants explanation. I suggest that only by seeing the emphasis as arising from a commitment to norms embedded in a collective practice

---

[9]Thus Hahn writes that

> [...] it cannot be denied that there is something scandalous in the spectacle of so many people refining the analyses of economic [equilibrium] states which they give no reason to suppose will ever, or have ever, come about. It probably is also dangerous. Equilibrium economics [...] is easily convertible into an apologia for existing economic arrangements and it is frequently so converted. (1970: 88–9)

Elsewhere, Hahn reveals in rather dramatic fashion what he feels should happen if people contemplate using such models for policy:

> When policy conclusions are drawn from such models, it is time to reach for one's gun. (Hahn 1982: 29)

can we make sense of it all. Of course, to provide a full explanation it is necessary to determine how the relevant set of norms became accepted in the first place and how challenges to its position/status are repelled. So it is to a sketch of these matters that I finally turn.

A Brief Overview of the History of Mathematical Modelling in Economics

Two things, at least, are clear in the history of mathematical modelling: (1) the modern emphasis on mathematical modelling did not arise as soon as attempts to mathematise the discipline started, but rather a long time later; and (2) the eventual positioning successes of the practice had nothing to do with any explanatory successes (which have notably been absent throughout).

The process of seeking to mathematise the subject, to get mathematical modelling methods into the toolbox of accepted practice, was well under way at least 200 years ago when, on observing the success of Newton in uniting heaven and earth with equations, Kant called for a social-scientific Newton. This stimulated much activity not least in France beginning with the Physiocrats.[10]

However, over most of the ensuing history of the discipline not only have most attempts to mathematise been singularly unsuccessful in terms of providing explanatory insight, but the efforts to render mathematical practices acceptable have most frequently been met with hostility and even derision (see Lawson 2003, chapter 10).

This was evident even in France where the project was pursued most actively. In particular, hostility derived from Laplace who, following the death of Lagrange (and on achieving near supremacy in scientific matters in France, especially at the Institut de France's Class of Geometry) set about actively purging any programme of mathematising society from the academy. In addition, Jean Baptiste Say (1767–1832) and the French Liberal school that he in effect founded (a school that was to dominate the field of social study for most of the nineteenth century) took much the same position as Laplace; indeed Say even (if somewhat idiosyncratically) made opposition to the mathematisation of social phenomena a central principle of the school's broader philosophy (see e.g., Ingrao and Israel 1990: 60; Arena 2000; Lawson 2003).

[10]Those French economists who early on accepted the baton and ran with it certainly included members of the Physiocratic 'sect', especially Quesnay (1694–1774); and also Turgot (1727–1781); Dupont de Nemours (1739–1817); Condorcet (1743–1794); Achylle-Nicolas Isnard (1749–1803); Canard (1750–1833); Dupuit (1804–1866); Cournot (1801–1877); and of course Walras (1834–1910). On all this see Lawson (2003, chapter 10) (Of course, the mathematical approaches of these contributors varied in numerous ways. For example Quesnay and the Physiocrats used simple arithmetic mainly aimed at simple accounting, whilst Cournot used the differential calculus that would drive the whole marginalist enterprise. See Nuno Martins (2014), especially chapter 5).

Attempts to get the use of mathematical methods accepted in the discipline lingered on, of course, but they were heavily constrained. Early contributions to the mathematising of economics were restricted to being analogous to successful formulations of the mathematical non-social sciences. The influence of Laplace in particular resulted mainly in a forced concentration on the strictly deterministic approach of mechanics based on methods of infinitesimal calculus. By the nineteenth century this essentially meant adhering to the 'classical reductionist programme' in physics, still applying the deterministic model of mechanics.

In other words, in order to be accepted amongst the variety or range of legitimate collective research practices in the economics academy, approaches to mathematical modelling were in effect treated as a sub-population with its own regulative norm, that of conforming in structure to the determinist methods of mechanics.

Eventually all was to change. But this was not at all because mathematical methods and practices were found to be explanatorily successful or otherwise capable of providing insight. Rather, fortunes were transformed in effect because of changes in the environment, first relating to the way mathematics itself became interpreted, and second in the environment of political practice. Let me very briefly explain.

Interpreting Mathematics

The fortunes of those who would mathematise the discipline of economics changed only in the early years of the twentieth century. At this point, as I say, a transformation took place in the manner that mathematics itself was interpreted. Basically the classical reductionist programme fell into disarray as developments in relativity theory and especially quantum theory caused the image of nature as continuous to be re-examined in particular. A result was that the role of infinitesimal calculus, which had previously been regarded as having almost ubiquitous relevance within physics, came to be re-examined even within that domain.

One result, facilitated by the contributions of David Hilbert in particular, was that mathematics became interpreted as no longer an attempt to apply the physics model, and specifically the mechanics metaphor, but rather as a discipline properly concerned with providing a pool of frameworks for *possible realities*. Mathematics was now viewed *not* as the language of (non-social) nature, abstracted from the study of the latter, but as a practice concerned with formulating systems comprising sets of axioms and their deductive consequences, with these systems in effect taking on a life of their own. The task of finding applications was henceforth regarded as being of secondary importance at best, and not of immediate concern.

This emergence of the axiomatic method removed many of the most severe constraints facing those who endeavoured to get mathematical practices accepted amongst the collective practices of the discipline of economics. For the time being, at least, researchers involved with mathematical projects in economics could postpone the day of interpreting their preferred axioms and assumptions. At this point mathematical modelling practices were included and able to compete amongst the accepted (collective) research practices of the discipline without the need to be formulated in ways that were analogous to the methods of mechanics, etc. Mathematical models indeed were created supposedly without carrying any necessary interpretation.

Consider for example Debreu's eventual (1959) axiomatic treatment of (the existence and uniqueness) of general equilibrium, a contribution that gained its author the Nobel Memorial Prize in economic science. Even today the language and symbolism of Debreu's *Theory of Value* is found in many axiomatic papers. Debreu's contribution rests for its legitimacy precisely on the claim that axioms are not in need of any interpretation. As Debreu expresses these matters himself:

> *Allegiance to rigor dictates the axiomatic form of the analysis where the theory, in the strict sense, is logically entirely disconnected from its interpretations.* In order to bring out fully this disconnectedness, all definitions, all the hypotheses, and the main results of the theory, in the strict sense, are distinguished by italics; moreover, the transition from the informal discussion of interpretations to the formal construction of the theory is often marked by one of the expressions: "in the language of the theory," "for the sake of the theory," "formally." Such a dichotomy reveals all the assumptions and the logical structure of the analysis. It also makes possible immediate extensions of that analysis without modification of the theory by simple reinterpretation of the concepts; [. . .]. (Debreu 1959, p. x, emphasis added)

This development in the interpretation of mathematics moreover fed into an arguably even more significant environmental shift, this time concerning the set of political practices. The latter include both the onset of World War II and most especially the post-war emergence of McCarthyite witch-hunts in the face of the ongoing Cold War. The story is long and detailed. Here I continue to provide but a brief sketch.

The Political Environment

With the decline in the classical reductionist program the project of mathematising economics received its greatest stimulus at this juncture in Austria and Germany, where the new physics, a revised conception of the role of mathematics and a specific emphasis upon axiomatic mathematics, had originated and now flourished. In particular, it was here that von Neumann, Wald, Morgenstern and other mathematicians made their initial contributions. Although approaches such as those of Wald and von Neumann were different in kind, they were later reconciled in the US, where many of the early contributors emigrated under the Nazi threat.

Of course countries that had been more wedded to the classical reductionist programme eventually witnessed significant related developments as well. This included France where attempts to mathematise economics in ways that were analogous to the mechanics model had perhaps been strongest. I have already commented upon the contribution of Debreu. Although Debreu's *Theory of Value* appeared after his move to the US Cowles Commission in the 1950s, Debreu was much influenced by the French Bourbaki 'school', a group of French mathematicians who argued that mathematical systems should be studied as pure structures devoid of any possible interpretations. It was at the École Normale Supérieure in the 1940s that Debreu came into contact with the Bourbaki teaching. And once trained in this maths, but with his interests aroused by economics, Debreu sought a suitable location to pursue an interest in reformulating economics in terms of this mathematics. It is noteworthy that his move to the Cowles Commission coincided with the latter's effective acceptance of Bourbakism.

So with attempts to mathematise economics freed from the burden of having to fit with reality, it is significant that many of the practitioners of this approach ended up being located in the US in the post war period. This is so for two reasons especially. First, it turned out that the US had the resources to dominate the post-world war II international academic scene in economics (as indeed it has done in so many other disciplines). Second, this emphasis on an economics without any necessary interpretation proved to be an attractive proposition in the context of the McCarthyite witch-hunts in the face of the Cold War.

At that time the nature of the output of economics faculties, traditionally the field that attracted those who sought a more humane system than capitalism, became a particularly sensitive matter. In such a context the project of mathematising economics proved to be especially attractive in that it carried scientific pretensions whilst being (especially when carried out in the spirit of the Bourbaki approach) significantly devoid of any necessary substantive, including political, content.

The group most feared or resented by the McCarthyites were the intellectuals (Reinert 2000). The mathematising project with its detached technicist emphasis, often to the exclusion of almost any critical or reflexive orientation, was clearly extremely convenient to those caught up in the situation. This was especially the case not just for insecure or fearful university administrators but also for the funding agencies of US social scientific research (who were especially important in this period – see for example, Coats 1992; Goodwin 1998; Yonay 1998).

It was in this way that the mathematising project (first allowed to compete openly following the change in the way mathematics itself was interpreted) came to dominate the discipline, initially in the US,[11] and eventually worldwide.

[11]Consider Debreu's own observations:

> As the Second World War was drawing near its resolution, economic theory entered a phase of intensive mathematization that profoundly transformed our profession. In several of its main features that phase had no precedent....
>
> While the professional journals in the field of mathematical economics grew at an unsustainably rapid rate, the *American Economic Review* underwent a radical change in identity. In 1940, less than 3 percent of the refereed pages of its 30th volume ventured to include rudimentary mathematical expressions. Fifty years later, nearly 40 percent of the refereed pages of the 80th volume display mathematics of a more elaborate type.
>
> At the same time, the mathematisation of economists proceeded at an even faster pace in the 13 American departments of economics labelled by a recent assessment of research-doctorate programs in the United States (Lyle V. Jones et al. 1982) as "distinguished" or

So it was also in this way that the notion that economics should be pursued mathematically, that proper or accepted economic practice necessitated the construction of mathematical models became in effect a norm of the discipline. Although power and contestation were clearly involved, much of the power-play occurred at the level of the environment of political practices that had a bearing in determining those research practices of economists that were able to survive, in the sense of receiving administrative back-up. With few exceptions only those individuals who accepted the norm of mathematical practices were institutionally supported. In due course, with equally few exceptions, only those whose practices were consistent with the norm were published in journals accepted as 'core'.

I am suggesting, then, that practices concerned with mathematising the discipline had been in play long before the twentieth century, albeit meeting with little explanatory success. These practices initially qualified as collective practices only when severely restricted by the norm of conforming to some model of physics. In the early to middle twentieth century, however, that project's fortunes, in terms of approval rating, started to improve remarkably. This occurred not as a result of any improved explanatory performance relative to that of any competing projects (or even in absolute terms). Rather, it was the climate of its reception that shifted. Fundamental here were changes in the way mathematics became interpreted, allowing a greater variety of mathematical practices amongst the positioned practices of the discipline. Equally fundamental, were changes in the political environment, especially in the US, which led to the mathematical component being not merely accepted but effectively required.

The account clearly does conform to a Darwinian natural-selection version of the evolutionary (PVRS) model in that the conditions responsible for the noted shifts in the environment (S) had little to do with the conditions generating the variety

"strong" according to the scholarly quality of their faculties. Every year the Fellows of the *Econometric Society* (ES) certify new members by election into their international guild, which increased in size from 46 in 1940 to 422 in 1990. For those 13 departments together, the proportion of ES Fellows among professors was less than 1 percent in 1940; it is now close to 50 percent. It equals or exceeds 50 percent for six of them, which were among those assessed as the eight strongest. So mathematized a faculty expects its students to have what it considers to be minimal mathematical proficiency, and knowledge of calculus and linear algebra is required, or forcefully recommended, for admission to all 13 graduate programs.

Several scholarly recognitions lay additional emphasis on the role that mathematical culture is now playing in our profession. Of the 152 members of the economics section of the American Academy of Arts and Sciences, 87 are Fellows of the Econometric Society; and of the 40 members of the economics section of the National Academy of Sciences of the United States, 34 are ES Fellows. From 1969 to 1990, 30 economics Nobel awards were made, and 25 of the laureates are, or were, ES Fellows. Since it was first presented to Paul Samuelson in 1947, the John Bates Clark medal of the *American Economic Association* has been given to 21 economists, of whom 20 are ES Fellows; and of the 26 living past presidents of our association, 13 are ES Fellows. (Debreu 1991: 1–2) of research practices (V) which economists followed. The conditions of variety generation and environmental selection were largely independent.

Of course, if I have suggested how practices of mathematical modelling came to dominate academic economics in the early post war period I have yet to discuss how they have been maintained in a position of dominance since. If the PVRS framework is appropriate, the answer will clearly include features of the environment. I very briefly list some of those that I take to be important.

Environmental Factors of Influence

The first factor of relevance is academic economists themselves. Here those who have been trained in mathematical methods have little incentive to experiment outside the bounds of mathematical modelling. This is the skill set acquired, and it is in terms of this skill set that promotion and other forms of academic success have been achieved.

With the rise of university research assessment exercises the tendencies just noted are simply reinforced. Evaluation committees in economics are made up of mathematical economists who highly rate only papers published in mathematical journals.

In making these observations I am not suggesting a conspiratorial note. Once the norm of mathematical reasoning is adopted, those most amenable to this orientation will themselves in a sense be selected. In addition, of course, various economists sooner or later internalise the norm of doing economics only mathematically. Once this happens, they can find the norm intrinsically motivating; their preferences adapt (Lawson 2015d). Many norms in all branches of society come to be in part "constitutive of the selfhood or identity of individual adherents." (Miller 2001). If internalization promotes reliable compliance, those who internalise it are found to care when someone else violates the norm, even if the violation does not (in any other sense) harm the norm adherents in question.[12]

[12]These issues relate back to the psychological need of individuals (often perhaps unconsciously) to control feelings of anxiety.

Certainly, it is clear that human beings are frequently disposed to engage in routinized forms of conduct even when there are no collective practices in place, and one obvious and common explanation of the noted phenomenon is a human need for, or one that is (or appears to be) satisfied by, a significant degree of continuity, stability and sameness in daily affairs, the avoidance of radical disruption. It would seem that at the level of the unconscious is a basic need for inner security grounding a generalised disposition towards the maintenance of trust in the world and the avoidance of anxiety, a disposition that is in practice fulfilled (or anyway met) through, if amongst other things, the doing of familiar things routinely. It can be argued (Lawson 1997) that the psychological origins of ontological security are to be found in basic anxiety-controlling mechanisms, hierarchically ordered as components of personality. The generation of feelings of trust in others, as the deepest element of the basic security system, depends substantially upon predictable and caring routines established by parental figures when the individual was an infant.

Second, there are the critics of the modern mainstream approach both within and outside of economics. However, there has long been a failure within this group to appreciate that the theories and policies they oppose as unrealistic are so in large part because of the emphasis on mathematical modelling. With the recent economic crisis there has been some (albeit far too little) soul searching within economics, but almost none of it oriented to the emphasis on mathematical modelling (see Lawson 2012a). Indeed, whilst this group is pluralistic in its rhetoric towards non-mathematical treatments, it too very often prioritises mathematical modelling, albeit seeking (always inevitably unrealistic) assumptions that allow conclusions to be drawn that are typically regarded as being somehow more progressive.

Third, there has been a tendency for all branches of social science to isolate themselves from each other and exaggerate the differences in order to shore up institutional power. This has afforded economists the opportunity of ignoring the undoubtedly valuable contributions that have been forthcoming in Sociology and elsewhere.[13] Moreover the belief of economists that mathematical methods are superior has led them actually to be dismissive of other branches of social science that proceed differently.

Finally, there is the wider environment, and in particular the political environment. Although the current political climate is generally speaking, not nearly as closed or oppressive as that of the McCarthy period in the US, I suspect that practices of mathematical modelling are sustained now for much the same reasons as they were able to rise to prominence in that earlier period: they do, and can do, nothing to challenge the status quo.

But there are alternative views. It can equally be argued that an over reliance on routines in an open world is ultimately as much a cause as a consequence of anxiety. The case of modern economics illustrates that many do choose to treat the open world as closed in conditions where it is quite inappropriate to do so. Yet most of us can easily refuse to rely on practices that (mis)treat open systems as closed. Indeed, acknowledging the openness of our world can be not only conducive to gaining awareness but also liberating and somewhat invigorating. For those modern economists for whom this is not so, it seems that a previous immersion in closed systems thinking has been so prolonged that the thought of letting go is met mostly by overwhelming anxiety. In a similar fashion, it is quite conceivable that in the social world more widely the (relatively) ontologically secure person will often participate in the following of routines without becoming anxious when routines are disrupted. And it is equally conceivable that those who most experience the disruption of routines as a direct threat to the self tend to be those that have previously immersed themselves most (and overly so) in routinized forms of conduct (on all this see Lawson 2015c; Willmott 1986).

This is not the place to develop or assess contending positions. I only note that there are competing conceptions of why unconscious motivations dispose us to engage in institutionalised or routinized forms of conduct. All I need note here is that they do.

Of course these remarks apply where, as in the case in question, existing collective practices are relatively shielded. Where this is not so the inevitable turn to increased reflexivity lead to very different outcomes (see e.g. Archer 2010).

[13]See the numerous highly relevant contributions of my colleagues on this morphogenesis project, most of whom are located in sociology departments, and all of whom are located outside of economics.

The point here is simply that the emphasis on event correlations or regularities (necessitated by a reliance on forms of mathematical modelling), and so the attachment to an implicit ontology of closure and atomism (see Lawson 1997, 2003), entails that any references to social relationality, and so to (relational) issues of power, discrimination, domination, oppression, and conflict generally, are effectively glossed over, masked or hidden, or at best trivialised. For the framework is ill-equipped even to allow such categories to be seriously contemplated. In short, the very emphasis on mathematical modelling renders impossible any meaningful analyses of real conflict, power relations and social transformation.

Thus, although the generalised malaise of modern economics does not reflect any significant ideological attachment to specific economic and/or political theories, the persistent irrelevance of academic mainstream economics, resulting from the emphasis on formal modelling, nonetheless inhibits any analysis capable of constituting meaningful constructive criticism of existing political-economic states of affairs. It is thus not unlikely that this consequence, if typically unintended, does contribute to explaining how the mathematical project persists in maintaining institutional power in the face of, and despite, its repeated failures and fictitious constructions. Government sponsored funding bodies and the like are actually less likely to withdraw funds from a project that provides no serious criticism of the government's actions.

I repeat, however, that in detailing all this I am not suggesting that those who contribute to the mathematising project in economics do so, in the main, opportunistically. Rather, I merely point out that whatever its advocates' intentions, the mainstream project (with its emphasis on mathematical deductivist modelling, and lack of criticality) may appear, and at times has indeed demonstrated itself to be (see Lawson 2003, chapter 10), conducive to those, especially outside the academy, seeking, for whatever reason, to deflect or minimise intellectual challenges to the underlying economic system. As such, this mathematical project, itself underpinned by norm-governed behaviour amounting to a methodological ideology, and not formulated by those pushing, or duped by, a politico-economic ideology, might nevertheless be said to contribute ultimately to sustaining the *status quo*.

Final Comments

In this short paper I have questioned how it is that in a context of turbulent change, including institutional transformation in all areas of society, stability of practices can yet be maintained, even in cases where the practices sustained do not seem especially desirable (amongst the possibilities imaginable).

At a fairly abstract level I have suggested that amongst the interesting structuring features of social reality there are (in addition to regulations imposed by relevant authorities, and restricted collective practices that are positioned in opposition to those of others situated differently) generalised collective practices in principle undertaken by all or most members of a given community. These intra-community collective practices often change in ways that are informal, shifting, slipping and sliding, and yet can be consistent with a degree a relative 'fixity'. I have suggested that an evolutionary or PVRS model is likely appropriate for their conceptual systematisation.

As a specific case study, I examined how the project of modern mainstream economics is able, even despite a (now widely recognised and reported) dearth of explanatory successes, to continue along its merry path almost unaffected. My assessment is that somewhere along the way the discipline, in effect, ceased to be an open academic intellectual venture concerned with furthering our understanding of social reality and instead (if largely unrecognised) morphed into little more than a norm-governed activity that exists more or less for its own sake, at least for the time being; a version of a collective practice, situated in an environment in which successful challenges to prevalent norms fail for various reasons to materialise.

At a deeper level, the focus of the paper is social positioning. Previously I have argued that amongst the factors incorporated as components of social totalities through positioning are human individuals, artefacts and communities. In the current paper I argue that this positioning activity, if in a manner that is usually no more than implicit and barely recognised, extends to the incorporation of certain individual practices as well. On being positioned, individual practices become versions of a collective practice with certain obligation-carrying aspects interpreted as norms. In social life, especially in times of rapid social change, competition amongst components of individual practices to be accepted as norms is likely fundamental. Equally it is the latter features that account for much of the social stability that is witnessed even in turbulent times.

Acknowledgements For helpful comments on an earlier draft of the paper I am grateful to Nuno Martins, Margaret Archer and to other members of the Workshop on Social Morphogenesis.

References

Archer, M. S. (2010). Routine, reflexivity, and realism. *Sociological Theory, 28*(3), 272–303.

Archer, M. S. (2015). How agency is transformed in the course of social transformation: Don't forget the double morphogenesis, chapter 7. In M. S. Archer (Ed.), *Generative mechanisms transforming the social order* (pp. 135–157). New York: Springer.

Archer, M. S. (2016). Morphogenesis and anormative social regulation. In M. Archer (Ed.), *Morphogenesis and the crisis of normativity*. Dordrecht: Springer.

Arena, R. (2000). Jean-Baptiste Say and the French liberal school of the nineteenth century: Outside the canon? In S. Peart (Ed.), *Reflections on the classical canon: Essays in honour of Samuel Hollander*. London: Routledge.

Coats, A. W. B. (1992). *On the history of economic thought: British and American economic essays, volume I*. London: Routledge.

Dawkins, R. (1976). *The selfish gene*. Oxford: Oxford University Press.

Dawkins, R. (1978). Replicator selection and the extended phenotype. *Zeitschrift für Tierpsychologie, 47*, 61–76.

Debreu, G. (1959). *The theory of value*. New York: Wiley.

Debreu, G. (1991). The mathematization of economic theory. *American Economic Review, 81*(1), 1–7.
Goodwin, C. D. (1998). The patrons of economics in a time of transformation. In S. Morgan Mary & M. Rutherford (Eds.), *From interwar pluralism to postwar neoclassicism. Annual supplement to volume 30, history of political economy*. Duke: Duke University Press.
Hahn, F. H. (1970, January). Some adjustment problems. *Econometrica, 38*. Reprinted as pp. 1–17 in Equilibrium and Macroeconomics. Oxford: Basil Blackwell.
Hahn, F. H. (1982). *Money and inflation*. Oxford: Basil Blackwell.
Hull, D., et al. (1981). Units of evolution: A metaphysical essay. In U. J. Jensen & R. Harré (Eds.), *The philosophy of evolution* (pp. 23–44). Brighton: Harvester Press.
Ingrao, B., & Israel, G. (1990). *The invisible hand*. Cambridge, MA: MIT Press.
Jones, L. V., Gardner, L., Porter, E., & Coggeshall (Eds.). (1982). *An assessment of research-doctorate programs in the United States: Social and behavioral sciences*. Washington, DC: National Academy of Sciences Press.
Lawson, T. (1997). *Economics and reality*. London: Routledge.
Lawson, T. (2003). *Reorienting economics*. London: Routledge.
Lawson, T. (2012a). Ontology and the study of social reality: Emergence, organisation, community, power, social relations, corporations, artefacts and money. *Cambridge Journal of Economics, 36*(2), 345–385. Reprinted in Stephen Pratten (ed.) (2015). *Social Ontology and Modern Economics*. London and New York: Routledge. pp. 413–64.
Lawson, T. (2012b). Mathematical modelling and ideology in the economics academy: Competing explanations of the failings of the modern discipline? *Economic Thought: History, Philosophy Methodology*, An open access journal of the *World Economic Association, 1*(1), 3–22.
Lawson, T. (2013a). Emergence, morphogenesis, causal reduction and downward causation. In M. S. Archer (Ed.), *Social morphogenesis* (pp. 61–84). New York: Springer.
Lawson, T. (2013b). What is this 'School' called neoclassical economics? *Cambridge Journal of Economics, 37*(5), 947–983. Reprinted in Lutfi Sunar (ed) (2014) *New Trends and Perspectives in Social Sciences*, published in Turkish by Nobel Publishing in their *Sociology and Social Theory series*. Also reprinted in Tony Lawson (2015f); and in Jamie Morgan (ed.) (2016).
Lawson, T. (2014). A speeding up of the rate of social change? Power, technology, resistance, globalisation and the good society. In M. S. Archer (Ed.), *Late modernity: Trajectories towards the morphogenetic society*. New York: Springer.
Lawson, T. (2015a). The nature of the firm, and peculiarities of the corporation. *Cambridge Journal of Economics, 39*(1), 1–32.
Lawson, T. (2015b). The modern corporation: The site of a mechanism of global social change, forthcoming. In M. Archer (Ed.), *Social morphogenesis: Generative mechanisms transforming the social order*. New York: Springer.
Lawson, T. (2015c). A conception of social ontology. In S. Pratten (Ed.), *Social ontology and modern economics* (pp. 19–52). London: Routledge.
Lawson, T. (2015d). What is an institution? In S. Pratten (Ed.), *Social ontology and modern economics* (pp. 553–557). London: Routledge.
Lawson, T. (2015e). Critical ethical naturalism: An orientation to ethics. In S. Pratten (Ed.), *Social ontology and modern economics* (pp. 359–387). London: Routledge.
Lawson, T. (Ed.). (2015f). *The nature and state of modern economics*. London/New York: Routledge.
Lazega, E. (2014). "Morphogenesis unbound" from the dynamics of multilevel networks: A non-structural perspective, chapter 8. In M. S. Archer (Ed.), *Late modernity: Trajectories towards Morphogenetic Society* (pp. 173–192). New York: Springer.
Maccarini, A. (2015). Turbulence and relational conjectures: The emergence of morphogenetic environments, chapter 8. In M. S. Archer (Ed.), *Generative mechanisms transforming the social order* (pp. 159–181). New York: Springer.
Maccarini, A. (2016). A tale of two wars: Universality and the normative tensions of the morphogenetic society. In M. Archer (Ed.), *Morphogenesis and the crisis of normativity*. Dordrecht: Springer.

Martins, N. (2014). *The Cambridge revival of political economy*. London: Routledge.
Miller, S. (2001). *Social action: A teleological account*. Cambridge: Cambridge University Press.
Morgan, J. (Ed.). (2016). *What is neoclassical economics? Debating the origins, meaning and significance*. London: Routledge.
Porpora, D. (2015). Why don't things change? The matter of morphostasis, chapter 9. In M. S. Archer (Ed.), *Generative mechanisms transforming the social order* (pp. 185–203). New York: Springer.
Porpora, D. (2016). The great normative changes of the twentieth century. In M. Archer (Ed.), *Morphogenesis and normativity*. Dordrecht: Springer.
Reinert, E. S. (2000). The Austrians and the other canon. In J. Backhaus (Ed.), *The history of evolutionary economics*. Aldershot: Edward Elgar.
Searle, J. R. (2010) *Making the social world: The structure of human civilization*. Oxford: Oxford University Press
Weiner, J. (1994). *The beak of the finch: A story of evolution in our time*. London: Jonathan Cape.
Wight, C. (2016). Emergence, development and death: Norms in International Society, chapter 4. In: Archer (Ed.), *Morphogenesis and the crisis in normativity*. Dordrecht: Springer.
Willmott, H. C. (1986). Unconscious sources of motivation in the theory of the subject; an exploration and critique of Giddens' dualistic models of action and personality. *Journal for the Theory of Social Behaviour, 16*(1), 105–122.
Yonay, Y. P. (1998). *The struggle over the soul of economics: Institutionalist and neoclassical economists in America between the wars*. Princeton: Princeton University Press.

Chapter 12
Ethics from Systems: Origin, Development and Current State of Normativity

Wolfgang Hofkirchner

This Chapter puts ethics in a system-theoretical perspective, gives an evolutionary account of how moral values came and still come into existence and analyses a deep moral-ideological crisis that is the outcome of the worldwide neoliberal project.

Here, normativity denotes the property of social systems to regulate human behaviour through norms, values and interests, through morals and through ethics. Morality is at the core and ethics is a meta-level phenomenon.

What, in that context, is meant by norms, values and interests, by morals and ethics (Haug 2004; Hörz and Hörz 2013; Klaus and Buhr 1974; Sandkühler 1990; Weingartner 1971)?

A norm is a collective expectation that represents an imperative to act in a determinate way and can be formulated as statement such as "you ought to do X (in circumstances Y)". An addressee of the imperative may or may not act accordingly.

A value is a collective attribution that represents the meaningfulness of an object and can be formulated as statement such as "Z is true", "Z is beautiful" or "Z is good". A given subject may or may not share any of these three evaluations.

An interest is a propensity for an individual intention that depends upon a collective entitlement, such that an actor is inclined to act in a way that is determined by the position the actor assumes and by the rights and obligations that go hand in hand with that position. An interest represents the directedness of the actor towards an object in accordance with the actor's location in the social relationships involved. It can be formulated as a statement of the kind, "I intend to appropriate Z in a way that is my proper right or obligation".

Morality is that part of normativity that implies a reference to goodness. Morals are about goodness. A norm is moral or morally relevant, if and when the expected action is considered as good, in terms of degrees of the good or of the evil. A value

W. Hofkirchner (✉)
Bertalanffy Center for the Study of Systems Science, Vienna, Austria
e-mail: wolfgang.hofkirchner@tuwien.ac.at

M.S. Archer (eds.), *Morphogenesis and the Crisis of Normativity*,
Social Morphogenesis, DOI 10.1007/978-3-319-28439-2_12

is moral or morally relevant, if and when the property that is attributed to something is "good", "more or less good" or "evil". An interest is moral or morally relevant, if and when the intention is good, more or less good or evil and the entitlement on which it is based is good, more or less good or evil.

Ethics is the philosophical, scientific, or every-day reflexion of morals or moral issues.

The first part of the Chapter discusses an epistemological issue: the most abstract knowledge of normativity, that is, philosophical accounts of normativity and their attempt to integrate themselves with scientific knowledge. It deals with ethics and the basic question ethics seeks to answer is: how are Is and Ought related to each other? Answers matter insofar as they provide different frames for analysing what goes wrong with morals in unbound morphogenesis. An answer is considered preferable here that connects ethics to systems philosophy and systems science.

The second part presents an ontological issue: Anthropological considerations about the origin of morals. Animals seem to have no morals, at least in the human sense. How then could human morality emerge? In this unresolved debate, empirical research can be of assistance, namely by specifying how it is aspects of human co-operation that make the difference. The Human species is deemed to be the species with the most sophisticated ability to co-operate. Morals are regarded here as epiphenomena of human co-operation.

The third part analyses a praxiological issue: the state of morals in today's societies. It observes a sharp contrast between the human potential to co-operate and the actuality of 30 years of neoliberal dictates on any societal level down to the individual. Individualism prevails to such an extent that it deserves the term "idiotism". Irresponsibility, kleptocracy, and corruption abound. Norms of behaviour and moral values are coupled in discretionary ways.

The Logical Foundation of Ought

The basic question ethics tries to answer can be considered as how to relate the factual with the normative. In the perspective of complexity and systems science, the factual is a property of systems, while the normative concerns the goal of a social system.

Ethical accounts can be classified along the four ways of thinking; those promoting reduction, projection, disjunction or integration. Bureaucracy as highlighted by Archer (Chap. 7) is framed by a reductionist account. In contradistinction to those accounts that fall prey to the so-called naturalistic, spiritualistic or postmodern fallacies, it is only the last account – the integrative one – that avoids problems of justification and the practical implications of universalism and relativism that are societally undesirable. Since 2010 I have termed the integrative account Emergent(ist) Ethics (Hofkirchner 2012), one that might be consonant with, or is at least close to, Realist Social theory (see Table 12.1).

Table 12.1 Ethical accounts

	Is	Ought
Naturalistic fallacy	Facts:	Norms:
	Sufficient conditions for norms	Results of facts
Spiritualistic fallacy	Facts:	Norms:
	Results of norms	Sufficient conditions for facts
	Facts	Norms
	Independent existents	
	Facts:	Norms:
	Necessary conditions for norms	Emergence of facts

The Naturalistic Fallacy

The naturalistic fallacy is only one kind of inference that does not hold. It is based on a reductionist way of thinking. It tries to derive prescriptions from descriptions, norms from facts, Ought from Is, thus levelling down a norm or an evaluation that is related to a fact to a proposition that only describes facts without making prescriptions or evaluating the facts (which is an implicit prescription). Reductionism, in general, reduces phenomena of higher complexity to those of less complexity. Insofar as norms or evaluations are not only, directly or indirectly, prescriptive but relate to facts they are more complex than descriptions of facts that lack the prescriptive element.

The Spiritualistic Fallacy

Another fallacy is wishful thinking, called here the 'spiritualistic fallacy'. It pretends that Is follows from Ought and projects the higher complexity given in prescriptions onto descriptions that are less complex. That is, projection presumes the existence of something in an area where it cannot be found.

The Postmodern Fallacy

A third fallacy might be called the postmodern one. As it is a feature of postmodernity to accept that grand narrative alone that states there are no great narratives any more, postmodern thinking deconstructs any and every consistency provided so far; things fall apart and so do Is and Ought. From that it follows there is no dependence of one on the other at all and every norm or value is as justified as any other. That is an expression of a way of thinking that disjoins things that are connected.

Emergentist Ethics

However, there is another possibility for conceptualisation: an ethics that is based upon emergentism. It is possible to look upon Is as a necessary, but not sufficient condition of Ought. In that way Is can be integrated with Ought. They are not rendered completely identical nor completely different. They are conceived of as being related by a certain connection that opens room to move between them. "Ought" can emerge as contingent upon a given basis. Thus reductionist, projectivist and disjunctivist ways of thinking are negated. Values, guidelines for actions, morals are seen as emerging in a historical context; they originate from, and depend on, history.

This is similar to modern views of laws of nature. Laws of nature that govern natural processes are not predeterminants that are given from outside nature or are unchangeable. It is hypothesised that laws of nature are time-dependent (Smolin 1997) and that the so-called fundamental constants of physics have, in fact, changed over cosmological time scales (Barrow 2002). Natural laws might "depend (at least to some extent) on what happens in the universe" (Davies 2010: 73): "the laws of physics are inherent in and emergent with the universe, not transcendent of it" (Davies 2010: 83). Physical laws seem to emerge along with matter and energy. Similarly, morals seem to develop with the circumstances in which they are embedded. System goals are construed on the basis of the actual interaction of the elements of that system. The former depend on the latter, but cannot be reduced to them. The former are a surplus that supervenes on the latter. Thus this position is called "Emergentist Ethics". Taking this position enables us to talk about ethical issues without being trapped in the naturalistic fallacy or any of the other fallacies discussed above.

Emergentist Ethics makes complex systems thinking compatible with critical thinking that supports criticism of current trends of societal development as measured against possibilities of improving the human condition. Goals need to be realistic in that there is a chance to realise them. Emergentist Ethics starts from here, stating that for the improvement of a social system one has to take into consideration that which is not only possible but also desirable and, in turn, not only what is desirable but also possible. This approach includes not only an account of the potential that is given with the actual but also enables an evaluation of those potentials that sort out the desirable. Thus, it embraces an ascendance from the potential given now in the actual to be established in the future as well as an ascendance from the less good now to the better-then, which together yield the Not-Yet in the sense of Ernst Bloch (1985).

Let us suppose a multistage scheme in which different phases and different levels can be distinguished such that each phase is marked by a leap in quality that introduces another level. Then the potential is a space of possibilities rooted in the conditions of the actual at a certain phase on a certain level. The future actual is a realisation of a certain possibility out of the range of possibilities and it adds a level to the existing ones. However, this is not the whole story. A value has to be assigned to the potential to discriminate whether or not it is better than the actual *hic et nunc*. Only in the case of improvement will the potential be realised. This constitutes an ascendance from the less good to the better. The 'Not-yet' is then the better future. It is anchored in the present potential. Thus, it is said to 'flash up' now. These flash-ups foreshadow the better future, or what Realists might term 'concrete utopias' – a term introduced by Bloch in 1937 (see Bloch 1972).

The Historical Origin of Morality

The existence of norms, values and interests, of morals and of ethics, is not only one out of many features of social systems. It is even considered by anthropologists, sociologists and evolutionary biologists as the distinctive feature of social systems in comparison with non-human living systems (see Niedenzu 2012).

A human is an *animale sociale* (*zoon politikon*) and not a Robinson Crusoe; her individual life depends on the integration with the collective, the connection to social groups and society, the inclusion in a social system. That sociality is the ontological ground for normativity and morality. Sciences that hypothesise the dynamics of anthropo-sociogenesis can provide an understanding of the emergence of morals.

As with any knowledge, anthropo-sociogenetic accounts come in reductionist, projectivist, disjunctivist and integrativist varieties. For the sake of simplicity, the relationship between nature and culture is presumed as the basic question of the emergence of social systems, including humans as their individual actors, in the course of the evolution of life on our planet – the first subsumed under the term "culture" (subsuming normativity), and the latter subsumed under the term "nature". Then we can differentiate between naturalist, culturalist-I and –II, and emergentist-systemist answers (see Table 12.2).

Naturalism

Reductionist accounts reduce the advent of human culture to the development of nature. The former is the necessary result of the latter. They have a monist view in which there is no room for decisively distinguishing culture and thus none for

Table 12.2 Anthropo-sociogenetic accounts

	Nature	Culture
Naturalism (monism)	Sufficient condition	Necessary result
Culturalism I (monism)	Necessary result	Sufficient condition
Culturalism II (dualism)	Independent existents	
Emergentist Systemism (dialects)	Necessary condition	Contigent emergent, dominant

normativity. Characteristics of culture are levelled down to being characteristics of nature. That view ignores that culture is of another quality than nature.

Culturalism I

Another monist view turns the tables. Human culture is not conceived as being as poor as nature, but nature is contended to be as rich as culture. Culture is projected onto nature, postulating that the features of cultural normativity occur in pre-human life, which, however, is far from evident.

Both anthropo-sociogenetic accounts of the naturalistic type and also of the type of culturalism I are conflationist and blur the distinction between nature and culture. They overemphasise the continuity from natural to cultural evolution.

Culturalism II

Another way to save the richness of culture and thus of normativity is to postulate a discontinuity between nature and culture and deny any comparability. Culture is disjointed from nature in this dualistic view. Both spheres are considered to be ontologically independent of each other, and therefore, on that basis they might interact. However, that view owes a scientific answer to the question, 'how did culture emerge?'

Emergentist Systemism

Since all three above accounts are flawed, only integration remains to promise to supply an acceptable conceptualization.

The integrativist view is neither monistic nor dualistic but dialectical. Nature is seen as the necessary condition upon which culture could emerge as an evolutionary contingency. In turn, as a supra-system, culture began to dominate, shape, re-ontologise the higher-order structure from which it had taken its departure.

Evolutionary systems thinking provides a multi-stage model as the heuristic for approaching qualitative leaps. That model also needs to be applied here.

The stage model combines the diachronic view with the synchronic view. The interactions of systems in a phase n prepare the ground for the transition to a meta-system in phase n+1. This step is accomplished once the interactions involved have actualised new organisational relations that inhered in the space of potentialities of phase n, such that these new organisational relations belong to a new level n+1. From there they exert a downward causal influence on the former systems as new elements on the level n of the new supra-system (which is the meta-system in hierarchical terms) (for more details see Hofkirchner 2013: 115–119).

Ludwig von Bertalanffy, one of the founders of General System Theory, had applied such thinking when he made obsolete the chasm between mechanism and vitalism in biology (see e.g. 1933).

In anthropo-sociogenesis, the qualitative leap from non-human biotic systems to human (social, cultural) systems is scrutinized. Which is the most plausible candidate for being the factor that, in non-human biotic systems, actualised a potential and fed back to the non-human biotic systems so as to transform them into a new – the human – system?

Vladimir I. Vernadsky, the founding father of biogeochemistry, applied the same thinking as Bertalanffy when promoting the analogy between the relationship of the biosphere to the non-biotic geosphere (life is the driver of the cycles of chemical substances through the atmo-, hydro- and lithosphere) and the relationship of what he called the noosphere – the sphere of human activity – to the non-human biosphere (human activity is the driver of the transformation of the biosphere and has an impact on our planet comparable to those that have changed the surface of our planet over geological periods of time) (see Vernadskij 1997).

Critical Psychologist Klaus Holzkamp (1983) developed a dialectical scheme of tipping-points to understand the transition from our ancestors to Homo sapiens. First, there is the emergence of some new feature under the dominance of old features. Second, there is the dominance of the new features over the old ones. That is, first, pre-human evolution finds a specific factor that transcends mere pre-human evolution but is still applicable in normal pre-human evolution; second, this works until a point in time when the new factor becomes so powerful that it takes the lead over pre-human evolution and sets human evolution going.

Usually, approaches to anthropo-sociogenesis name the following factors:

- Anatomic ones like the cerebral growth, the descent of the larynx, bipedalism and the opposed thumb and the fingers etc. Those traits, if significant, are biological in nature. They do not seem to transcend their biological origin. Should we believe that by happenstance all those single developments resulted in an anatomy that makes sense for humans? Of course, all of them are necessary. But some of these developments seem not to be the adjacent necessary condition. And those which might be – were perhaps adaptations due to another factor?
- Psychic functions like thought and others. But how did human thinking emerge? Should we believe that this psychic function came about by happenstance? Maybe human cognitive capabilities were not centre stage then?
- The ability to speak – language. But how did human language emerge? Should we believe that this human ability came about by happenstance? Maybe human communicative capabilities were important, but not centre stage?
- The ability to devise and manufacture artefacts, in particular, tools. But how did that ability emerge? Should we believe that this came about by happenstance too? Maybe productive capabilities do not have an individual but a collective origin?

Vernadsky identified the sought-after factor as work, the deliberative change of the environment as a collective enterprise that embraced all the other factors above – the production of tools, language and thought, including science. And, going beyond

Vernadsky, one could hypothesise that some of the anatomic developments listed above were instigated by the fact that work established social relations that through downward causation also demanded changes in the anatomy.

How can this be conceptualised? Norms, values, interests, morals and ethics are all human (social) information phenomena, phenomena of cognition, communication and co-operation.

The Triple-C Model that I have put forward myself (Hofkirchner 2013) contends that a hierarchy of information processes is located in the processes that bring about evolutionary, self-organising, systems or reproduce or transform them. At the bottom you have elemental activity that conveys cognitive information processes; elemental activities then couple with interaction that conveys communicative information processes; and on top there are systemic relations that convey co-operative information processes. With social systems you have at the bottom actions of actors that are capable of human (social) cognition; interaction of actors that are capable of human (social) communication; and on top social relations by which the actors are made capable of human (social) co-operation.

Human thought is part of human cognition and can be found on the bottom level; human language is part of human communication and is situated at the intermediate level; human tools are part of work that belongs to human co-operation and resides at the topmost level.

This hierarchy means the lower level is a necessary condition for the functioning of the higher level. Starting with work at the top, it is about setting common goals and reaching common goals. Work is consensual. Co-operation involves finding and building consensus. What is needed here, are shared intentions. Shared intentionality provides the perspective of the whole We, the perspective of the social system.

Consensuality, in turn, presupposes a certain collaboration that designs specific tasks for reaching the shared goals and assigns these tasks to certain actors. That is done on the level below, on the level of language. Communication functions as the means to realise that kind of collaboration that is needed for the upper level. That is, taking the perspective of the other facilitates collaboration. However, taking the perspective of the other is promoted by taking the perspective of the whole in which one's own and the others' roles are included.

Collaboration, in turn, presupposes a certain co-ordination that devises certain operations for fulfilling the tasks and guides certain actors in performing the operations. That is worked out on the lowermost level, on the level of thought. Cognition allows the actors to understand what form of co-ordination is needed by the upper level. It enables the actors to reflect upon the relationship between operations, tasks and goals.

According to that model, the dissimilarity of human (social) information processes, compared with pre-human information processes, has to do with the kind of co-operation humans are practicing in contradistinction to the behaviour of nonhuman species.

Now, if the Triple-C hierarchy is plausible from the synchronic perspective, what does it tell us about the diachronic perspective? The crucial development that is the candidate for the historical origin of mankind and social systems needs to be sought in the context of what – in the course of the decisive transition to real human life – turned into the building blocks of the uppermost level in the Triple-C hierarchy. The key idea is that it is conditions of co-operation that made the difference in evolution. Evolutionary pressure unfolded a ratchet effect that yielded ever higher complex co-operation. Thus children show a higher degree of social intelligence than adult chimpanzees or orang-utans. That is, in short, what the *American Scientist* calls perhaps the most remarkable approach towards explaining the unique cognitive capabilities of humans and, as can be added, the unique communicative and co-operative capabilities too – the article describes the research programme of Michael Tomasello, the psychologist, who does empirical research on primates and infants (Stix 2014). Since 1998, Tomasello, has been Director at the Max Planck Institute of Evolutionary Anthropology in Leipzig, Germany. He is well-known for his publications on cognition, communication and co-operation. In his most recent book *A Natural History of Human Thinking* (2014) he sums up his position substantiated by evidence found over long years of research carried out at his Department of Developmental and Comparative Psychology.

Tomasello contends that the so-called "shared intentionality" hypothesis provides an evolutionary and structural explanation of the difference yielded by human co-operation, and presupposes different human communicative and, as a consequence, different human cognitive capabilities as well.

According to Michael Tomasello, our great ape ancestors were social beings, but "they lived mostly individualistic and competitive lives" (Tomasello 2014: 4), they were "individually intentional and instrumentally rational" (Tomasello 2014: 30) as great apes are still today. Early humans began to speciate only when they took advantage of going beyond "individual intentionality" and adopted "more complex forms of cooperative sociality" (Tomasello 2014: 31), which enabled them to achieve shared goals and brought about "shared intentionality".

Tomasello hypothesises two steps towards shared intentionality. A first step occurred "in the context of collaborative foraging" (Tomasello 2014: 33), that is the hunting of large game and gathering of plant foods, around 2 million years ago and culminating 400,000 years ago. This was a step from individual to joint intentionality, from the competitive sociality of Great Ape ancestors to ad-hoc dyadic relationships with a "significant other" (G. H. Mead). Multiple and vanishing dyadic relationships formed in which early humans shared a joint goal.

In order to support the negotiation of joint goals and the coordination of collaboration, human communication originated with "a commitment to informing others of things honestly and accurately, that is, truthfully" (Tomasello 2014: 51); "being committed to informing others of things honestly, for *their* not *our* benefit, is the starting point" (Tomasello 2014: 51–52). Cognitively, "when early humans began engaging in obligatory collaborative foraging, they schematized a cognitive model of the dual-level collaborative structure comprising a joint goal with individual roles and joint attention with individual perspectives" (Tomasello 2014: 69). Triangulation began.

The most striking point is that we not only have here the origins of humanity but also of morality, since early humans not only felt committed to help others through giving truthful information that was relevant to them. They "could also view the world at the same time from the perspective of the other, which might also include her perspective on my perspective" (Tomasello 2014: 78). Thus they "self-regulated their behavioural decisions with others' evaluations in mind. Now we may talk of something that is socially regulated, that is, socially normative, albeit only in second-person (as opposed to agent-neutral) form" (Tomasello 2014: 75).

Thus,"[e]arly humans simulated the evaluative judgments that others made of them with regard to their cooperative proclivities – precursors to norms of morality – and also with regard to the intelligibility of their communicative acts – precursors to norms of rationality "(Tomasello 2014: 76). The importance of the first step lies in the fact that social selection started it off. It did so because the evaluation of others as good or bad co-operative partners began.

The second step is that from early to modern humans who became "thoroughly group-minded individuals" (Tomasello 2014: 80) in larger groups, in which they "had to be prepared to coordinate with anyone from the group, with some kind of generic other" (Tomasello 2014: 81) some 200,000 years ago. This was a step from joint intentionality to collective intentionality, a step to the co-operation within a larger group organisation (culture) as the "generalised other" (G. H. Mead, see Aboulafia 2012).

With culture, says Tomasello, it is not "one individual evaluating another individual" any more but, rather, "modern group-minded humans" evaluating all others "in agent-neutral, transpersonal mode" (Tomasello 2014: 87). Social norms, which are mutual expectations, now operate in that new mode. That implies "an objective standard against which an individual's behaviour is evaluated and judged", i.e. the "group's agreed-upon evaluations", and a target that is in principle applicable to anyone belonging to the group (Tomasello 2014: 88–89). This new mode is a generalisation. Group members self-monitor and self-regulate their individual actions via group norms so as to co-ordinate with the expectations of the group.

Accordingly, communication started to involve discourses about "objective" facts and needed compelling arguments, and so cognition turned into full-blown human reasoning; "the individual no longer contrasted her own perspective with that of a specific other [. . .]; rather, she contrasted her own perspective with some kind of generic perspective of anyone and everyone about things that were objectively real, true and right from any perspective whatsoever" (Tomasello 2014: 122). The importance of the second step is that social selection took over.

Cognition and communication are shaped for co-operation, and morals go hand in hand with co-operation.

The State of Morals After 30 Years of Neoliberalism

The state of morals can best be demonstrated by an analysis of the role (1) of morals in dominant means-end relationships, (2) of concomitant interests and (3) of the underlying kind of reflexivity.

A categorisation of means-end relationships can be based upon the categorisation of is-ought relationships. The end is a kind of Ought, because it presents a desired state; the means is a kind of Is, because it presents a state of possible dynamics the initiation of which might bring about the desired state.

The end has a moral dimension, since what is desired is good, more or less good, or evil. The means as a means it has, at first glance, no moral dimension, since the dynamics work in one way or another. It is appropriate to reach the end, or it is inappropriate or it is even counterproductive, which is a matter of fact. As such the means is right or wrong in relation to the end.

However, the means is not only a means to a given end but, it also has an independent existence. As an imperative to act it is subject to moral judgements. In itself, the required action is good, more or less good, or evil, and this property is dependent on its consequences. Those consequences can be close-range or long-range effects, short-term or long-term effects, or side effects, and they can be intended or unintended, and, most importantly, they can be desired or undesired. If the consequences are desired or undesired, that is, if they can be evaluated with regard to goodness, then that degree of goodness can be conferred from the consequences to the action that causes the consequences, and the means acquires a moral dimension.

If the end is the only consequence of the action, and if the end is good and the means is proper, then goodness can be conveyed from the end to the means. As a matter of fact, actions usually do not have one single consequence alone. They have several; and each of those would need evaluating and all of them an overall weighing up against each other in order to reach a substantive moral judgement. That is the means-end relationship seen from a moral perspective.

Applying the general Is-Ought categories of relationship, we can also find the four ways of thinking (reductionism, projectivism, disjunctivism, integrativism) in means and ends too (see Table 12.3) and the tendencies of amoralisation, of hyper-moralisation, a tendency towards a moral disconnect, and a new-cosmopolitan tendency.

Table 12.3 Accounts of means-ends relationships, interests and reflexivity from a moral perspective

	Means-ends relationship	Interests	Reflexivity
Amoralisation (pragmatism)	The means shall lead to the end	Universal claim of partialities	Restriction: myopia
Hyper-moralisation (fundamentalism)	The end justifies the means		
Moral Disconnect (indifferentism)	Means and ends are independent	Relativist claim of partialities	
New Cosmo-politanism (convergentism)	Means and ends are balanced by a step by step formation of global	Unity through diversity	Extension: self- and community-concern

Amoralisation

1. The naturalistic fallacy yields a tendency towards amoralisation. The moral end is camouflaged and reduced to pretended real necessities, to the "Sachzwang" of technocracy, of punditocracy (German "Expertokratie"), of bureaucracy (see Margaret Archer Chap. 7 in this volume), that represent mere means.

   A good example is the current conflict around Greece. The institutions of the former Troika demand realism from the newly established Greek government and require reforms as if social reality could offer only one option. They hide the fact that the measures they advocate have morally disputable social consequences, such as the redistribution of public goods to private ownership, redundancies and further cuts in social security. "There is no alternative" (TINA) is the credo of the neoliberal "Institutions". Jürgen Habermas writes that the crux of the problem is that politicians in Brussels and Berlin refuse to encounter their colleagues from Athens as politicians. They look like politicians but speak only in their economic role of creditors. The purpose of this transformation into "Zombies" is to make the protracted insolvency of a state appear as a non-political issue, an issue to be disputed before the courts under private law (Habermas 2015). Whereas the sociologists of the 1960s and 1970s talked about "state-embedded markets", the new paradigm seems to be "market-embedded states" (Brunkhorst 2015) according to the political requirements of democracy to conform to the markets, as Chancellor Merkel put it, and not the other way round. The ideology of the Social Democrats has no influence anymore, and the model of a social market economy has lost its Christian Democratic foundation.

   Thus, norms are stripped of their moral values. That kind of pragmatism makes a universal claim. Since capitalism has penetrated the economies of almost all cultures and countries, that claim has a self-evident basis. Capitalism, in its current neoliberal development, seems to be the only possible economic reality.

   "The fact is that 'contemporary man has not been trained to use power well'", says Pope Francis in his recent Encyclical Letter "Laudato si'" quoting Romano Guardini's *The End of the Modern World* (pp. 82–83), "because our immense technological development has not been accompanied by a development in human responsibility, values and conscience. [...] in effect, 'power is never considered in terms of the responsibility of choice which is inherent in freedom' since its 'only norms are taken from alleged necessity, from either utility or security'" (Franciscus 2015, #105). "We have too many means and only a few insubstantial ends", says Francis (#203).
2. The pursuit of neoliberal, capitalist interests goes without saying. There is no need to say that those interests are neoliberal, capitalist ones. The behaviour is in no need of justification. The superficial reality suffices.

   In the case of Greece, the representatives of the 18 Eurogroup states pretended to act in the interest of the whole EU. However, they did not do so, camouflaging their own national interests that, in the last resort, are the interests of several fractions of financial capital. Above all, the intransigence of Greece's negotiating partners shows that it is not about a fight over money, since there can be no doubt that Greece cannot pay back those loans, while the IMF is going to bend its own rules and concede to Ukraine what is not conceded to Greece, and despite Germany's debts having been cut in 1953 by 50 %. It is about a fight for power and defending hegemony (Milne 2015). It is about the political decision to socialise private debts and it is about the unequal economic relationships practiced within the EU. Moreover, the political scientist Gesine Schwan, former president of the European University Viadrina Frankfurt (Oder) and presidential candidate of the SPD in 2004 and 2009, concluded in an interview that those who have power head for regime change in Greece. Only after regime change would they be willing to agree to a rescheduling of the debts. Schwan bemoans the fact that they address their national publics alone. This reanimation of nationhood within Europe made the European Council lose sight of the whole and give up its willingness to compromise (Pfaff 2015).

3. The ruling out of any questioning of the ends, the moral loading of the ends and of the positions produced by social relations, make the incumbents of those positions inclined to behave in the way they behave, one characterised by a state of restricted reflexivity, that is one of restricted cognitivity, communicativity and co-operativity, limited to individual self-concern and suppressing any concern for the community. Cognition deteriorates into self-censorship, communication into propaganda and co-operation into an egoistic We-against-Them behaviour.

In the struggle with Greece, those who exercise the arrogance of power are not able and not willing to understand that the resistance of the Syriza-led government to the imposition of further austerity measures is not only morally demanded but is also a possible trigger for Europe finding a way out of its crises. It is the Spanish protest party Podemos that understands what is at stake. Interestingly, non-European experts such as Nobel laureates Paul Krugman, Joseph Stiglitz and Amartya Sen or Jeffrey Sachs, director of Columbia University's Earth Institute, but also French economist Thomas Piketty have a view of the crisis surrounding Greece that is radically different from the propaganda campaigns conducted in Europe. Even the Washington Post provides refreshing comments (O'Brien 2015). Inside Greece you find the same propaganda; media coverage shows that in the week before the referendum, private network stations did not report on activities of the "no"-proponents as much as on those of the "yes"-proponents (Aswestopoulos 2015).

Hyper-Moralisation

The spiritualistic fallacy turns into a hyper-moralisation tendency.

1. A particular moral end is preached in a fundamentalist way and projected onto particular measures such that the end justifies the means. That is particularism.

   This is not only true of Islamic State but also of the United States of America or Israel. Whereas the former is guilty of cruel decapitations and other atrocities intended to lead to the build-up of the praised theocratic State, the latter two share two different varieties of exceptionalism that counterbalances their violations of international law. The USA, irrespective of the administration in office, has been waging wars all over the world in the name of freedom, democracy and human rights just as Israeli governments have been proclaiming the just cause of the Jews to exonerate acts of aggression against the Palestinians. "Illegal but legitimate" is the motto for the priority of certain values over certain norms.

In every case the actors deem themselves to be good, such that whatever they do cannot be other than good too, even in case of doing bad things such as the Obama administration's "dirty wars" with drones. But in every case it is particular moral values that are passed off as universal.

2. Accordingly, it is particular interests that are pursued. As long as positions are antagonistic and each fights to prevail over those who contradict them, they cannot be generalised and cannot become valid in a universal sense (see Hofkirchner 2015).

   US-President Obama made that very clear in his West Point speech on 28 May, 2014. "Here's my bottom line: America must always lead on the world stage." And he made clear that he will stick to the principle of unilateralism he put forward at the outset of his presidency: "the United States will use military force, unilaterally if necessary, when our core interests demand it – when our people are threatened; when our livelihood is at stake; or when the security of our allies is in danger. In these circumstances, we still need to ask tough questions about whether our action is proportional, effective and just. International opinion matters. But America should never ask permission to protect our people, our homeland, or our way of life" (Traywick 2014).
3. The reflexive quality connected with values and interests that are linked to fundamentalism are just as particularistic as is the case with pragmatism – albeit not disguised but unveiled – and is a restricted one too. The quest for commonness of interests is extraneous.

Moral Disconnect

The postmodern fallacy at large tends towards a secular disconnect.

1. That is the disconnect of means and ends, of norms and morals, of the micro and the macro (see Douglas Porpora in Chap. 2). The argument here is that morals of the ends (macro) are neither reduced to nor projected onto the norms governing the means (micro), but that either side is disjointed from the other. Norms are without morals and morals without norms. Norms are not grounded in morals and morals do not support norms. Neither norms nor morals can be criticised by reference to the other. Hence the change of norms or morals becomes a matter of accidental or arbitrary action. In turn, that fosters overall indifference, because the disconnect leads inevitably to pluralism – a diversity of zero or equal moral values; any norm or morals goes.

For purposes of illustration, consumerism provides a variety of different norms to perfect your body; ideology provides you with a variety of different moral offers, including even universal ones. But in both cases it is up to one's individual decision which alternative to take.

2. In any case those decisions are again subject to individual interests, to interests that are particularistic, to parochialism.
3. And reflexivity faces restrictions again, since there is no corrective against the pursuit of self-concerned interests.

A New Cosmopolitanism as Global Imperative

The only exception is integrativism based upon the Emergentist Ethics approach. Amidst all those tendencies of a- or hyper-moralisation or towards a disconnect, there is a step-by-step convergent tendency too that orients towards the formation of a global conscience as part of a global consciousness, a tendency that comes along with cosmopolitanism, leading to the quest for what can be called a global sustainable information society.

1. Regarding the means-end relationship, a permanent adjustment of the means to the end and of the end to the means is assumed to be feasible and mandatory. The means is open to critique, if it does not lead to the desired moral end, and the end is open to critique too, if it turns out to frustrate a higher moral end.

   Such is the doctrine of just war, which has always been debatable from a moral point of view. But now that mankind possesses weapons of mass destruction, the military factor cannot be considered as a norm accounting for neither building nor keeping peace any more. Means and ends are made appropriate for each other in a historical process of development and evolution of social systems. That is the process of shaping morals in a humane way – the humanisation of morals.
2. Interests are compelled to replace myopia and self-concern by a view that does justice to far-sightedness and concerns of the (generalised) other too. Individual interests need not be particularistic. They can balance the personal concern of and for one's own with the public concern and can be coherent with social relations that care for all individuals.
3. Reflexivity itself is compelled to make reference to commonalities. Those promptings qualify the reflexivity in question, the interestedness in question, the morality in question and the view of the means-ends relationship in question as fitting for a new cosmopolitanism.

In contradistinction to pragmatism and fundamentalism that yield unity without diversity, and in contradistinction to indifferentism that yields diversity without unity, the new cosmopolitanism is defined by yielding unity through diversity.

Given the four logical categories of reduction, projection, disjunction and integration, and given the examples from contemporary history for each of the categories, the hypothesis is that currently, in times some call unbound morphogenesis, the presence of instantiations of all categories is a marker of a deep ideological crisis, a crisis in normativity, basically in morality, in the following sense: ideological hegemony is given to the trinity pragmatism–fundamentalism–indifferentism, all three positions still have vitality in late modernity, and in the case of neoliberalism even taken to extremes, yielding on the micro-level an acceleration of mental fluctuations that, eventually, on the macro-level serve as obstacle to a qualitative systemic change, since any and all fundamental relationships remain unaffected. Conversely, new cosmopolitanism is *ante portas* – an idea whose time has come. The latter can serve as the indicator of the grounds being prepared for another Great Transformation.

Conclusion

In conclusion, 30 years of neoliberal dominance did not make the most of the human potential to co-operate, it made the least – if not even less: a historical, developmental and evolutionary regress lagging behind potentials already reached. It is time to reverse that trend and to live up to the actualisation of humanity's potential needed for survival in dignity. "No system can completely suppress our openness to what is good, true and beautiful", says Pope Francis in his recent Encyclical (Franciscus 2015, #205). "Human beings, while capable of the worst, are also capable of rising above themselves, choosing again what is good, and making a new start, despite their mental and social conditioning. We are able to take an honest look at ourselves, to acknowledge our deep dissatisfaction, and to embark on new paths to authentic freedom."

We are witnesses to, and maybe participants in, the emergence of a new morality. The values of the new cosmopolitanism are the response to the real challenges to our common future. According to Emergentist Ethics, those values are emergent, and that means they are contingent. You can have different moral responses to the factual. You can celebrate the last party and end up in extermination or you can try to be committed to each other, as we all share the same fate. The first argument boils down to the breakdown of the system. The second, however, can give hope and add to the secular evolutionary trend towards more understanding and less violence (Pinker 2011), the collective enterprise of a breakthrough to a system of higher order. Thus morality in an appropriate sense is the remedy in a situation of increasing complexity.

References

Aboulafia, M. (2012). George Herbert Mead. *Stanford Encyclopedia of Philosophy*. http://plato.stanford.edu/entries/mead/. Accessed 5 July 2015.

Aswestopoulos, W. (2015, July 4). Warnung an alle Fotografen, bleibt den Kamerateams der Sender fern. *Telepolis*.http://www.heise.de/tp/artikel/45/45348/1.html. Accessed 4 July 2015.

Barrow, J. D. (2002). *The constants of nature*. New York: Random House.

Bertalanffy, L. v. (1933). *Modern theories of development: An introduction to theoretical biology*. Oxford: Clarendon.

Bloch, E. (1972). *Vom Hasard zur Katastrophe. Politische Aufsätze aus den Jahren 1934–1939*. Frankfurt: Suhrkamp.

Bloch, E. (1985). *Das Prinzip Hoffnung* (Vol. 3). Frankfurt: Suhrkamp.

Brunkhorst, H. (2015). *Weil Europa sich ändern muss*. Wiesbaden: Springer VS.

Davies, P. (2010). Universe from Bit. In P. Davies & N. H. Gregersen (Eds.), *Information and the nature of reality, from physics to metaphysics* (pp. 65–91). New York: Cambridge University Press.

Franciscus. (2015). *Encyclical Letter Laudato Si' on Care for our Common Home*. http://w2.vatican.va/content/francesco/en/encyclicals/documents/papa-francesco_20150524_enciclica-laudato-si.html. Accessed 27 June 2015.

Habermas, J. (2015, June 22). Warum Merkels Griechenland-Politik ein Fehler ist. *Süddeutsche Zeitung*. http://www.sueddeutsche.de/wirtschaft/europa-sand-im-getriebe-1.2532119. Accessed 25 June 2015.

Haug, W. F. (2004). *Historisch-Kritisches Wörterbuch des Marxismus* (Vol. 6/II). Berlin: Argument.

Hofkirchner, W. (2012). Sustainability and self-organisation: Sustainability in the perspective of complexity and systems science and ethical considerations. In T. Nishigaki & T. Takenouchi (Eds.), *Information ethics* (pp. 190–217). Nagoya City: V2 Solution Publisher.

Hofkirchner, W. (2013). *Emergent information*. Singapore: World Scientific.

Hofkirchner, W. (2015). "Mechanisms" at work in information society. In M. Archer (Ed.), *Generative mechanisms transforming the social order* (pp. 95–112). Cham: Springer.

Holzkamp, K. (1983). *Grundlegung der Psychologie*. Frankfurt: Campus Verlag.

Hörz, H. E., & Hörz, H. (2013). *Ist Egoismus unmoralisch? Grundzüge einer neomodernen Ethik*. Berlin: Trafo.

Klaus, G., & Buhr, M. (1974). *Philosophisches Wörterbuch*. Leipzig: VEB Bibliographisches Institut.

Milne, S. (2015, July 1). *Syriza can't just cave in. Europe's elites want regime change in Greece, the guardian*. http://www.theguardian.com/commentisfree/2015/jul/01/syriza-cave-in-elites-regime-change. Accessed 3 July 2015.

Niedenzu, H.-J. (2012). *Soziogenese der Normativität. Zur Emergenz eines neuen Modus der Sozialorganisation*. Weilerswist: Velbrück.

O'Brien, M. (2015, June 25). *Europe strikes back: It seems to be trying to push Greece out of the euro, Washington Post*. http://www.washingtonpost.com/blogs/wonkblog/wp/2015/06/25/europe-strikes-back-it-seems-to-be-trying-to-push-greece-out-of-the-euro/. Accessed 1 July 2015.

Pfaff, J. (2015, July 1). *Politik wird durch Zwang ersetzt, Freitag*. https://www.freitag.de/autoren/jan-pfaff/politik-wird-durch-zwang-ersetzt. Accessed 4 Jul 2015.

Pinker, S. (2011). *Gewalt. Eine neue Geschichte der Menschheit*. Frankfurt (Main): S. Fischer.

Sandkühler, H. J. (1990). *Europäische Enzyklopädie zu Philosophie und Wissenschaften*. Hamburg: Meiner.

Smolin, L. (1997). *The life of the cosmos*. New York: Oxford University Press.

Stix, G. (2014). What makes human different than any other species. *Scientific American, 311*(3), 73–79.

Tomasello, M. (2014). *A natural history of human thinking*. Cambridge, MA: Harvard University Press.

Traywick, C. (2014, May 28). *President Obama at West Point: Watch the speech, read the transcript, foreign policy*. http://foreignpolicy.com/2014/05/28/president-obama-at-west-point-watch-the-speech-read-the-transcript/. Accessed 5 July 2015.

Vernadskij, V. I. (1997). *Der Mensch in der Biosphäre. Zur Naturgeschichte der Vernunft*. Wien: Peter Lang.

Weingartner, P. (1971). *Wissenschaftstheorie I*. Stuttgart: Frommann Holz.

MIX
Papier aus verantwortungsvollen Quellen
Paper from responsible sources
FSC® C105338

If you have any concerns about our products,
you can contact us on
ProductSafety@springernature.com

In case Publisher is established outside the EU,
the EU authorized representative is:
Springer Nature Customer Service Center GmbH
Europaplatz 3, 69115 Heidelberg, Germany

Printed by Libri Plureos GmbH
in Hamburg, Germany